Practical Old Age Psychopharmacology: a multi-professional approach

Edited by

Stephen Curran
Consultant in Old Age Psychiatry and Visiting Professor of Old Age Psychopharmacology
School of Human and Health Sciences
University of Huddersfield
Huddersfield

and

Roger Bullock
Consultant Psychiatrist
Kingshill Research Centre
Victoria Hospital
Swindon

Foreword by
Alistair Burns

Radcliffe Publishing
Oxford • Seattle

Radcliffe Publishing Ltd
18 Marcham Road
Abingdon
Oxon OX14 1AA
United Kingdom

www.radcliffe-oxford.com
Electronic catalogue and worldwide online ordering facility.

British Library Cataloguing in Publication Data

A catalogue record for this book is available from the British Library.

ISBN 1 85775 958 3

Typeset by Anne Joshua & Associates, Oxford
Printed and bound by TJ International Ltd, Padstow, Cornwall

Contents

Foreword

This book is long overdue. The increased awareness of drugs in psychiatry in general, and old age psychiatry in particular, means that a summary of the key drugs and their main indications will be well received by everyone involved in the prescription and monitoring of medications. Psycopharmacology is a field which develops quickly, and it is hard to keep up with every new initiative or ruling by a regulatory agency. Notwithstanding that, this collection of contributions serves as a super addition to the literature, and provides an excellent summary of the situation at present.

The main areas covered include all those which an old age psychiatrist will encounter in practice. After introductory chapters on basic science issues, there is an admirable summary of each of the main fields, both organic and functional illness, which summarises information available to date.

As with many projects, the trick is to get a niche in the market, and the editors and their authors are to be congratulated for putting together such a fine number of contributions. This book will serve as a baseline for everything else in this area of work – not just a baseline but a gold standard. It should be welcomed by all clinicians working in the area, and will serve as an excellent book for continuing professional development.

Professor Alistair Burns
Professor of Old Age Psychiatry
University of Manchester
April 2005

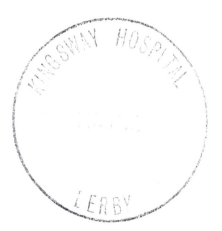

Preface

In this book we have brought together findings from recent research with a multi-disciplinary perspective into the practical aspects of old age psychopharmacology. We strongly believe in the importance of bringing together the best in research and practice. When these are divorced, researchers may lose the vision of the real purpose of their work, and practitioners may not have access to the most recent advances in knowledge. We hope that this book will help to bridge this gap.

If we ever develop a mental illness in later life we would like people to notice it early. We would like them to respect our autonomy but steer us quickly in the direction of the best help available. We would like to be seen by appropriately qualified people who could make a diagnosis and provide any useful medical treatment and social, psychological, nursing and therapy support and advice to ourselves and our families. We would like a truly personal approach to our needs. We believe that this applies equally to drug treatments, but in our experience this is not always the case.

Psychotropic drugs have an important role to play in the management of older people with mental illness. We hope that this book will help clinicians to use psychotropic drugs more appropriately so as to maximise their undoubted clinical benefits while minimising some of their unwanted effects.

Stephen Curran
Roger Bullock
April 2005

About the editors

Stephen Curran works as a Consultant Old Age Psychiatrist in Wakefield, and is a Visiting Professor in Old Age Psychopharmacology at the University of Huddersfield. He graduated in psychology in 1983 and completed his undergraduate medical training in 1986. He then worked as a Research Fellow and Lecturer in Old Age Psychiatry at the University of Leeds before moving to Wakefield in 1998. His research interests include old age psychopharmacology, particularly the use of qualitative methods to assess drug effects, and he leads the Ageing and Mental Health Research Group at the University.

Roger Bullock completed his medical and psychiatric training at Oxford and St Bartholomew's Hospital, London. In 1993 he was appointed Consultant in Old Age Psychiatry in Swindon, and two years later he founded the Kingshill Research Centre. The work of the centre is to study psychopharmacology and neuropsychology in the elderly, and to apply research from both fields to mainstream clinical practice. Roger is now Clinical Lead of the Swindon services and Director of the Research Centre, which is now affiliated to the University of Bath, where he is a Reader in Geriatric Psychopharmacology.

List of contributors

Robert C Baldwin, Consultant in Old Age Psychiatry and Honorary Professor, Manchester Mental Health and Social Care Trust, Manchester Royal Infirmary, Manchester

Roger Bullock, Consultant Psychiatrist, Kingshill Research Centre, Victoria Hospital, Swindon, Wiltshire

E Jane Byrne, Senior Lecturer/Honorary Consultant Psychiatrist, University of Manchester, School of Psychiatry and Behavioural Sciences, Education and Research Centre, Wythenshawe Hospital, Manchester

Richard J Clibbens, Nurse Consultant, Older People's Services, Fieldhead Hospital, Wakefield, West Yorkshire

Mary Crabb, Pharmacist, St Luke's Hospital, Huddersfield, West Yorkshire

Stephen Curran, Consultant in Old Age Psychiatry and Visiting Professor of Old Age Psychopharmacology, School of Human and Health Sciences, University of Huddersfield, Huddersfield, West Yorkshire

Owen P Dempsey, General Practitioner and Lead Researcher, Lockwood Research Practice, Huddersfield, West Yorkshire

Alison Diaper, Research Student, HPRU Medical Research Centre, School of Biomedical and Molecular Sciences, University of Surrey, Guildford, Surrey

Margaret M Esiri, Professor of Neuropathology, The Radcliffe Infirmary, Oxford

Paul Hardy, Pharmacist, Pinderfields General Hospital, Wakefield, West Yorkshire

David Healy, Honorary Consultant Psychiatrist/Director, North Wales Department of Psychological Medicine, University of Wales, College of Medicine, Hergest Unit, Gwynedd Hospital, Bangor, Gwynedd

Ian Hindmarch, Professor of Human Psychopharmacology and Head of HPRU Medical Research Centre, School of Biomedical and Molecular Sciences, University of Surrey, Guildford, Surrey

Clive Holmes, Senior Lecturer/Honorary Consultant in Old Age Psychiatry, Memory Assessment and Research Centre, Moorgreen Hospital, Southampton

Naila Jawaid, Specialist Registrar in Old Age Psychiatry, Manchester Mental Health and Social Care NHS Trust, Manchester Royal Infirmary, Manchester

James Lindesay, Professor of Psychiatry for the Elderly, University of Leicester, Leicester General Hospital, Leicester

Michelle C McCulley, Research Fellow, Human Genetics Division, University of Southampton, Southampton

Sharon Nightingale, Consultant in Old Age Psychiatry, Asket Croft Community Unit for the Elderly, Leeds

Andrew W Procter, Consultant Psychiatrist, Manchester Royal Infirmary, Manchester

Srinivas Suribhatla, Consultant in Old Age Psychiatry, Bennion Centre, Glenfield Hospital, Leicester

John P Wattis, Consultant and Visiting Professor of Old Age Psychiatry, School of Human and Health Sciences, University of Huddersfield, Huddersfield

Chapter 1

Psychopharmacological history through the looking-glass of advancing years

David Healy

Introduction

In 1956, Roland Kuhn described the effects of imipramine in a 56-year-old woman, Paula J F, who had a severe delusional melancholic disorder. Imipramine was subsequently demonstrated to be effective in a patient group suffering from vital depression with psychomotor retardation and often psychotic developments in older individuals. At the time, this condition was regarded by many as the distinct diagnostic entity of involutional melancholia. The success of imipramine led to an almost immediate disappearance of this syndrome.

It might not be thought surprising that an effective psychotropic agent should lead to the disappearance of a syndrome, on the basis that most people assume this is what effective agents should do. What was astonishing about this disappearance was that, far from imipramine being effective in the sense that penicillin was for general paralysis of the insane (GPI), imipramine seemed to be a treatment that validated the existence of the syndrome and the need for its possible ongoing maintenance treatment. Yet a few years later the diagnostic category of involutional melancholia had effectively disappeared.

This disappearance is at odds with the mainstream of psychopharmacological history, in which classification has been driven largely by the response (or otherwise) to psychotropic drugs rather than by the clinical criteria that drove classification in the pre-psychotropic era. The disappearance of involutional melancholia gives a first hint that the history of psychotropic agents given to older individuals might be radically different to conventional histories of the psychotropic era. Unfortunately, there are few histories of what happens when psychotropic drugs are given to older individuals.[1,2] The usual assumption appears to have been that what happens in the elderly will only reflect what is happening in a general adult group. However, there are good grounds to think that, in future, the books may reflect a quite different history, as this brief chapter seeks to illustrate.

The conventional history of the antidepressants

The conventional origin of the antidepressant was when Roland Kuhn discovered the effects of imipramine in 1956. Unpersuaded of his reports, Geigy sought confirmation elsewhere. At a time when compounds could be synthesised in the laboratory and could enter mainstream clinical use within 3 months, imipramine took 2 years to market. A major reason for Geigy's reluctance appears to have stemmed from the perception that depression was a relatively rare condition.[3]

At almost the same time as Kuhn reported on the effects of imipramine to Geigy, Nathan Kline made the discovery that one of two recently synthesised anti-tubercular agents, iproniazid, had psychic energising properties. It later became known as one of the first of the monoamine oxidase inhibitor (MAOI) antidepressants. Roche were not interested in such a compound.

Yet even before Kline or Kuhn, in 1952, Max Lurie had discovered that isoniazid, another anti-tubercular agent, had antidepressant properties. This discovery was replicated in Paris in the same year. However, none of the pharmaceutical companies that Lurie approached were interested in the idea of an antidepressant. The very term was new, having probably been coined by Lurie.

There had indeed been yet another discovery of a drug with antidepressant properties before Kuhn and Kline. In 1955, researchers from the Institute of Psychiatry demonstrated in an article published in the *Lancet* that reserpine was an antidepressant. However, Ciba, the makers of reserpine, were not interested in developing an antidepressant.

It was not until the discovery of amitriptyline and its marketing by Merck that any pharmaceutical company showed an interest in developing an antidepressant. Merck realised that if they were going to market this new class they would also have to sell the illness, so they purchased 50 000 copies of Frank Ayd's *Recognising the Depressed Patient*.[4] Despite this, sales of the antidepressants remained flat during the 1960s and 1970s.

The antidepressant market only truly developed when the benzodiazepine tranquillisers ran into difficulties in the 1980s. Concerns about dependence on these drugs steered the marketing development of a new generation of drugs that acted on the serotonin system towards an antidepressant route.

Thus the selective serotonin reuptake inhibitors (SSRIs) were developed in 1971 from a conjunction of clinical observations by Paul Kielholz and neuro-scientific observations by Arvid Carlsson. Kielholz noted that not all of the tricyclic and MAOI antidepressants did the same things to people who were depressed, and he categorised 'antidepressants' according to whether they were energy enhancing or whether they produced 'cognitive' changes. Reviewing Kielholz's classification in the late 1960s, Carlsson, one of the key pioneers of neuroscience, noted that the antidepressants which Kielholz stated were more energy enhancing acted on the catecholamine system, whereas those with cognitive effects acted on the serotonergic system. This led Carlsson to create the first SSRI, namely zimelidine, to see what the effects of such a drug would be. Zimelidine was launched in 1982, but was later withdrawn because of toxicological problems. It was succeeded by fluvoxamine, fluoxetine, sertraline, paroxetine and citalopram.

The unconventional history of the antidepressants

Following the emergence of the SSRIs, the antidepressant market mushroomed. If antidepressants are effective, this should not have happened, and indeed this is not what happened in the case of involutional melancholia. The most parsimonious explanation of what happened was that a process was initiated whereby cases of Valium were converted into cases of Prozac. This did not happen in Japan and many other parts of the world where the SSRIs did not emerge as antidepressants so early on. In these countries the antidepressant market remains a comparatively small one compared with the market for tranquillisers.

The development of the SSRIs was predicated on the notion that agents which act on catecholamine systems were energy enhancing whereas agents which act on the serotonin system appeared to do something else that was either anxiolytic or produced some other cognitive effect. The SSRIs were therefore designed as drugs that were different from the tricyclic antidepressants, rather than 'cleaned-up' versions of the same (which is how they had originally been marketed).

In fact the SSRIs have proved singularly ineffective for hospital depressions or depressions of the kind that Paula J F suffered from. In contrast, selective catecholamine reuptake inhibitors such as reboxetine have proved very effective in hospital depressions, but apparently much less effective in community depressions of the more anxious depressive type. This suggests that there may well be a distinctive component to the kinds of depression cases who end up in hospital, particularly those who end up in hospital in their middle to later years.

There remains a consensus of opinion that electroconvulsive therapy (ECT) is an effective treatment for the kinds of vital depression for which imipramine was first thought to be useful. ECT is not regarded as a treatment for those kinds of anxious depressions which are found in the community. Broadly speaking, the conditions thought to be responsive to ECT are the ones that in the 1980s were thought to be characterised by dexamethasone non-suppression, a set of depressions in which there is thought to be substantial elevation of cortisol levels, possibly brought about by escape from circadian control. This is not found in the depression cases in the community, and SSRIs in general appear to be less effective in dexamethasone non-suppression.[5]

Recently, however, mifepristone, which was previously used as an abortifacient agent, has been demonstrated to have an effect on severe or psychotic depressions.[6] It also appears to have effects on cortisol systems that are comparable to the effects of agents such as dexamethasone or ECT. Should the clinical efficacy of mifepristone be replicated, it will be an interesting test of pharmaceutical company perceptions of the depressive market to see whether it, unlike reboxetine, is developed further. If this were to happen, there might be a need to reinvent melancholia (if not involutional melancholia) and redesignate the SSRIs as anxiolytics, a process that is arguably well under way.

There are alternative frameworks within which to place such a development. While involutional melancholia may never have been the distinctive entity it was once thought to be, this clinical classification arguably embodied some clinical insights of substance. The distinctive response of this syndrome to some agents and not to others points to different physiological underpinnings. One possibility is that a constitutional or temperamental component shapes the differential response to selective agents seen in these vital depressions. Alternatively, a constitutional or temperamental component may shape clinical presentations so that some affective disorders in older years have features of anxiety, while others have features of a vital syndrome. Older age may in fact be a key setting in which some of these issues that seem irresolvable in younger populations may be teased out.

The conventional history of the antipsychotics

The conventional history of the antipsychotics has it that the discovery of chlorpromazine was first interpreted as the discovery of a new form of sleep treatment. The subsequent synthesis of a number of non-sedative phenothiazine agents, such as proclorperazine, led to a recognition that these new agents might have neuroleptic rather than just sedative effects.[7]

This created two schools of thought. One school based in Lyon argued for a classification of neuroleptic drugs ranging from the sedative to the incisive, and for a recognition that different agents would suit different clinical syndromes and different constitutional types. This notion underpinned the development of sedative neuroleptics such as thioridazine and levomepromazine, in addition to perphenazine and other more incisive agents. In Paris, in contrast, Deniker and Delay argued that a neuroleptic effect was the common therapeutic effect of all of these agents, and that other properties such as sedative properties were simply side-effects. The notions of Delay and Deniker led to a research and drug development agenda that focused on optimising the core neuroleptic effect.

The battle between Lyon and Paris was brief but bitter, with Paris triumphing. The development in 1958 of haloperidol, a non-sedative agent, appeared to endorse the insights of the Paris school. Haloperidol became the ultimate neuroleptic, and subsequent antipsychotics were developed on the basis of a set of laboratory tests aimed at replicating its effects.

The development of haloperidol almost led to the abortion of clozapine. On a number of the emerging tests of neuroleptics the latter drug, which had first been synthesised in 1958, failed. This failure led to a relatively half-hearted development programme, which was abandoned once the propensity of clozapine to produce agranulocytosis was recognised. However, a number of European clinicians, including Jules Angst, Raymond Battegay and Hanns Hippius, objected and argued that clozapine was indeed an effective antipsychotic even though it appeared not to have standard neuroleptic properties. The protest kept clozapine alive.

With the discovery of the effect of the neuroleptic drugs on dopamine systems, the development pathway focused on producing more selective and more potent D_2-receptor antagonists. This culminated in the benzamide group of drugs, namely sulpiride, amisulpiride and remoxipride, which arguably had somewhat fewer side-effects than other agents but were in general no more potent. With the re-emergence of clozapine, arguments were offered that the additional $5HT_2$ blockade which this compound offered might account for its apparently better effects than standard neuroleptics in schizophrenia.

The unconventional history of the antipsychotics

In the mid-1960s, concerns emerged about the propensity of neuroleptics to produce tardive dyskinesia. This syndrome, which is sometimes present in untreated older patients with psychoses, appeared to occur with a much greater frequency and severity in patients who were taking neuroleptics. At a time of rising antipsychiatric discontent with orthodox psychiatry, tardive dyskinesia provided a lightning rod to focus this discontent. In 1974, SmithKline and French settled their first million-dollar legal action with regard to tardive dyskinesia, and a subsequent generation of antipsychotic drug development was abandoned.

Apart from the benzamides, which were not developed in the USA, drug development in this area was only renewed in the wake of the re-emergence of clozapine. Contrary to popular mythologies, the re-emergence of clozapine stemmed not from any superior clinical efficacy, but rather from the fact that this was a compound that did not cause tardive dyskinesia. The agents that came in the wake of clozapine, namely sertindole, olanzapine, quetiapine and risperidone, were also developed primarily as agents that would minimise the risk of tardive dyskinesia.

Apart from a lower incidence of tardive dyskinesia, especially for quetiapine, none of these newer agents are more effective than the older agents. Risperidone and olanzapine both produce dose-dependent extrapyramidal side-effects, and are in fact rather typical neuroleptics. The non-extrapyramidal spectrum of side-effects of these agents in general suggests that they may in many ways be less safe than the older agents. Olanzapine and clozapine are associated with elevated lipid levels, the production of diabetes and weight gain, all of which can be expected to elevate cardiovascular mortality.

The new agents differ in their propensity to block D_2 receptors and also in terms of their sedative properties. Amisulpiride and risperidone are most like conventional neuroleptics, while clozapine and quetiapine are more like sedative neuroleptics such as thioridazine or levomopromazine. Recent studies which tested the ability of agents such as amisulpiride to augment the effects of clozapine in clozapine-refractory patients suggest that this cycle of drug development has returned us to the position that faced clinicians from Lyon in 1958, namely that antipsychotic agents vary across a spectrum, and while there may be some key elements in common, such as D_2-receptor blockade, the differences between agents are also significant. Classical neuroleptics may be effective in particular conditions, while others of a more sedative type may be more effective for other conditions.

What is clear is that this new generation of agents has brought an increased interest in the use of antipsychotics in the elderly. The elderly population would seem to be the best population in which to test out the competing visions of Lyon and Paris, in that the onset of psychoses in older age throws up a set of quite different syndromes to those that are found in younger populations. For example, will typical agents be more effective in systematised paranoid states, with atypical or sedative agents being more effective in disorganised states?

There are in fact some historical pointers that might guide clinical observations in this area. In addition to being effective for psychoses, the early results obtained with chlorpromazine suggested that this agent was effective in both manic and delirious states. Although the neuroleptics in general are not seen as agents that cure psychoses, they can effectively cure delirious states.

The contributions of neuroleptic pharmacology to the management of delirious states were explored during the 1990s in an interesting set of clinical experiments in Japan, which demonstrated that mianserin was an effective agent in the treatment of delirium.[8] The significance of this lies in the fact that mianserin is an agent devoid of dopamine receptor-blocking effects. Its efficacy in the treatment of delirious states appears to stem from its $5HT_2$-blocking properties. This has been confirmed by subsequent demonstrations of the efficacy of trazodone in delirious states.

These findings suggest in general that agents with significant $5HT_2$-blocking properties, such as clozapine and quetiapine, may be particularly effective for disorganised or confusional psychoses in the elderly, whereas the more selective paranoid psychoses may respond better to agents with potent D_2-blocking properties, such as amisulpiride or risperidone.

The conventional history of cognitive enhancing agents

The current role of cholinomimetic drugs in the dementias arose somewhat by default. Early neuroscientific research indicated that antidepressants might act on both catecholamine and serotonergic systems, while the antipsychotics acted on dopamine systems. This left one major brain system without either a pathology or a set of drugs. The cholinergic system by default became the system that was linked to dementia. This linkage was helped by the fact that anticholinergic drugs can produce cognitive effects.

This default option was arguably a mistake of historic proportions, in that anticholinergic agents produce confusion or delirium in high doses, rather than dysmnesias.[2] The amnestic effects of anticholinergic agents seem to be less clear-cut than the amnestic effects of the benzodiazepines. For example, many older patients with chronic obstructive pulmonary disease have always been maintained on anticholinergic agents without difficulty. There were accordingly few grounds for thinking that cholinomimetic agents would be of significant utility in the dementias.

However, the cholinomimetic research paradigm led to a development programme which successively worked through a variety of cholinomimetic principles, from replacement strategies with choline and lecithin to acetylcholine-releasing agents, such as piracetam and acetyl cholinesterase (ACE) inhibitors, to early ACE inhibitors such as physostigmine and tacrine, and finally to a later generation of cholinesterase inhibitors such as galantamine and donepezil.

Some recent cholinomimetic agents appear to have marginal efficacy across the dementia spectrum. At present, this efficacy seems to be best interpreted in terms of these drugs having significant effects in particular individuals or for particular syndromes, such as dementia with Lewy bodies (DLB). This makes sense given that DLB appears to have a greater cholinergic deficit compared with other dementing syndromes.

In parallel with these developments in the pharmacotherapy of the dementias, there has been an increasing awareness of the possibilities of cognitive enhancement in patients with conditions other than dementia. This option opened up with early work by Kral in the late 1950s on senescent forgetfulness,[9] and has proceeded through to concepts such as age-associated memory impairment.

The unconventional history of cognitive enhancing agents

Latterly, with the emergence of drugs that act on cholinergic systems, a greater appreciation of the potential role of such drugs has developed. This is perhaps best exemplified by examining one of the enduring myths of psychopharmacology. With the emergence of the monoamine theories of depression, antidepressants were supposed to act on either catecholamine or serotonergic systems, according to different schools of thought. However, common to both schools of thought was the notion that other actions, such as the anticholinergic effects of the tricyclics, could only contribute side-effects. Chief among these anticholinergic-induced side-effects was urinary retention. However, it is now clear that the urinary retention produced by tricyclic agents stems from their catecholamine reuptake-inhibiting properties. Anticholinergics do not cause urinary retention.

In fact any clinical trials undertaken with anticholinergic agents suggest that these drugs, which clearly cause a relatively rapid onset of euphoria when given in modest doses, may in fact be antidepressant. Modulating the cholinergic system has the potential to produce a range of quality-of-life-enhancing effects, as the marketing of ACE inhibitors as quality-of-life-enhancing antihypertensives helps to demonstrate. Restricting considerations of the role of drugs that act on the cholinergic system to their possible effects in memory enhancement or memory compromise is an unduly restrictive way of viewing their use.

Further evidence for this thesis can be seen in the increasing use of drugs such as donepezil in trials for childhood disorders such as attention deficit hyper-activity disorder (ADHD). Conversely, classic remedies for ADHD, such as methyl-phenidate, have found increasing use in the behavioural management of dementing conditions in the elderly in recent years.

A further recent development has been the demonstration that agents which act on glutamate systems, and in particular on the N-menthyl-D-aspartate (NMDA) receptor, may have effects in the dementing disorders. Glutamate was in fact recognised as a neurotransmitter before dopamine, and almost as early on as noradrenaline and serotonin.[10] However, despite its widespread availability in the brain, where it is the commonest neurotransmitter, a range of misconceptions about the nature of neurotransmission prevented an appreciation of its role, as did subsequent difficulties in generating agents that modulate this system effectively. In recent years this picture has changed, and increasing numbers of agents are being developed, with the potential to help both as cognitive enhancers and as agents which might prove useful in the management of cerebral insults.

The first agent of this type to come on stream was memantine, which has been widely available on many European markets from the early 1990s. There is in fact a body of evidence stemming back prior to the development of specific NMDA-active agents, indicating that agents such as ketamine or phencyclidine had promnestic effects.[11] Future generations of such agents offer interesting prospects because these actions on the NMDA receptor may also offer the possibility of neuroprotective effects.

The issues of neuroprotection and cognitive enhancement potentially frame a new vision of psychopharmacotherapy. There is every chance that the answers to the problems posed by the affective or schizophrenic psychoses will emerge from efforts to arrest neurodegeneration, rather than from the direct attack on these disorders that governs current drug development. The issue of cognitive enhancement in individuals who may not have frank disease opens up the prospects of *smart drugs*. At a time when almost all previous grounds for discrimination in our societies have been made illegal, we still discriminate on the basis of intellectual advantage. However, smart drugs are likely to erode advantages, and therefore there may well be considerable debate surrounding the use of such compounds in the future. Should they be restricted to 'medical' conditions such as age-associated memory impairment, or should they be more freely available? Some of these agents may well be life prolonging,[12] – and what then?

The increasing usage of 'drugs for the elderly' in other areas, such as donepezil for children, and the reciprocal use of methylphenidate in the elderly, suggests that the 'permafrost' that has encased established notions of psychotropic drug use in the elderly for so long is now 'melting'. The new clinical realities will also in due course lead to a new set of histories.

Conclusions

The impact of treatment with psychotropic agents in old age psychiatry differs in many significant respects from that found in other areas of psychiatry. Researchers interested in the history of psychotropic drugs will in future years probably learn more about the true place of these drugs in psychiatry from studying the impact of treatment on the clinical syndromes found in old age psychiatry, and the classification of those syndromes, than they will from studying the impact of treatment on syndromes manifest in any other age group.

Key points

- The use of antidepressants, antipsychotics and cognitive enhancing agents in old age psychiatry demonstrates interactions between syndromes and treatments that are not seen as readily in other areas of psychiatry.
- The notion that dementia involves a cholinergic deficit is probably a historically grounded mistake.

References

1 Ban TA (1980) *Psychopharmacology for the Aged*. Karger, Basel.

2 Ban TA (1995) Bridging the gap between psychogeriatric practice and research: a personal review. *Neurol Psychiatry Brain Res.* **3**: 155–60.

3 Healy D (1997) *The Antidepressant Era*. Harvard University Press, Cambridge, MA.

4 Ayd F (1961) *Recognising the Depressed Patient*. Grune & Stratton, New York.

5 Young EA, Altemus M, Lopez JF *et al.* (2004) HPA axis activation in major depression and the response to fluoxetine. *Psychneuroendocrinology.* **29**: 1198–204.

6 Belanoff JK, Flores BH, Kalezhan M, Sund B and Schatzberg AF (2002) Rapid reversal of psychotic depression using mefipristone. *J Clin Psychopharmacol.* **21**: 516–21.

7 Healy D (2002) *The Creation of Psychopharmacology*. Harvard University Press, Cambridge, MA.

8 Uchiyama M, Tanaka K, Isse K and Toru M (1996) Efficacy of mianserin on symptoms of delirium in the aged. *Prog Neuropsychopharmacol Biol Psychiatry.* **20**: 651–6.

9 Kral VA (1962) Senescent forgetfulness: benign and malignant. *J Can Med Assoc.* **86**: 257–60.

10 Watkins J (1998) Excitatory amino acids: from basic science to therapeutic applications. In: D Healy (ed.) *The Psychopharmacologists. Volume 2.* Arnold, London.

11 Harborne GC, Watson FL, Healy D and Groves L (1996) The effects of sub-anaesthetic doses of ketamine on memory, cognitive performance and subjective experience in healthy volunteers. *J Psychopharmacol.* **10**: 134–40.

12 Knoll J (2000) The psychopharmacology of life and death. In: D Healy (ed.) *The Psychopharmacologists. Volume 3.* Arnold, London.

Chapter 2

Neuropathology

Margaret M Esiri

Brain anatomy

The extraordinary complexity of the brain's structure can hardly be appreciated from its naked-eye appearance. Weighing approximately 1.5 kg, when viewed from the outside it is made up of three main components, namely the paired *cerebral hemispheres* with their deeply corrugated surfaces, below them the paired *cerebellar hemispheres*, and between these the *brainstem* (*see* Figure 2.1a and b).

More hints of complexity of structure emerge as a result of cutting across the cerebral hemispheres and brainstem (*see* Figure 2.2a, b, c and d), when it can be seen that there are distinct grey and white matter regions variously distributed around a central fluid-filled ventricular cavity. This cavity forms the paired lateral ventricles in the cerebral hemispheres communicating with the single midline third and fourth ventricles below. The grey matter contains the nerve cells and their synaptic connections, and the white matter contains the long axons that interconnect them, surrounded by their fatty myelin sheaths.

The alterations in naked-eye structure of the brain that occur in mental illness in older people are relatively slight, and mainly affect the regions that have been stippled in Figures 2.1 and 2. These are listed according to the numbers indicated in Figures 2.1 and 2 in Box 2.1. It is therefore with these regions that we are concerned, and they will be considered in more detail below. Not all of these regions are affected in all of the diseases to be considered here. Rather, different diseases are relatively selective in the regions that they damage, as indicated later. In this chapter the anatomy of the relevant brain regions is outlined, followed by a brief account of the changes in these regions that occur with ageing, and finally by summaries of the pathology of the various mental illnesses that will be considered in this volume.

(a)

(b)

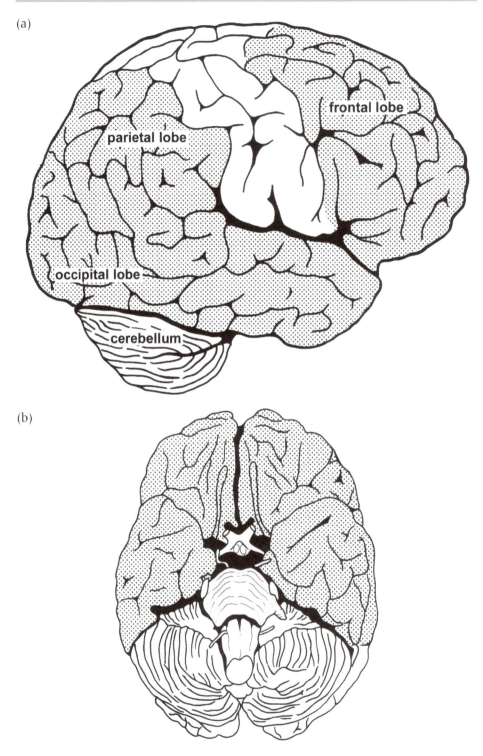

Figure 2.1 (a) Lateral and (b) inferior views of the human brain. Stippling indicates structures affected in mental disorders in older people.

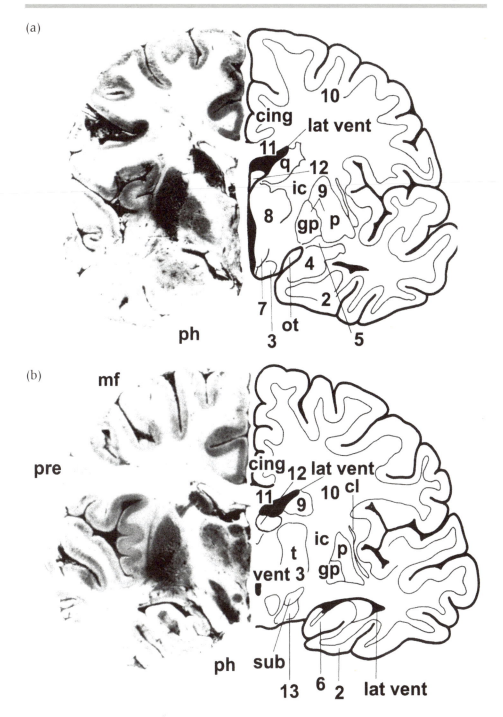

Figure 2.2 Slices across the mid-cerebrum at two adjacent levels, displaying (a) the cut slices and (b) a diagrammatic representation. (c) Myelin-stained transverse section across the midbrain. (d) Myelin-stained transverse section across the mid-pons. The white matter appears black in the left-hand section, depicted in diagrammatic form on the right. (For areas indicated by numbers, see Box 2.1, which indicates structures affected in mental disorders in older people.)

(c)

(d)

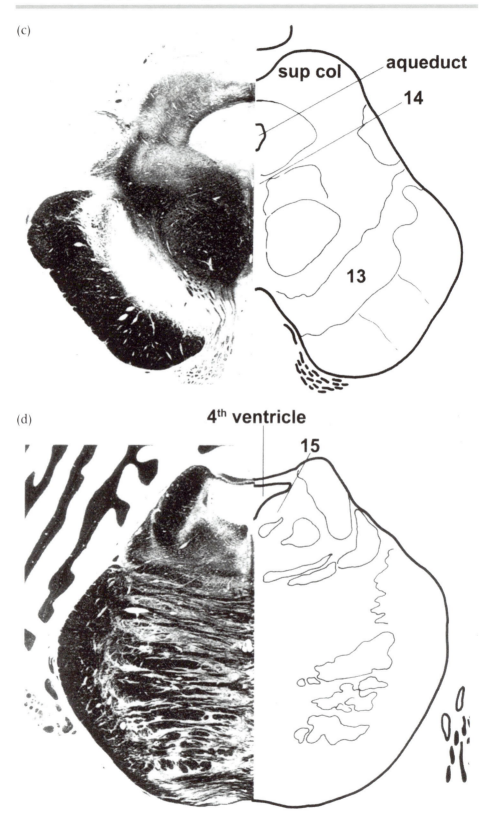

Box 2.1 Summary of brain structures relevant to mental disorders in older people

Grey-matter structures
1 Cerebral cortex – note especially particular subregions, stippled in Figure 2.1, association cortex, cingulate cortex (cing)
2 Parahippocampal gyrus
3 Mamillary body
4 Amygdala
5 Basal nucleus of Meynert
6 Hippocampus
7 Hypothalamus
8 Thalamus
9 Basal ganglia
13 Substantia nigra
14 Raphe nuclei
15 Locus ceruleus

White-matter structures
10 Cerebral white matter
11 Corpus callosum
12 Fornix

Grey-matter structures

Cerebral cortex

The cerebral cortex consists of a layer of grey matter of relatively uniform thickness (a few millimetres) that lies beneath the meninges and covers the whole surface of the corrugations, or *gyri*, of the cerebral hemispheres, also extending into the gaps, or *sulci*, that separate the gyri. Within this layer are nerve cells (*neurons*) orientated perpendicular to the surface, arranged in six strata that differ slightly in their relative thickness and cellular content from one part of the cortex to another. Specialisation of function is found in different regions of the cortex, from reception of sensory information to generation of impulses responsible for voluntary movement and execution of higher mental functions including decision making, generation and reception of language, memory and calculation. These higher mental functions are largely carried out in what is termed *association cortex*, which is found in all the main cerebral lobes, but particularly the frontal, temporal and parietal lobes. Another important part of the cortex for the execution of these functions, and for their integration with emotions, is the *cingulate gyrus*, which lies in the medial aspect of the cerebral hemisphere, just above the corpus callosum. In carrying out its functions the cerebral cortex does not act on its own, but in concert with impulses conveyed to it from subcortical structures such as the thalamus, amygdala, raphe nuclei, locus ceruleus and nucleus basalis of Meynert (see below).

Activity in the cortex is dependent on the transmission of impulses across wide networks of connections from one region of cortex to another, which travel through the white matter within each cerebral hemisphere and also from one hemisphere to the other through a wide band of white-matter nerve fibres called the *corpus callosum*. Additional impulses from the cortex also reach many subcortical structures, with which each area is specifically and selectively connected. These form complex communication circuits that return to the cortex or are relayed to further subcortical groups of neurons, or nuclei. Electrical impulses conveyed along nerve axons are eventually converted to chemical signals that exert their influence across narrow synaptic junctions between nerve cells, the chemical released differing according to the nerve-cell type from which the impulse originates. Some chemicals transmit an inhibitory signal to the post-synaptic neuron, and others are excitatory. Cortical neurons are of two main types, namely pyramidal (the majority) and non-pyramidal. Pyramidal neurons convey excitatory signals expressed mainly by release of the neurotransmitter chemical *glutamate*. Non-pyramidal neurons are in general inhibitory and release the chemical transmitter gamma-aminobutyric acid (GABA), in some cases also accompanied by the release of a peptide such as substance P, vasoactive intestinal peptide (VIP) or corticotropin-releasing factor (CRF). To exert their influence on postsynaptic neurons, these neurons need to express specific receptors for the neurotransmitter or neuropeptides.

Hippocampus

The hippocampus is a folded layer of relatively simplified cortex situated in the medial part of the temporal lobe (*see* Figure 2.2b). It is a three-layered structure containing, like the rest of the cerebral cortex, pyramidal and non-pyramidal neurons. The hippocampus is closely connected with the adjacent entorhinal cortex and parahippocampal gyrus and, via the fornix, with the septal area of the frontal lobe and mamillary body in the hypothalamus. It has a unique function in enabling new memories to be formed. It is damaged relatively early in the course of Alzheimer's disease, in which impaired ability to form new memories is often a correspondingly early clinical feature.

Amygdala

The amygdala is a closely interconnected cluster of neuronal nuclei lying in the anterior temporal lobe just in front of the hippocampus. It is closely connected with the hippocampus, the olfactory sensory system, neighbouring regions of cerebral cortex and the cingulate cortex. It has a key role in emotional responses and feelings. It is damaged in Alzheimer's disease and dementia with Lewy bodies.

Basal nucleus of Meynert

The basal nucleus of Meynert and some related neurons lying more anteriorly, in the diagonal band of Broca, are the neurons that supply the cerebral cortex and hippocampus with the neurotransmitter acetylcholine. These clusters of large neurons do not form a well-defined grey-matter structure, but are distributed in the substantia innominata which lies just below the anterior commissure and external segment of the globus pallidus, part of the basal ganglia. These clusters of neurons assumed importance in our understanding of dementia when it was discovered that acetylcholine deficiency is an early and conspicuous neurotransmitter deficiency in the cerebral cortex in Alzheimer's disease (*see* Chapter 3).

Hypothalamus

This is a key centre of autonomic control in the brain. It lies in the wall of the third ventricle beneath the thalamus. It has many different constituent nuclei that subserve different functions. One region, the median eminence, has connections with the pituitary gland. Another portion is the mamillary body, which as we have already seen has close connections with the hippocampus. The mamillary bodies are damaged in Korsakov's psychosis, most commonly seen as a complication of alcoholism. A third component is the suprachiasmatic nucleus, which controls sleep rhythms and develops pathology in Alzheimer's disease. Other nuclei control water and food intake and sexual function.

Thalamus

The thalamus is a large mass of grey matter lying in the walls of the third ventricle and extending as far laterally as the internal capsule, a large white-matter tract that conveys axons to and from all parts of the cerebral cortex. There are many different nuclei in the thalamus, some of which are concerned with relaying sensory information from the periphery, while others are concerned with motor function and yet others with memory function.

Basal ganglia

The basal ganglia form the other large subcortical group of nuclei, lying in front of the thalamus. The three major subdivisions of the basal ganglia are the *caudate nucleus* (which abuts the lateral wall of the frontal horn of the lateral ventricle), the *putamen* (which merges with the lateral aspect of the caudate nucleus anteriorly and is separated from it by the anterior limb of the internal capsule more posteriorly) and the *globus pallidus* (which lies medial to the posterior portion of the putamen and lateral to the internal capsule). The basal ganglia are mainly functionally concerned with control of movement. However, functional activity in this region is altered in obsessive-compulsive disorder, and addictive behaviour is related to excess dopamine stimulation in the nucleus accumbens in the inferior part of the caudate nucleus. The caudate nucleus is relatively selectively damaged in Huntington's disease.

Raphe nuclei

The raphe nuclei are a group of nuclei situated in the medial part of the upper brainstem (midbrain) in the floor of the aqueduct, the narrow channel linking the third and fourth ventricles. Their neurons have axons projecting to all parts of the cerebrum, particularly the cortex and hippocampus. The neurotransmitter used by raphe neurons is serotonin (5-HT). Damage to these nuclei occurs in Alzheimer's disease.

Locus ceruleus

The locus ceruleus is a tightly localised column of pigmented neurons lying in the upper and mid pons, just beneath the floor of the upper part of the fourth ventricle. It is the source of the transmitter noradrenalin, which it supplies through axonal connections to most parts of the cerebrum and cerebellar cortex. As with the substantia nigra, the pigment in its neurons is melanin, which accumulates as a by-product of noradrenalin synthesis. The locus ceruleus is damaged in Alzheimer's disease and to a lesser extent in Parkinson's disease.

White-matter structures

The white matter consists almost exclusively of axons, many of which are surrounded by myelin sheaths, and the blood vessels needed to nourish them. Relatively short axons linking local regions of cortex run in the immediately subcortical white matter, while longer connections linking more distant parts of cortex of the same or the contralateral hemisphere, or linking cerebral cortex with subcortical structures, run more deeply in the white matter. A reduction in the density of nerve fibres in white matter can arise as a result of directly inflicted damage, usually by ischaemia, but it can also occur secondarily to loss of parent nerve cells in cortex or subcortical nuclei.

Changes in brain structure with normal ageing

The pathology of specific diseases that affect the brain towards the end of life needs to be distinguished from changes that occur as an inevitable consequence of ageing. These are found even in the brains of older people known to have had well-preserved mental function when they were alive.[1] These changes chiefly consist, at the macroscopic level, of the following:

- a slight but significant reduction in brain weight
- slight enlargement of the lateral ventricles
- slight fibrous thickening of the leptomeninges that cover the brain
- a slight reduction in the volume of the cerebral white matter.

The main microscopic changes that occur are as follows:

- accumulation of dense spherical structures called corpora amylacea which develop mainly in the processes of glial cells (the cells that nurture and support nerve cells)
- a reduction in the size of neurons at some sites, including the cerebral cortex
- a reduction in the number of synapses in the cerebral cortex
- a reduction in the number of neurons at some sites, including the cerebral cortex and hippocampus
- the appearance in the association cortex of argyrophilic (silver-staining) plaques of the type also seen in Alzheimer's disease (see below)
- the appearance in the hippocampus and adjacent cortex of small numbers of neurofibrillary tangles of the type also seen in Alzheimer's disease (see below).

The first two of these microscopic changes are not clearly correlated with degeneration of neurons. The reduction in the size of neurons is likely to be related to the reduction in the number of synapses, since the size of a nerve-cell body is related to the extent of its processes and the number of synapses on those processes that it needs to support. The reduction in the number of neurons with age is of the order of 1% per year after the age of 70 years for cerebral cortex[2] and for some subregions of the hippocampus.[3]

The most likely reason for the changes seen in the brain with ageing is progressive damage to neuron constituents (mitochondria, DNA and cell membranes) caused by free radicals, coupled with progressive failure of the mechanisms normally intended to protect cell constituents from such damage.[4]

Neuropathology of dementia

Alzheimer's disease

About 75% of cases of progressive dementia in the elderly are due to Alzheimer's disease occurring either alone or with vascular or Lewy body disease. It is therefore not surprising that a major research effort has been under way for some decades to enable a full understanding of the disease to be acquired. However, there are still many aspects of this complex disease that need to be clarified. Recently, animal models based on genetic mutations that cause familial disease have helped to elucidate some of the multiple factors that contribute to the disease.[5]

In elderly sufferers from Alzheimer's disease the brain may show only mild and non-specific changes to the naked eye, namely a mild degree of cerebral cortical and hippocampal atrophy, mild ventricular enlargement and loss of pigment from the locus ceruleus. In early-onset disease these changes tend to be more severe. However, in both age groups the distinctive pathology is only seen at the microscopic level.

It was mentioned earlier that even in normal elderly people's brains, substantial numbers of argyrophilic plaques may be present in microscopic sections of association cortex. These plaques consist of abnormal fibrillary material deposited in clumps within the neuropil (the tissue that occupies the space between cells in the cerebral cortex). However, detailed study of prospectively assessed elderly subjects has shown that a particular subtype of these plaques, when present in large numbers, is associated with dementia and occurs alongside the other hallmark microscopic feature of Alzheimer's disease, namely neurofibrillary tangles. The subtype of plaque that is associated with dementia is the *neuritic plaque* – one in which there are abnormal neuritic processes caught up in the structure (*see* Figure 2.3).

Plaques that lack this feature are referred to as *diffuse plaques* (*see* Figure 2.4), and these are the ones that are frequently abundant in the brains of undemented elderly people. It is thought likely that diffuse plaques are converted into neuritic ones over the course of time as additional pathological reactions take place in them. This view is supported by the observation that in subjects with Down's syndrome, in whom the pathology of Alzheimer's disease invariably develops by late middle age, diffuse plaques are seen at an earlier age than neuritic ones.[6]

Many neuritic plaques have at their centre a dense core of amyloid surrounded by a cluster of microglial cells (glial cells that are of the macrophage lineage). Beyond them lies a corona of neuritic and glial cell processes. Within the neuritic processes in such plaques can be found, at the ultrastructural level, abnormal mitochondria and abnormal paired, helically wound filaments that are structurally and chemically identical to the abnormal filaments that make up the inclusions in neuron cell bodies that are called *neurofibrillary tangles* (*see* Figure 2.5). It was tangles that Alzheimer particularly associated with dementia,

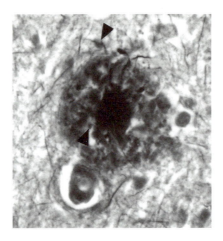

Figure 2.3 Microscopic appearance of a neuritic plaque stained with silver. The black granules (indicated by arrowheads) represent neuritic processes. At the centre is an amyloid core.

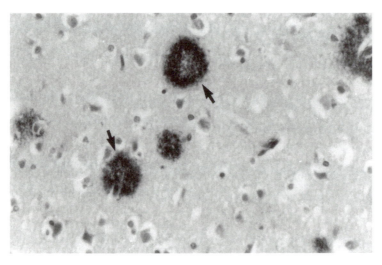

Figure 2.4 Microscopic appearance of diffuse plaques stained with silver (indicated by arrows). There are no neuritic processes, and no amyloid core is present.

and more recent studies fully corroborate this association by demonstrating that the severity of dementia in an individual with Alzheimer's disease is closely correlated with the numbers of tangles that are present in the brain.[7,8] In contrast, the correlation of dementia severity with the number of neuritic plaques is only modest, and the correlation with the number of diffuse plaques is insignificant.[8]

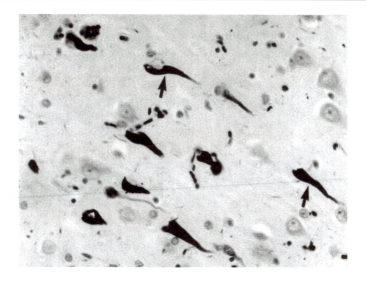

Figure 2.5 Microscopic appearance of neurons containing neurofibrillary tangles (indicated by arrows). Section stained with Gallyas silver stain.

Thus, in brief, Alzheimer's disease is characterised by a complex pathology in which there is deposition of plaques *outside* cells in regions of grey matter that are known to be important for cognitive function (association cortex and hippocampus), coupled with the appearance of tangles *inside* neurons in similar areas of the brain. At the start of the process, plaques are widespread but diffuse in type whereas tangles are restricted to the hippocampus and adjacent entorhinal cortex. This small amount of tangle formation does not initially interfere with memory and cognitive function, but as the process continues and more tangles are formed, impaired memory starts to make an appearance. Later, plaques become neuritic and tangles become more widespread, occurring mainly in pyramidal neurons of the association cortex but also in subcortical nuclei that project to the cortex, particularly the nucleus basalis of Meynert, the raphe nuclei and the locus ceruleus. Tangles also develop in other nuclei in, for example, the amygdala, the suprachiasmatic nucleus and some other hypothalamic nuclei, and in some parts of the thalamus. Plaques may also appear in subcortical nuclei such as the amygdala, caudate nucleus and putamen.

It has been noted that populations of neurons that are prone to develop tangles also lose a substantial proportion of their neurons, probably by an apoptotic-like process. Some neurons that harbour tangles die, leaving an insoluble 'ghost' tangle marking their place, but other neurons seem to die without developing tangles. Even tangle-bearing neurons that remain alive are unable to function normally because their cytoskeleton collapses. This is because the filamentous protein accumulations that form tangles are composed of a protein, *tau*, that is normally present in non-fibrillar form, helping to maintain the cytoskeleton of microtubules and neurofilaments in normal alignment. Filamentous tau is hyperphosphorylated by abnormally expressed enzymes, although exactly why this occurs and how it is related to the deposition of plaques, which probably occurs initially at synapses, is not fully understood. Plaques themselves are composed of a different protein, β-amyloid, which is a polypeptide product of the enzymatic digestion of the amyloid precursor protein, a membrane protein of unknown function. β-amyloid, in the fibrillar form in which it is deposited in plaques, has been shown to have toxic effects on neurons in culture, although it is by no means clear whether tangle formation in nerve cells in most cases of sporadic Alzheimer's disease is simply a consequence of the production of excess amounts of β-amyloid. One difficulty with this hypothesis is that, while transgenic mice that express disease-causing mutations in the gene coding for amyloid precursor protein develop large numbers of cortical plaques, they do not develop tangles.[9] However, the processes that are thought to give rise to Alzheimer's disease in humans operate over very long periods, of the order of many years, which may make a short-lived rodent an unsuitable animal on which to model the disease.

There are a number of risk factors for Alzheimer's disease other than the main one of advancing age. Apart from the minority of cases in which gene mutations in the amyloid precursor protein gene or in the genes for presenilin 1 and 2 are responsible for (usually) early-onset disease, these include the epsilon-4 polymorphism in the gene for apolipoprotein E, some other less well-established gene polymorphisms, hypertension and exposure to head trauma. Exactly how such risk factors operate is as yet unclear. Discussion of them can be found in recent reviews.[10,11]

Some of the symptoms of Alzheimer's disease, and indeed some of the most troublesome symptoms to deal with, are caused by changes in behaviour rather than in cognition. Although the pathological basis of such behavioural changes is much less well understood than that of cognitive decline, there has been some research conducted on these aspects of the disease in the hope that increased understanding of the basis of these symptoms may lead to an improvement in their alleviation (*see* Chapter 13). In general, changes in behaviour in Alzheimer's disease relate to changes in subcortical nuclei or to attempts by the brain to overcome the effects of subcortical pathology. Thus depression in the disease has been correlated with loss of serotonin in the cortex secondary to loss of and tangle formation in raphe neurons. Anxiety has been correlated with relatively good preservation of $5HT_{2a}$ receptors in cortex,[12] aggression has been linked to loss of locus ceruleus neurons[13] or relative preservation of substantia nigra neurons,[14] and psychotic symptoms have been linked to changes in muscarinic acetylcholine receptors in the cortex.[15]

With regard to dealing with the problem of Alzheimer's disease in ageing world populations, it is worth noting that at present only treatment that ameliorates (albeit incompletely) the cholinergic transmission deficit, or that alleviates behavioural changes, is available. Such treatment does not prevent the disease from progressing. Much more effective would be a means of preventing or reversing the abnormal fibrillar protein deposits that accumulate inside and outside neurons, especially the intracellular tangles that are so closely related to defective cognition and neuron drop-out. Although there is some experimental evidence that plaques may be removable,[16] there has been no sign as yet of a mechanism to remove tangles.

Vascular disease and dementia

There has been considerable confusion over several decades as to the role of cerebrovascular disease in dementia, but some clarification has emerged more recently. One of several difficulties that researchers have had to contend with is that cerebrovascular disease takes diverse forms, some of which occur together, and some of which are difficult to quantify with regard to their severity. One convenient way to classify cerebrovascular disease is into two subdivisions as follows:

- *lobar infarction* – involving cerebral cortex and contiguous white matter, usually the result of obstruction to blood flow in a major artery or its branches, and classically giving rise to 'stroke'
- *subcortical infarction* – involving mainly white matter in a relatively diffuse distribution and deep grey matter in the form of *lacunes*. Subcortical infarction is commonly incomplete, producing attenuation rather than obliteration of tissue, particularly in white matter (*see* Figure 2.6). It is associated with inadequate blood perfusion through arterioles and small arteries that have had their lumens narrowed but not usually obstructed. The vessel walls are thickened by fibrosis. These changes are often consequent upon longstanding hypertension.

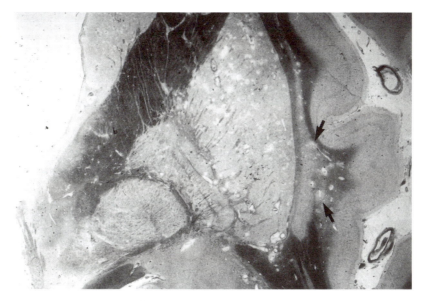

Figure 2.6 Low-power view of a section of basal ganglia and white matter stained for myelin. The 'lacy' appearance is due to widening of perivascular spaces around small arteries and arterioles. Myelin, which is stained black, is pale around some of these vessels (see arrows), indicating loss of myelin.

Initial studies on the role of cerebrovascular disease in dementia suggested that the latter was related to large volumes of lobar infarction. However, recent studies have shown that dementia is more closely correlated with subcortical vascular disease.[17] This is the type of disease which, in advanced form, has long been recognised as *Binswanger's disease*. A recently recognised familial disease with similar pathology is referred to as CADASIL (cerebral arteriopathy with dementia and subacute ischaemic encephalopathy), and tends to present with early-onset dementia.[18] These diseases produce a type of dementia that is characteristic of subcortical pathology, with poor concentration and slowed responses. In general, it is unusual for vascular disease to be the sole cause of dementia.

Cerebrovascular disease and Alzheimer's disease can combine to cause dementia. It has been recognised for many years that cerebrovascular disease and Alzheimer's disease commonly occur together. There are several common risk factors for the two diseases, including possession of the ApoE ϵ4 gene polymorphism, hypertension, and elevated levels of cholesterol and homocysteine in the blood. One specific type of vascular disease, namely β-amyloid deposition in the walls of leptomeningeal and cortical vessels, does indeed occur in over 90% of cases of Alzheimer's disease, but it is unclear whether this significantly compromises blood supply to the brain. However, it can give rise to small and large lobar or subarachnoid haemorrhages.

One form of dementia occurs shortly after a stroke. Although initially it was thought that 'post-stroke' dementia was likely to be due to vascular disease, it now seems probable that some cases are due to subclinical Alzheimer's disease which has been 'unmasked' by an additional insult to the brain in the form of a stroke. Pathological study of prospectively assessed elderly subjects has shown that those who were found at autopsy to have relatively mild degrees of Alzheimer-type pathology with neurofibrillary tangles confined to the entorhinal cortex and hippocampus were not clinically demented in life unless they were also found to have additional cerebrovascular disease.[19] Subcortical lacunes also distinguished demented subjects among elderly nuns with abundant plaques in another study.[20] Thus Alzheimer's disease, particularly in its early stages, can summate with cerebrovascular disease to cause dementia. The important implication is that prevention of cerebrovascular disease has the potential to reduce clinical expression of Alzheimer's disease in its common early stages.

Dementia with Lewy bodies

The classical disease associated with the presence of Lewy bodies in the brain is Parkinson's disease, in which a movement disorder characterised by bradykinesia, cogwheel rigidity and tremor is attributable to loss of pigmented neurons from the substantia nigra and the presence of inclusions, termed *Lewy bodies*, in some surviving pigmented neurons. Lewy bodies are rounded, frequently spherical structures composed of granular and filamentous components that occur in the cytoplasm of neurons (*see* Figure 2.7). Their principal chemical constituent is a protein called α-synuclein, whose normal function is uncertain. Although they are most commonly found in the substantia nigra and locus ceruleus in Parkinson's disease, Lewy bodies also occur at several other sites, including the

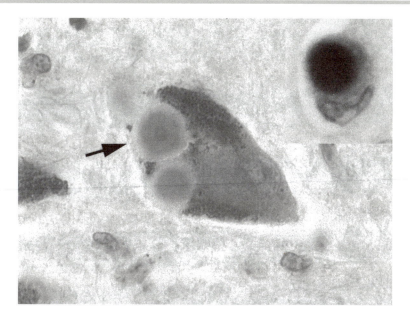

Figure 2.7 Microscopic appearance of Lewy bodies in a pigmented neuron in the substantia nigra (haematoxylin and eosin stain). Inset shows cortical Lewy body stained with an antibody to α-synuclein.

amygdala, nucleus basalis and hypothalamus, in that disease. A few may also be found in the cerebral cortex.

Dementia is more common in people with Parkinson's disease than in healthy individuals of similar age. The pathology in some cases of dementia with Parkinson's disease combines that of Alzheimer's disease with that of Parkinson's disease, but in many cases Alzheimer-type pathology, if present, is only mild in extent and insufficient on its own to explain the dementia. Such cases also have considerable numbers of Lewy bodies in cerebral cortical neurons, most commonly in the parahippocampal gyrus and cingulate gyrus. It is now recognised that a form of dementia can occur in which the main burden of Lewy body pathology falls on the cerebral cortex, rather than on subcortical nuclei such as the substantia nigra. These changes result in dementia without very many, if any, Parkinsonian features, although at autopsy the substantia nigra does show some neuron loss and Lewy body formation. This condition is known as *dementia with Lewy bodies*.[21] It has certain characteristic clinical features that make it recognisable, namely fluctuation in the severity of dementia, visual hallucinations and, often, mild parkinsonian features. It has been shown that in dementia with Lewy bodies the cortical cholinergic deficit is more severe than in Alzheimer's disease, probably because the nucleus basalis is damaged by both pathologies.[22] Thus such patients may respond well to drugs that augment cholinergic function. They are also unduly sensitive to neuroleptic medication, which can cause significant clinical deterioration. For these reasons it is important to recognise dementia with Lewy bodies clinically and to distinguish it from 'pure' Alzheimer's disease.

Pick's disease and other forms of frontal lobe dementia

These diseases are much less common than Alzheimer's disease, and tend to present initially with altered behaviour, reflecting impaired frontal lobe function, or with language deficits rather than with memory problems. Some cases present in middle age, but others present later. About 50% of the cases have a family history of dementia. In Pick's disease the naked-eye changes in the brain are usually more severe than in Alzheimer's disease, with marked atrophy of the poles of the frontal and/or temporal lobes (*see* Figure 2.8), and marked expansion of the frontal and inferior horns of the lateral ventricles. The caudate nuclei may also be moderately atrophied.

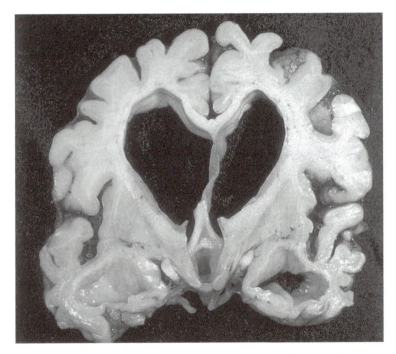

Figure 2.8 Macroscopic appearance of the brain from a case of Pick's disease. Note the narrowing of cortex and widening of sulci (reflecting cortical atrophy) in the frontal and temporal lobes, with massive compensatory dilation of the lateral ventricles.

The microscopic features of Pick's disease are a dramatic loss of neurons from the atrophic cortical regions, reactive enlargement and an increase in the number of glial cells (astrocytes), and the presence in some remaining neurons of fibrillary rounded inclusions known as *Pick bodies* (*see* Figure 2.9). These bodies are composed of the same protein, tau, that accumulates as tangles in Alzheimer's disease, although it has a slightly different molecular conformation in Pick bodies to that in tangles. Some neurons are greatly expanded to form 'ballooned' neurons by the intracytoplasmic tau filaments – these are called *Pick cells*. These inclusions are found principally in frontal and temporal lobe cortex and hippocampus. A few inherited cases of Pick's disease have been shown to be due to mutations in the tau gene on chromosome 17.

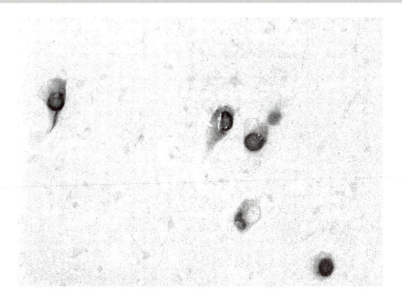

Figure 2.9 Microscopic appearance of Pick bodies in a frontal lobe section stained with an antibody to tau protein.

Some cases with a clinical presentation similar to that of Pick's disease have much less severe frontal and temporal lobe atrophy and lack the tau inclusions characteristic of that disease. Such cases frequently show little in the way of specific microscopic pathology (mild neuron loss in the cortex of frontal and anterior temporal lobes, mild reactive astrocytosis and the presence of vacuoles in the second layer of the cortex). In these regions it may be possible to demonstrate small distorted neuritic processes that react with the protein ubiquitin, a protein that binds to cytoplasmic proteins destined for degeneration. (Ubiquitin antibodies also bind to the proteins in Lewy bodies and neurofibrillary tangles.) This condition is frequently termed *non-specific frontal lobe dementia*.

Dementia caused by alcohol misuse

There are both reversible and irreversible effects of excess alcohol intake on brain structure. The reversible effect is atrophy of the frontal lobes, particularly the white matter. This is probably due to removal of water from the tissue. The irreversible effects are thought to be due in part to a direct toxic influence on the cerebellum, which leads to patchy loss of Purkinje cells, particularly in the vermis (midline region), and to loss of some cerebral cortical nerve cells. The other irreversible pathology is due to vitamin B_1 (thiamine) deficiency, to which severe alcoholics are prone, possibly because the cerebral metabolism of alcohol requires a high level of consumption of the vitamin, and alcoholics tend to have a diet deficient in vitamins. Vitamin B_1 deficiency causes damage to the capillaries in the regions of the brain close to the third ventricle, particularly the mamillary bodies and dorsomedial nucleus of the thalamus. This damage to the endothelial cells allows leakage of red blood cells into the neuropil, where they are phagocytosed by macrophages, lysed and metabolised to haemosiderin. Neurons are not the primary target of damage in this vitamin deficiency, but are damaged secondarily to the vascular damage, haemorrhage and iron deposition.

Other causes of dementia

The three conditions of Alzheimer's disease, cerebrovascular disease and dementia with Lewy bodies alone, or in combination, account for the great majority of cases of dementia in the elderly. However, there are many other diseases that are occasionally encountered and which should be borne in mind, particularly when there are atypical features in the clinical presentation. These include cerebral tumours (gliomas, metastases and meningiomas), normal-pressure hydrocephalus, HIV/AIDS, Creutzfeldt–Jakob disease, progressive supranuclear palsy, Huntington's disease, leucodystrophies, and chronic subdural haematomas. For accounts of the pathology of these conditions, the reader is referred to Graham and Lantos[23] and Esiri et al.[24]

Neuropathology of depression in older people

The relatively effective treatment of depression with selective inhibitors of serotonin reuptake (see Chapter 8) implicates the raphe nuclei and their projections in this condition. Until relatively recently there had been very little study of the neuropathology of depression, but there have now been neuroimaging and neuropathological studies of unipolar depression and of bipolar disorder in subjects of various ages, and of depression in the elderly, which are beginning to cast some light on this subject. In familial unipolar depression and bipolar disorder, attention was directed to the subgenual cortex, the most anterior and inferior part of the cingulate cortex, by positron emission topography (PET) studies that found a reduced volume of cortex here.[25] Subsequent neuropathological study of this area showed a reduced number of glial cells, but no change in the neurons.[26] Neuroimaging studies of depression in the elderly have demonstrated changes in the frontal lobe white matter suggestive of vascular damage,[27] and pathological studies have reported non-specific inflammatory changes in adjacent dorsolateral prefrontal cortex consistent with reaction to vascular damage.[28] Other neuropathological studies, in these instances directed at the brainstem nuclei sending serotonergic and noradrenergic projections to the cortex, the raphe nuclei and locus ceruleus, have reported reduced[29] or unaltered[30] numbers of neurons in these nuclei in depression. Although these initial studies of depression present a somewhat bewildering picture of disparate pathology in the cortex, cerebral white matter and brainstem, it could be the case that these reflect impaired delivery of serotonin to the cortex, which could conceivably influence glial cell numbers (since glial cells have receptors for 5-HT on their surface), interruption of serotonergic and noradrenergic axons in white matter by subcortical vascular disease, and a reduction in the number of raphe and locus ceruleus neurons in old age associated with Alzheimer-type pathology or age-related change. These possibilities will need to be investigated further in future studies.

Neuropathology of psychotic disorders

Psychotic symptoms sometimes develop in demented individuals who may be suffering from either Alzheimer's disease or dementia with Lewy bodies. The pathology of such symptoms has been touched upon in the section on dementia above. The neuropathology of schizophrenia is beyond the scope of this chapter, but those who wish to read about it are referred to reviews by Harrison[31] and Esiri and Crow.[32]

Key points

- Brain structure and chemistry are subtly altered in mental disorders of old age. Many widespread areas of the brain can show changes, with the region affected depending on the disease.
- In Alzheimer's disease the hallmark changes are microscopic – principally the formation of extracellular plaques composed mainly of β-amyloid protein, and intraneuronal tangles composed of tau protein. These deposits are accompanied by neuron and synapse loss, particularly in the cerebral cortex and hippocampus.
- In vascular dementia, subcortical small-vessel disease is more significant than major lobar infarction. Vascular disease on its own only rarely causes dementia, but it commonly summates with mild Alzheimer-type pathology to do so. It may also cause depression in old age.
- Dementia with Lewy bodies represents a form of dementia in which pathology of the type seen in Parkinson's disease participates. It deserves clinical recognition because it responds relatively well to cholinesterase inhibitor drugs, but is adversely affected by neuroleptics.
- Although Alzheimer's disease, cerebrovascular disease and dementia with Lewy bodies are (in that order) the commonest causes of dementia in the elderly, there are many other causes which should be considered, particularly in clinically atypical cases.

References

1 Esiri MM (1994) Dementia and normal aging. In: FA Huppert, C Brayne and DW O'Connor (eds) *Dementia and Normal Aging*. Cambridge University Press, Cambridge.

2 Anderson JM, Hubbard BM, Coghill GR and Slidders W (1983) The effect of advanced old age on the neurone content of the cerebral cortex. Observations with an automatic image analyser point counting method. *J Neurol Sci*. **58**: 235–46.

3 West MJ, Coleman PD, Flood DG and Troncoso JC (1994) Differences in the pattern of hippocampal neuronal loss in normal ageing and Alzheimer's disease. *Lancet*. **344**: 769–72.

4 Halliwell B and Gutteridge JMC (1999) *Free Radicals in Biology and Medicine*. Oxford University Press, Oxford.

5 Borchelt D (2003) Transgenic mouse models of dementia. In: MM Esiri, VM-Y Lee and J Trojanowski (eds) *The Neuropathology of Dementia* (2e). Cambridge University Press, Cambridge.

6 Lemere CA, Blusztajn JK, Yamaguchi H, Wisniewski T, Saido TC and Selkoe DJ (1996) Sequence of deposition of heterogeneous amyloid beta-peptides and Apo E in Down syndrome: implications for initial events in amyloid plaque formation. *Neurobiol Dis.* **3**: 16–32.

7 Wilcock GK and Esiri MM (1982) Plaques, tangles and dementia. A quantitative study. *J Neurol Sci.* **56**: 343–56.

8 Nagy Z, Esiri MM, Jobst KA *et al.* (1995) Relative roles of plaques and tangles in the dementia of Alzheimer's disease: correlations using three sets of neuropathological criteria. *Dementia.* **6**: 21–31.

9 Games D, Adams D, Alessandrini R *et al.* (1995) Alzheimer-type neuropathology in transgenic mice overexpressing V717F beta-amyloid precursor protein. *Nature.* **373**: 523–7.

10 Ritchie K and Lovestone S (2002) The dementias. *Lancet.* **360**: 1759–66.

11 Kawas CH and Katzman R (1999) Epidemiology of dementia and Alzheimer disease. In: RD Terry, R Katzman, KL Bick and SS Sisodia (eds) *Alzheimer Disease.* Lippincott, Williams and Wilkins, Philadelphia, PA.

12 Esiri MM (1996) The basis for behavioural disturbances in dementia. *J Neurol Neurosurg Psychiatry.* **61**: 127–30.

13 Matthews KL, Chen CP, Esiri MM, Keene J, Minger SL and Francis PT (2002) Noradrenergic changes, aggressive behavior, and cognition in patients with dementia. *Biol Psychiatry.* **51**: 407–16.

14 Victoroff J, Mack WJ, Lyness SA and Chui HC (1995) Multicenter clinicopathological correlation in dementia. *Am J Psychiatry.* **152**: 1476–84.

15 Lai MK, Lai OF, Keene J *et al.* (2001) Psychosis of Alzheimer's disease is associated with elevated muscarinic M_2 binding in the cortex. *Neurology.* **57**: 805–11.

16 Bard F, Cannon C, Barbour R *et al.* (2000) Peripherally administered antibodies against amyloid beta-peptide enter the central nervous system and reduce pathology in a mouse model of Alzheimer disease. *Nat Med.* **6**: 916–19.

17 Esiri MM, Wilcock GK and Morris JH (1997) Neuropathological assessment of the lesions of significance in vascular dementia. *J Neurol Neurosurg Psychiatry.* **63**: 749–53.

18 Morris JH and Kalimo H (2003) Vascular dementia. In: MM Esiri, VM-Y Lee and J Trojanowski (eds) *The Neuropathology of Dementia* (2e). Cambridge University Press, Cambridge.

19 Esiri MM, Nagy Z, Smith MZ, Barnetson L and Smith AD (1999) Cerebrovascular disease and threshold for dementia in the early stages of Alzheimer's disease (letter). *Lancet.* **354**: 919–20.

20 Snowdon DA, Greiner LH, Mortimer JA, Riley KP, Greiner PA and Markesbery WR (1997) Brain infarction and the clinical expression of Alzheimer disease. The Nun Study. *JAMA.* **277**: 813–17.

21 McKeith IG, Galasko D, Kosaka K *et al.* (1996) Consensus guidelines for the clinical and pathologic diagnosis of dementia with Lewy bodies (DLB): report of the consortium on DLB international workshop. *Neurology.* **47**: 1113–24.

22 Perry EK, Haroutunian V, Davis KL *et al.* (1994) Neocortical cholinergic activities differentiate Lewy body dementia from classical Alzheimer's disease. *Neuroreport.* **5**: 747–9.

23 Graham DI and Lantos PL (eds) (2002) *Greenfield's Neuropathology* (7e). Arnold, London.

24 Esiri MM, Lee VM-Y and Trojanowski J (eds) (2004) *The Neuropathology of Dementia* (2e). Cambridge University Press, Cambridge.

25 Drevets WC, Price JL, Simpson JR Jr *et al.* (1997) Subgenual prefrontal cortex abnormalities in mood disorders. *Nature.* **386**: 824–7.

26 Ongur D, Drevets WC and Price JL (1998) Glial reduction in the subgenual prefrontal cortex in mood disorders. *Proc Natl Acad Sci USA.* **95**: 13290–5.

27 O'Brien J, Ames D, Chiu E, Schweitzer I, Desmond P and Tress B (1998) Severe deep white matter lesions and outcome in elderly patients with major depressive disorder: follow-up study. *BMJ.* **317**: 982–4.

28 Thomas AJ, O'Brien JT, Davis S *et al.* (2002) Ischemic basis for deep white matter hyperintensities in major depression: a neuropathological study. *Arch Gen Psychiatry.* **59**: 785–92.

29 Chan-Palay V and Asan E (1989) Alterations in catecholamine neurons of the locus coeruleus in senile dementia of the Alzheimer type and in Parkinson's disease with and without dementia and depression. *J Comp Neurol.* **287**: 373–92.

30 Syed A, Chatfield M, Matthews F, *et al.* (2005) Depression in the Elderly: pathological study of raphe and locus ceruleus. *Neuropathol Appl Neurobiol.* In press.

31 Harrison PJ (1999) The neuropathology of schizophrenia. A critical review of the data and their interpretation. *Brain.* **122**: 593–624.

32 Esiri MM and Crow TJ (2002) Psychiatric disorders. In: DI Graham and PL Lantos (eds) *Greenfield's Neuropathology* (7e). Arnold, London.

Chapter 3

Neurochemical changes in old age

Andrew W Procter

Introduction

Effective drug treatments for depression and psychosis have been available since the 1950s. Much is known about the pharmacological actions of such drugs, but the precise nature of the underlying neurochemical pathology in these conditions remains unknown. Conversely, effective neurotransmitter-based therapies for the major neurodegenerative disease causing dementia in old age, namely Alzheimer's disease (AD), have only become available in recent years, despite nearly three decades of study of this condition. The model for such treatment of a neurodegenerative condition has been Parkinson's disease, the neurochemical pathology of which was described in the 1960s. Understanding of monoamine and other neurotransmitter systems developed at around the same time and led to therapies for this condition. Thus, with this exception, it is broadly true to say that we are currently in the position of having effective treatments for those conditions for which we have a poor understanding of the neurobiology, yet few treatments for those conditions about which we know much more.

In part this may be true because the neurodegenerative disorders tend to be fatal after a relatively short period, and many studies have therefore been made of *post-mortem* brain tissue. The investigation of the biology of functional psychiatric disorders has been dependent on techniques which can be applied in life, when these conditions are relatively uncomplicated by other disorders and conditions. For many years the investigation of *post-mortem* brain tissue has been a standard against which other studies have been compared, and these neurochemical studies have provided information about neurotransmitter function and other metabolic processes. However, such studies need to be interpreted carefully and conducted in such a way as to take account of the potential artefacts and epiphenomena which have often complicated studies of AD. This disorder provides a model of how the effects of these factors may be taken into account.

Nonetheless, our present understanding of neurotransmitter systems, their receptors and second-messenger systems in the human brain and their relevance to the psychiatric disorders of old age is largely informed by such *post-mortem* studies. It is these neurotransmitter systems which form the site of action of most of the drugs in use at present for psychiatric disorders, and their involvement in the pathology of neurodegenerative disorders will be the focus of this chapter.

The neurochemical study of *post-mortem* brain

Many neurochemical studies have been undertaken of relatively small numbers of subjects using *post-mortem* tissue. Such studies were often conducted on patients previously resident in institutions, and thus are likely to have over-represented subjects with prominent behavioural symptoms. In AD, behavioural symptoms frequently determine whether patients come to medical attention and the care that they subsequently require. Yet conclusions have often been drawn about patients in general, even though the clinical characteristics of these subjects do not represent those of all patients with AD.

Studies that have been based upon more epidemiologically sound samples,[1] including subjects assessed during life for the range of clinical features of AD, are likely to be able to resolve these issues and demonstrate which biochemical features are characteristic of AD, and which are those of subsets with particular behavioural syndromes.

Similarly, control subjects must definitely be free from the condition. Although it may be relatively easy to ensure that they are free from advanced disease, it may be more difficult to be confident that they are free from early or pre-symptomatic stages of the disorder. If neurochemical changes that occur early in the course of the disease and which may be of possible pathogenic significance are to be examined, it may be necessary to screen potential control subjects before death to confirm that they are genuinely asymptomatic.

Studies of many aspects of the biochemistry of human brain have demonstrated an apparent inherent variability compared with the situation in experimental animals. While demographic factors such as age and sex, and other factors such as drug treatment must be taken into account, the mode of the patient's death is a factor of particular note, indicated by measures such as the duration of terminal coma.[2] As the precise details of this are rarely available to the biochemist working with *post-mortem* samples, the pH value of brain tissue homogenates[3,4] may be a valid index.

Particularly in neurodegenerative conditions, tissue atrophy may confound interpretation of biochemical data because it is normal practice to report results per unit mass. This does not make allowance for any reduction in the volume of brain structure. Therefore shrinkage or loss of some structures but not others may lead to reports of an increase in the markers in unaffected structures, such as increased γ-aminobutyric acid (GABA) content of frontal cortex from Alzheimer biopsy tissue.[5]

Although conditions such as AD are progressive disorders, this is rarely acknowledged in *post-mortem* studies, which almost invariably examine patients dying at an advanced stage of disease. It has been possible to study samples removed earlier in the course of the disease, as neocortical tissue is occasion-ally removed surgically for diagnostic purposes. These samples have been compared with comprehensive control data obtained from neurosurgical pro-cedures in which the removal of neocortical tissue of normal appearance was a necessary part of the surgical procedure.[6] In general, *post-mortem* studies reveal more extensive and severe neurochemical pathology than is found in biopsy material.

Neurotransmitter systems in human brain

The cholinergic system

Anatomy and function of the neocortical cholinergic system

The cerebral cortex receives two major distally projecting cholinergic pathways.[7] One of these originates in the basal forebrain, comprising the nuclei of the septum, diagonal band and Meynert. This terminates in all areas of the cortex, with particularly dense innervation of the hippocampus as well as the amygdala. The other pathway originates in the brainstem, and while it innervates the thalamus in particular, it also terminates in selected areas of the cortex, notably the frontal and occipital cortex. This cholinergic projection is thought to have a major role in processes such as attention and arousal. The basal forebrain cholinergic system is thought to have a role in regulating the activity of the entire cerebral cortex, and to maintain the cortex in its operative mode.[7,8] The practical manifestation of this is that acetylcholine (ACh) is thought to have a role in the control of selective attention,[9] by affecting discriminatory processes, the reception and evaluation of stimuli, and the modification of cortical responsiveness. Cholinergic mechanisms therefore appear to govern many brain functions associated with different cortical regions, such as perception, learning, cognition and judgement.

Neurochemistry

ACh is synthesised in nerve terminals from its precursor, choline, which is transported to the brain via the bloodstream. Choline enters cholinergic nerve cells via a high-affinity uptake system which is specific to these neurons. In the cytoplasm, choline reacts with acetyl-coenzyme A, a process that is catalysed by the enzyme choline acetyltransferase (ChAT). This enzyme is synthesised in the nerve-cell bodies and transported to the nerve terminals.

The ACh thus synthesised is not uniformly distributed in the neurons. About 20% appears to be in solution in the cytoplasm, and the remaining 80% is stored in a particulate component of the nerve endings. Morphological studies have shown that there are ACh-containing vesicles in the presynaptic terminal, and it is these vesicles which probably correspond to the particulate component of the ACh. It is generally accepted that the vesicles represent an intracellular organelle in which neurotransmitter is stored prior to being released by neuronal stimulation.

Released ACh is not removed from the synaptic cleft by active reuptake systems, as is the case with many other neurotransmitters, but is broken down by a membrane-bound enzyme, acetylcholinesterase (AChE). This is an enzyme specific to ACh and can generally be distinguished from a plasma enzyme, butyrylcholinesterase, which also metabolises ACh but is not specific to synapses. The latter enzyme is often referred to as 'pseudocholinesterase'.

Two distinct types of receptor, *nicotinic* and *muscarinic*, mediate the postsynaptic actions of ACh. Nicotinic receptors occur at the neuromuscular junction and in the central nervous system (CNS). It is difficult to distinguish subtypes of nicotinic receptors using drugs, but molecular biology studies have shown distinct differences. All nicotinic receptors consist of five protein subunits arranged around a trans-membrane ion channel. It is the opening of this ion channel which mediates the postsynaptic actions of the transmitter. The muscarinic receptors mediate slower neuronal responses by activation of second-messenger systems. The drug pirenzepine distinguishes two subclasses of muscarinic receptors, those blocked by this drug being designated M_1 and all others being designated M_2. Molecular biology studies of these receptors have since confirmed the existence of further subgroups, M_3 and M_5, which show similarities to M_1, and M_4, which shows similarities to M_2.

Cholinergic system in Alzheimer's disease

Early demonstrations of substantial losses of ChAT from the brain tissue of patients with AD *post mortem*[10–14] and *ante mortem*[15] have stimulated much subsequent research on this neurotransmitter. This cholinergic deficit is one of the most prominent features of AD.[6] Neuropathological studies have shown that there is usually considerable loss of the neurons which give rise to the cortical cholinergic innervation, the neurons of the nucleus basalis of Meynert,[16–20] which is associated with loss of nucleolar volume of the cells.[20]

Biochemical measures of cholinergic function have shown consistent and extensive losses of those biochemical activities which are associated with cholinergic terminals. In particular, ChAT activity seems to be reduced *post mortem* in all areas of the cerebral cortex of patients with AD.[10–14,21] Early in the course of the disease, neurosurgical specimens confirm this loss of activity and a reduced ability of the tissue to synthesise acetylcholine.[15,22]

It is generally accepted that there is probably little alteration in the M_1 subtype of postsynaptic receptor, at least until late in the disease, and the M_2 subtype is at most only moderately affected,[23,24] and probably only in the frontal cortex.[25] The involvement of M_2 receptors may be involved in the pathogenesis of psychotic symptoms in AD.[25] However, loss of nicotinic receptors is a consistent finding,[26,27] and has led to the proposition that this may be an early and important aetiological event.[23]

The magnitude of the cholinergic dysfunction is correlated with the severity both of the cognitive impairment assessed on global measures of cognitive function,[28–31] and of the neuropathological changes, including senile plaque formation[21,30,32] and loss of neurons.[21] Considerable emphasis has been placed on the significance of this cholinergic deficit, and it has been suggested that the dementia of AD is due primarily to this.[33] Other conditions associated with cognitive impairment are also associated with cholinergic pathology. These include Parkinson's disease, progressive supranuclear palsy and cerebrovascular dementia, as well as head injury[34] and dementia with Lewy bodies (DLB),[35] and they are associated with such pathology independently of the severity of Alzheimer pathology. However, AD is probably not solely a disorder of the cholinergic system. The neocortical cholinergic deficit probably only explains part of the cognitive decline, as has been suggested by neuropsychological studies of the effects of cholinergic antagonists.[36] The clinical syndrome of AD consists of more than just cognitive impairment, and frequently includes behavioural and psychiatric symptoms such as wandering, aggression and depression. Although the extent to which these disorders of conduct and personality have been found in AD could be an overestimate, especially in the presenium, these symptoms are almost certainly related to non-cholinergic transmitter pathologies. However, some non-cognitive symptoms may have a cholinergic basis.[37] Visual hallucinations are related to the severity of the cholinergic deficits in DLB,[38] a condition in which the cholinergic deficits are generally more severe and visual hallucinations more common than in AD.[39]

Monoamine neurotransmitters

In addition to the cholinergic innervation, the cortex receives inputs from at least three other populations of subcortical neurons, each using a different transmitter. These are the catecholamine neurotransmitters, noradrenaline and dopamine, and the indoleamine 5-hydroxytryptamine (5-HT).

Anatomy and function of monoamine neurotransmitter systems

Within the CNS the cell bodies of 5-HT neurons are located in the midline of the upper brainstem, forming distinct nuclei, the raphé nuclei. The inferior group of these project to the brainstem, cranial nerve nuclei and spinal cord. The superior group project rostrally and innervate the limbic and sensory areas of the forebrain. This group of nuclei shows a degree of topographic organisation of their projections such that the fibres of the dorsal raphé nuclei innervate the basal ganglia and cerebellum, whereas the fibres of the median raphé nuclei innervate the hippocampus and septum. As a result of its presence in these structures of the CNS, 5-HT plays a role in a great variety of behaviours, such as food intake, activity rhythms, sexual behaviour and emotional states. The serotonergic system is also thought to play a significant role in learning and memory,[40,41] in particular by interacting with the cholinergic, glutamatergic, dopaminergic or GABA-ergic systems.

The locus coeruleus (LC) is the major nucleus of origin of noradrenergic fibres in the mammalian brain. Rostral and dorsal LC neurons innervate forebrain and cortical structures, whilst the caudal and ventral neurons project to the cerebellum and spinal cord.[42,43] It has been proposed that this noradrenergic system, together with other sympathetic systems, yields rapid adaptive responses to urgent stimuli,[44] although other proposed roles of LC-noradrenaline neurons include those in sleep, attention, memory and vigilance.

Neurochemistry of monoamine neurotransmitter systems

The neurotransmitter 5-HT is synthesised from the amino acid tryptophan by the enzyme tryptophan hydroxylase. This enzyme has many features in common with tyrosine hydroxylase, which converts tyrosine to l-dopa during the synthesis of dopamine and noradrenaline. The synthesised transmitters are found primarily in storage vesicles. The uptake of transmitter into these vesicles is an energy-dependent process which can be disrupted by such drugs as methylenedioxymethamphetamine (MDMA, 'ecstasy'). Release of transmitter from the vesicles and nerve endings is regulated by the released transmitter via a number of autoreceptors, as well as other neurotransmitters by way of heteroreceptors. Released transmitters are inactivated by presynaptic active uptake systems.

Monoamine neurotransmitter systems in AD

Catecholamines

Studies of dopamine neurotransmitter function in AD have not shown any consistent pattern of involvement.[6] Not surprisingly, therefore, there seems to be little relationship between measures of dopamine innervation and the clinical features of the syndrome.[45]

The LC is known to be significantly damaged in AD,[46–49] and a decreased noradrenaline content is found in the cerebral cortex.[50–54] Concentrations of the major metabolite are unaltered or even elevated,[6,52,53,55,56] probably reflecting increased turnover of NA. In the LC itself, alterations in neuronal morphology, neurofibrillary tangle (NFT) formation and loss of pigmented noradrenaline neurons in topographically distinct regions have been observed.[49,57] The clinical significance of changes in the noradrenaline system in AD is unclear. The extent of LC neuron loss has been reported to relate to disease duration[58] and severity of cognitive decline,[47,48] as has loss of neurotransmitter.[59] Studies have also found greater LC neuron loss in depressed[60–62] and aggressive[59] subjects with AD, although this may not be a consistent finding.[63]

5-HT

Biochemical determinations of neurons containing 5-HT in AD have mostly relied on determinations of the concentrations of 5-HT and its major metabolite, 5-hydroxy-indoleacetic acid (5-HIAA), in *post-mortem* samples. The content of these in many areas of the neocortex of AD subjects may be reduced,[52,53,55,56] and neurofibrillary degeneration and neuronal loss in the raphé nucleus has been reported.[64] However, this is by no means a consistent finding, and even in AD brains at autopsy half of the cortical areas may have no selective reduction of presynaptic 5-HT activity.

As discussed above, this discrepancy between studies may in part be explained by the inadvertent selection of hospitalised subjects with marked behavioural symptoms. In studies of epidemiologically representative samples of community-based AD patients assessed in life, presynaptic cortical markers of 5-HT neurons were not uniformly affected in AD. Thus although the density of 5-HT uptake sites in AD temporal cortex was significantly reduced (61% of control), there was no significant alteration in the frontal cortex. Reduced 5-HT concentrations in the frontal cortex were also found to indicate those subjects with the most rapid cognitive decline.

Patients judged to be aggressive during life showed more severe loss of both 5-HT concentration and postsynaptic receptors in both retrospectively[64,65] and prospectively assessed[66] subjects. Disorders of 5-HT innervation have also been implicated in the aetiology of depression, anxiety and overactivity in AD.[66,67] Aggressive behaviour has been linked to more advanced disease, suggesting that loss of both 5-HT_2[65] and 5-HT_{1A}[67] receptors is a feature of more extensive pathology found towards the end stage of the disorder. However, brain imaging studies in healthy subjects also implicate 5-HT_{1A} in aggressive traits,[68] so the loss of cortical 5-HT_{1A} receptors may well be particularly associated with aggressive tendencies in AD.[67]

Inhibitory amino acid neurotransmitters and neuropeptides

The principal inhibitory neurotransmitters in the central nervous system are the amino acids γ-aminobutyric acid (GABA) and glycine. GABA appears to act as a transmitter in virtually all areas of the CNS, and glycine is largely confined to the caudal part of the brain and spinal cord.[69]

GABA in AD

Within the cortex there are large numbers of interneurons containing GABA, often co-localised with one or more of a variety of neuropeptides. The balance of evidence indicates that loss of these substances is not a fundamental characteristic of AD. *Post-mortem* assessment of GABA-releasing neurons has been complicated by artefacts and epiphenomena.[5] Thus no change in the activity of the enzyme responsible for GABA synthesis, glutamate decarboxylase (GAD), was found in a careful study in which AD and control subjects were matched for the nature of the terminal illness.[56] Normal GAD activity and GABA content have been confirmed with cortical biopsy tissue.[6] Another presynaptic measure of GABA innervation, namely the GABA transporter GAT-1, was similarly unaltered in AD.[70] Perhaps not surprisingly, an attempt to treat AD with a GABA agonist was unsuccessful.[71]

Other amino acids and peptides in AD

Both glycine and taurine are also thought to function as inhibitory neurotransmitters, and their content is unchanged in AD, based on both *post-mortem* and biopsy tissue.[5,72] The neuropeptides cholecystokinin, vasoactive intestinal polypeptide and neuropeptide Y are unchanged in AD,[73,74] as is probably corticotropin-releasing factor.[75]

Many studies have indicated that somatostatin is reduced, but this was not confirmed in biopsy samples.[6] Larger reductions in somatostatin and GABA content have been reported in *post-mortem* studies that included only subjects displaying severe histopathology than in those where no such selection criteria were employed.[5] The loss of somatostatin correlates with the severity of cognitive impairment.[76,77]

Excitatory amino acid neurotransmitters

Anatomy and function of excitatory amino acid neurotransmitters

The amino acid glutamate has been known for some time to be the major transmitter of excitatory signals of the long axonal projections of the CNS. In addition, a large proportion of sensory fibres contain glutamate and aspartate, as is also the case for nerve cells linking different areas of the brain. However, because glutamate has an important role in the metabolism of all cells, and is also the precursor of the inhibitory transmitter GABA, the precise localisation of the transmitter glutamate has been difficult. Nevertheless, a combination of techniques, including histochemistry for glutamate and its putative synthetic enzyme and retrograde transport of radiolabelled glucose (GLU), has provided strong evidence for a transmitter role for glutamate in a number of pathways.[78] This has been convincingly demonstrated for cortico-fugal fibres, the projections of pyramidal neurons of layer V of the cerebral cortex. There is less definitive evidence available establishing a role for glutamate as a transmitter of other cortical pyramidal neurons, in particular the cortico-cortical association and transcallosal fibres (typically found in cortical layers II and III). However, results obtained using a variety of techniques are consistent with glutamate being the major neurotransmitter of these groups of neurons.

There is much evidence that the initiation and maintenance of epileptic seizures involve the release of glutamate, and drugs which block the NMDA receptor have anticonvulsant actions. Excitatory amino acids are found in most sensory fibres and probably contribute to the transmission of pain stimuli.

It is widely accepted that the phenomenon of long-term potentiation (LTP) is fundamentally involved in the formation of memories. LTP is a long-lasting enhancement of synaptic effectiveness which follows prolonged stimulation of hippocampal input pathways. Types of glutamate receptor appear to be involved in this process. Prolonged activation of glutamate receptors can cause neuronal damage due to excessive calcium entry, a phenomenon known as excitotoxicity. This appears to have a major role in ischaemic brain damage. Brief periods of ischaemia can interrupt glutamate reuptake by neurons and glia. This causes excessive stimulation of postsynaptic receptors and calcium entry, which can cause osmotic and metabolic damage to the neuron.

Neurochemistry of excitatory amino acid neurotransmitters

Glutamate has many important functions in the body. It is a component of proteins and is involved in a key step in cellular energy production. However, that of the glutamate which has a neurotransmitter role may be formed by a different metabolic pathway to that which is involved in metabolism. Once glutamate is released, there are high-affinity uptake sites in terminals and glia which remove it from the synaptic cleft.

Studies with selective agonists and antagonists have indicated that there are four major classes of glutamate receptors. These are the N-methyl-D-aspartate (NMDA), kainate, α-amino-3-hydroxy-5-methyl-4-isoxazole proprionate (AMPA) and metabotropic classes. The AMPA receptors consist of four protein subunits that form a trans-membrane ion channel.

The majority of AMPA receptors control sodium ion influx and thus cellular depolarisation, although some also regulate calcium entry. Thus the AMPA receptors probably mediate a fast depolarisation response to glutamate release. Many kainate receptors appear to occur presynaptically, and probably therefore have a role in regulating glutamate release. The metabotropic receptors are least well understood, but act by way of a second-messenger system coupled through G-proteins to potassium and calcium channels.

The NMDA receptor is probably the best studied of the glutamate receptors. Activation produces a slow, prolonged depolarisation, so these receptors do not mediate the fast transmission of excitation and the initiation of nerve impulses. Activation of the receptor controls an ion channel that is permeable to sodium and calcium. However, the entry of calcium alters intracellular pathways and this is probably the means by which NMDA-receptor activation alters neuronal activity. The receptor is complex, with recognition sites for several distinct groups of compounds which seem to have a regulatory role. In addition to the recognition site for glutamate, there are also sites for glycine.

Excitatory amino acids in AD

The pyramidal cells of the temporal and parietal lobes of the cerebral cortex use glutamate as a neurotransmitter and are major and early sites of pathological changes in AD. Severity of cognitive impairment is correlated with the pyramidal cell counts in layer III[28] and the number of synapses in layer III.[79]

Synaptosomal Na^+-dependent D-[^3H] aspartate uptake (ASP uptake) has been used as a marker of the relative density of glutamate nerve terminals. ASP uptake may be reliably measured in tissue from promptly performed autopsies, and in such specimens was reduced by 50% in the temporal cortex of AD patients,[80] indicating a loss of glutamate synapses. The most likely interpretation is that this reflects loss of synapses of corticocortical fibres, since loss of the cells of origin of these fibres is the major pathology. Studies in hippocampus have indicated that all the major input and output pathways (except the septohippocampal cholinergic pathway) use glutamate as transmitter.[78] There was cell loss and tangle formation in the entorhinal cortex and in CA1 in AD patients at post-mortem.

Glutamatergic pathways are considered to be involved in memory,[81] and it follows that this loss of presynaptic glutamatergic innervation is likely to contribute to the memory dysfunction in AD. This may be compounded by postsynaptic and other regulatory factors.[82]

Cell death and the other pathological hallmarks of AD may be brought about through glutamate-mediated mechanisms. However, the distribution of pathology does support the idea that the disease spreads along cortical glutamate pathways[83–85] which may share the common property of synaptic plasticity.[86] The effects of reduced glutamatergic activity might include the promotion of the formation of senile plaques.[87] Hypoactivity of glutamatergic neurons is also implicated in aberrant mechanisms of tau and thereby possible neurofibrillary tangle formation.[6,82]

Key points

- It has been generally assumed that the neurochemical study of *post-mortem* brain tissue reveals information of relevance to the understanding of that condition in life. However, many factors need to be considered for this to be a valid assumption. It is probably true to say that the rigorous demonstration of reliability and validity which is normally expected in many other areas of psychiatry has rarely been applied to biological measures.
- Studies controlling for confounding factors, and using epidemiologically sound samples of subjects, have indicated that early in the course of the disease abnormalities of relatively few neurotransmitters are obvious. This is in contrast to the situation late in the disease, which is usually examined in *post-mortem* tissue.
- Thus the most reliable and consistent changes are those seen in the cholinergic innervation of the cortex and the cortical pyramidal neurons. However, by the time of death there is usually considerable involvement of other neurons. The clinical effect of this appears to be to cause some aspects of the cognitive dysfunction characteristic of AD. However, it is most likely that disorders of other (especially monoamine) neurotransmitters cause most of the behavioural and other non-cognitive symptoms.

References

1 Hope T, Keene J, Gedling K *et al.* (1997) Behaviour changes in dementia. 1. Point of entry data of a prospective study. *Int J Geriatr Psychiatry.* **12:** 1062–73.

2 Harrison PJ, Procter AW, Barton AJL *et al.* (1991) Terminal coma affects messenger RNA detection in *post mortem* human brain tissue. *Mol Brain Res.* **9:** 161–4.

3 Kingsbury AE, Foster OJF, Nisbet AP *et al.* (1995) Tissue pH as an indicator of mRNA preservation in human *post mortem* brain. *Mol Brain Res.* **28:** 311–18.

4 Yates CM, Butterworth J, Tennant MC *et al.* (1990) Enzyme activities in relation to pH and lactate in *post mortem* brain in Alzheimer-type and other dementias. *J Neurochem.* **55:** 1624–30.

5 Lowe SL, Francis PT, Procter AW *et al.* (1988) Gamma-aminobutyric acid concentration in brain tissue at two stages of Alzheimer's disease. *Brain.* **111:** 785–99.

6 Procter AW (2002) Neurochemical pathology of neurodegenerative disorders in old age. In: R Jacoby and C Oppenheimer (eds) *Psychiatry in the Elderly*. Oxford University Press, Oxford.

7 Mesulam MM (1995) The cholinergic contribution to neuromodulation in the cerebral cortex. *Neuroscience.* **7:** 297–307.

8 Wenk GL (1997) The nucleus basalis magnocellularis cholinergic system: one hundred years of progress. *Neurobiol Learn Mem.* **67:** 85–95.

9 Voytko ML (1996) Cognitive functions of the basal forebrain cholinergic system in monkeys: memory or attention? *Behav Brain Res.* **75:** 13–25.

10 Bowen DM, Smith CB, White P *et al.* (1976) Neurotransmitter-related enzymes and indices of hypoxia in senile dementia and other abiotrophies. *Brain.* **99:** 459–96.

11 Davies P (1979) Neurotransmitter-related enzymes in senile dementia of the Alzheimer type. *Brain Research.* **171:** 319–27.

12 Davies P and Maloney AJF (1976) Selective loss of central cholinergic neurons in Alzheimer's disease. *Lancet.* **ii:** 1403.

13 Perry EK, Gibson PH, Blessed G *et al.* (1977) Neurotransmitter enzyme abnormalities in senile dementia. Choline acetyltransferase and glutamic acid decarboxylase activities in necropsy brain tissue. *J Neurol Sci.* **34:** 247–65.

14 Perry EK, Perry RH, Blessed G *et al.* (1977) Necropsy evidence of central cholinergic deficits in senile dementia. *Lancet.* **i:** 189.

15 Bowen DM, Benton JS, Spillane JA *et al.* (1982) Choline acetyltransferase activity and histopathology of frontal neocortex from biopsies of demented patients. *J Neurol Sci.* **57:** 191–202.

16 Nagai R, McGeer PL, Peng JH *et al.* (1983) Choline acetyltransferase immunohistochemistry in brains of Alzheimer's disease patients and controls. *Neurosci Lett.* **36:** 195–9.

17 Whitehouse PJ, Price DL, Struble RG *et al.* (1982) Alzheimer's disease and senile dementia: loss of neurons in the basal forebrain. *Science.* **215:** 1237–9.

18 Mann DMA and Yates PO (1982) Is the loss of cerebral cortical choline acetyltransferase activity in Alzheimer's disease due to degeneration of ascending cholinergic nerve cells. *J Neurol Neurosurg Psychiatry.* **45:** 936.

19 Arendt T, Bigl V, Tennstedt A *et al.* (1985) Neuronal loss in different parts of the nucleus basalis is related to neuritic plaque formation in cortical target areas in Alzheimer's disease. *Neuroscience.* **14:** 1–14.

20 Mann DM, Yates PO and Marcyniuk B (1984) Presenile Alzheimer's disease, senile dementia of Alzheimer type and Down's syndrome of middle age all form an age-related continuum of pathological changes. *Neuropathol Appl Neurobiol.* **10:** 185–207.

21 Mountjoy CQ, Rossor MN, Iversen LL *et al.* (1984) Correlation of cortical cholinergic and GABA deficits with quantitative neuropathological findings in senile dementia. *Brain.* **107:** 507–18.

22 Sims NR, Bowen DM, Allen SJ *et al.* (1983) Presynaptic cholinergic dysfunction in patients with dementia. *J Neurochem.* **40**: 503–9.

23 Perry EK (2000) The cholinergic system in Alzheimer's disease. In: J O'Brien, D Ames and A Burns (eds) *Dementia.* Arnold, London.

24 Roberson MR and Harrell LE (1997) Cholinergic activity and amyloid precursor protein metabolism. *Brain Res Brain Res Rev.* **25**: 50–69.

25 Lai MK, Lai OF, Keene J *et al.* (2001) Psychosis of Alzheimer's disease is associated with elevated muscarinic M_2 binding in the cortex. *Neurology.* **57**: 805–11.

26 Aubert I, Araujo DM, Cecyre D *et al.* (1992) Comparative alterations of nicotinic and muscarinic binding sites in Alzheimer's and Parkinson's diseases. *J Neurochem.* **58**: 529–41.

27 Perry EK, Morris CM, Court JA *et al.* (1995) Alteration in nicotine-binding sites in Parkinson's disease, Lewy body dementia and Alzheimer's disease: possible index of early neuropathology. *Neuroscience.* **64**: 385–95.

28 Neary D, Snowden JS, Mann DMA *et al.* (1986) Alzheimer's disease: a correlative study. *J Neurol Neurosurg Psychiatry.* **49**: 229–37.

29 Palmer AM, Francis PT, Bowen DM *et al.* (1987) Catecholaminergic neurones assessed *ante mortem* in Alzheimer's disease. *Brain Res.* **414**: 365–75.

30 Perry EK, Tomlinson BE, Blessed G *et al.* (1978) Correlation of cholinergic abnormalities with senile plaques and mental test scores in senile dementia. *BMJ.* **2**: 1457–9.

31 Minger SL, Honer WG, Esiri MM *et al.* (2001) Synaptic pathology in prefrontal cortex is present only with severe dementia in Alzheimer disease. *J Neuropathol Exp Neurol.* **60**: 929–36.

32 Perry EK, Blessed G, Tomlinson BE *et al.* (1981) Neurochemical activities in human temporal lobe related to aging and Alzheimer-type changes. *Neurobiol Aging.* **2**: 251–6.

33 Coyle JT, Price DL and DeLong MR (1983) Alzheimer's disease: a disorder of cortical cholinergic innervation. *Science.* **219**: 1184–90.

34 Murdoch I, Perry EK, Court JA *et al.* (1998) Cortical cholinergic dysfunction after human head injury. *J Neurotrauma.* **15**: 295–305.

35 Samuel W, Alford M, Hofstetter CR *et al.* (1997) Dementia with Lewy bodies versus pure Alzheimer disease: differences in cognition, neuropathology, cholinergic dysfunction and synapse density. *J Neuropathol Exp Neurol.* **56**: 499–508.

36 Kopelman MD and Corn TH (1988) Cholinergic 'blockade' as a model for cholinergic depletion. *Brain.* **111**: 1079–110.

37 Minger SL, Esiri MM, McDonald B *et al.* (2000) Cholinergic deficits contribute to behavioral disturbance in patients with dementia. *Neurology.* **55**: 1460–7.

38 Perry EK, Haroutunian V, Davis KL *et al.* (1994) Neocortical cholinergic activities differentiate Lewy body dementia from classical Alzheimer's disease. *Neuroreport.* **5**: 747–9.

39 Perry EK, Marshall E, Thompson P *et al.* (1993) Monoaminergic activities in Lewy body dementia: relation to hallucinosis and extrapyramidal features. *J Neural Transm Park Dis Dement Sect.* **6**: 167–77.

40 Buhot MC, Martin S and Segu L (2000) Role of serotonin in memory impairment. *Ann Med.* **32**: 210–21.

41 Meltzer CC, Smith G, DeKosky ST *et al.* (1998) Serotonin in aging, late-life depression, and Alzheimer's disease: the emerging role of functional imaging. *Neuropsychopharmacology.* **18**: 407–30.

42 Waterhouse BD, Lin CS, Burne RA *et al.* (1983) The distribution of neocortical projection neurones in the locus coeruleus. *J Comp Neurol.* **217**: 418–31.

43 Loughlin SE, Foote SL and Fallon JH (1982) Locus coeruleus projections to cortex: topography, morphology, and collateralisation. *Brain Res Bull.* **9**: 1–16.

44 Aston-Jones G, Shipley MT and Grazanna R (1995) The locus coeruleus, A5 and A7 noradrenergic cell groups. In: G Paxinos (ed.) *The Rat Nervous System. Academic Press, Sydney.*

45 Bierer LM, Knott PJ, Schmeidler JM *et al.* (1993) *Post-mortem* examination of dopaminergic parameters in Alzheimer's disease: relationship to noncognitive symptoms. *Psychiatr Res.* **49:** 211–17.

46 Mann DMA, Lincoln J, Yates PO *et al.* (1980) Changes in the monoamine-containing neurones of the human CNS in senile dementia. *Br J Psychiatry.* **136:** 533–41.

47 Bondareff W, Mountjoy CQ and Roth M (1981) Selective loss of neurones of origin of adrenergic projection to cerebral cortex (nucleus locus coeruleus) in senile dementia. *Lancet.* **i:** 783–4.

48 Bondareff W, Mountjoy CQ and Roth M (1982) Loss of neurons of origin of the adrenergic projection to cerebral cortex (nucleus locus coeruleus) in senile dementia. *Neurology.* **32:** 164–8.

49 Chan-Palay V and Asan E (1989) Alterations in catecholaminergic neurones of the locus coeruleus in senile dementia of the Alzheimer type and in Parkinson's disease and amyotropic lateral sclerosis. *J Comp Neurol.* **287:** 373–92.

50 Francis PT, Palmer AM, Sims NR *et al.* (1985) Neurochemical studies of early-onset Alzheimer's disease. Possible influence on treatment. *NEJM.* **313:** 7–11.

51 Adolfsson R, Gottfries CG, Roos BE *et al.* (1979) Changes in brain catecholamines in patients with dementia of Alzheimer type. *Br J Psychiatry.* **135:** 216–23.

52 Arai H, Kosaka K and Iizuka R (1984) Changes of biogenic amines and their metabolites in postmortem brains from patients with Alzheimer-type dementia. *J Neurochem.* **43:** 388–93.

53 Gottfries CG, Adolfsson R, Aquilonius SM *et al.* (1983) Biochemical changes in dementia disorders of Alzheimer type (AD/SDAT). *Neurobiol Aging.* **4:** 261–71.

54 Palmer AM, Wilcock GK, Esiri MM *et al.* (1987) Monoaminergic innervation of the frontal and temporal lobes in Alzheimer's disease. *Brain Res.* **401:** 231–8.

55 Cross AJ, Crow TJ, Johnson JA *et al.* (1983) Monoamine metabolism in senile dementia of Alzheimer type. *J Neurol Sci.* **60:** 383–92.

56 Reinikainen KJ, Paljarvi L, Huuskonen M *et al.* (1988) A *post-mortem* study of noradrenergic serotonergic and GABAergic neurons in Alzheimer's disease. *J Neurol Sci.* **84:** 101–16.

57 Iversen LL, Rossor MN, Reynolds GP *et al.* (1983) Loss of pigmented dopamine-β-hydroxylase positive cells from locus coeruleus in senile dementia of Alzheimer's type. *Neurosci Lett.* **39:** 95–100.

58 German DC, Manaye KF, White CL III *et al.* (1992) Disease-specific patterns of locus coeruleus cell loss. *Ann Neurol.* **32:** 667–76.

59 Matthews KL, Chen CP, Esiri MM *et al.* (2002) Noradrenergic changes, aggressive behavior, and cognition in patients with dementia. *Biol Psychiatry.* **51:** 407–16.

60 Zubenko GS and Moossy J (1988) Major depression in primary dementia. Clinical and neuropathologic correlates. *Arch Neurol.* **45:** 1182–6.

61 Forstl H, Burns A, Luthert P *et al.* (1992) Clinical and neuropathological correlates of depression in Alzheimer's disease. *Psychol Med.* **22:** 877–84.

62 Zweig RM, Ross CA, Hedreen JC *et al.* (1988) The neuropathology of aminergic nuclei in Alzheimer's disease. *Ann Neurol.* **24:** 233–42.

63 Hoogendijk WJ, Sommer IE, Pool CW *et al.* (1999) Lack of association between depression and loss of neurons in the locus coeruleus in Alzheimer disease. *Arch Gen Psychiatry.* **56:** 45–51.

64 Palmer AM, Stratmann GC, Procter AW *et al.* (1988) Possible neurotransmitter basis of behavioral changes in Alzheimer's disease. *Ann Neurol.* **23:** 616–20.

65 Procter AW, Francis PT, Stratmann GC *et al.* (1992) Serotonergic pathology is

not widespread in Alzheimer patients without prominent aggressive symptoms. *Neurochem Res.* **17:** 917–22.

66 Chen CPL, Alder JT, Bowen DM *et al.* (1996) Presynaptic serotonergic markers in community-acquired cases of Alzheimer's disease: correlations with depression and neuroleptic medication. *J Neurochem.* **66:** 1592–8.

67 Lai MK, Tsang SW, Francis PT *et al.* (2003) Reduced serotonin 5-HT$_{1A}$ receptor binding in the temporal cortex correlates with aggressive behavior in Alzheimer disease. *Brain Res.* **974:** 82–7.

68 Parsey RV, Oquendo MA, Simpson NR *et al.* (2002) Effects of sex, age, and aggressive traits in man on brain serotonin 5-HT$_{1A}$ receptor-binding potential measured by PET using [C-^{11}]WAY-100635. *Brain Res.* **954:** 173–82.

69 Farrant M (2001) Amino acids: inhibitory. In: RA Webster (ed.) *Neurotransmitters, Drugs and Brain Function*. John Wiley and Sons, Chichester.

70 Nagga K, Bogdanovic N and Marcusson J (1999) GABA transporters (GAT-1) in Alzheimer's disease. *J Neural Transm.* **106:** 1141–9.

71 Mohr E, Bruno G, Foster N *et al.* (1986) GABA-agonist therapy for Alzheimer's disease. *Clin Neuropharmacol.* **9:** 257–63.

72 Lowe SL, Bowen DM, Francis PT *et al.* (1990) *Ante-mortem* cerebral amino acid concentrations indicate selective degeneration of glutamate-enriched neurons in Alzheimer's disease. *Neuroscience.* **38:** 571–7.

73 Beal MF, Clevens RA, Chatta GK *et al.* (1988) Galanin-like immunoreactivity is unchanged in Alzheimer's disease. *J Neurochem.* **51:** 1935–41.

74 Gabriel SM, Davidson M, Haroutunian V *et al.* (1996) Neuropeptide deficits in schizophrenia vs. Alzheimer's disease cerebral cortex. *Biol Psychiatry.* **39:** 82–91.

75 DeSouza EB, Whitehouse PJ, Kuhar MJ *et al.* (1986) Reciprocal changes in corticotropin-releasing factor (CRF)-like immunoreactivity and CRF receptors in cerebral cortex of Alzheimer's disease. *Nature.* **319:** 593–5.

76 Minthon L, Edvinsson L and Gustafson L (1997) Somatostatin and neuropeptide Y in cerebrospinal fluid: correlations with severity of disease and clinical signs in Alzheimer's disease and frontotemporal dementia. *Dementia Geriatr Cogn Disord.* **8:** 232–9.

77 Grouselle D, Winsky-Sommerer R, David JP *et al.* (1998) Loss of somatostatin-like immunoreactivity in the frontal cortex of Alzheimer patients carrying the apolipoprotein epsilon-4 allele. *Neurosci Lett.* **255:** 21–4.

78 Ottersen OP (1991) Excitatory amino acid neurotransmitters: anatomical systems. In: BS Meldrum (ed.) *Excitatory Amino Acid Antagonists*. Blackwell Scientific Publications, Oxford.

79 DeKosky S and Scheff SW (1990) Synapse loss in frontal cortex biopsies in Alzheimer's disease: correlation with cognitive severity. *Ann Neurol.* **27:** 457–64.

80 Procter AW, Palmer AM, Francis PT *et al.* (1988) Evidence of glutamatergic denervation and possible abnormal metabolism in Alzheimer's disease. *J Neurochem.* **50:** 790–802.

81 Hyman BT, Van Hoesen GW and Damasio AR (1990) Memory-related neural systems in Alzheimer's disease: an anatomic study. *Neurology.* **40:** 1721–30.

82 Francis PT (2003) Glutamatergic systems in Alzheimer's disease. *Int J Geriatr Psychiatry.* **18:** S15–21.

83 Esiri MM, Pearson RC, Steele JE *et al.* (1990) A quantitative study of the neurofibrillary tangles and the choline acetyltransferase activity in the cerebral cortex and the amygdala in Alzheimer's disease. *J Neurol Neurosurg Psychiatry.* **53:** 161–5.

84 Pearson RC and Powell TP (1989) The neuroanatomy of Alzheimer's disease. *Rev Neurosci.* **2:** 101–23.

85 Pearson RCA, Esiri MM, Hiorns RW *et al.* (1985) Anatomical correlates of the distribution of the pathological changes in the neocortex in Alzheimer's disease. *Proc Natl Acad Sci USA.* **82:** 4531–4.

86 Arendt T, Bruckner MK, Gertz HJ *et al.* (1998) Cortical distribution of neurofibrillary tangles in Alzheimer's disease matches the pattern of neurons that retain their capacity of plastic remodelling in the adult brain. *Neuroscience.* **83:** 991–1002.

87 Bowen DM, Francis PT, Chessell IP *et al.* (1994) Neurotransmission – the link integrating Alzheimer's research. *Trends Neurosci.* **17:** 149–50.

Chapter 4

Practical issues in assessing and prescribing psychotropic drugs for older people

Stephen Curran, Sharon Nightingale and John P Wattis

Introduction

The management of older people with mental illness invariably needs an integrated approach, with pharmacological, social and psychological interventions working together. However, this chapter will focus mainly on pharmacological treatments. Drug treatments have an important role to play alongside psychological and social interventions, but these broad approaches are not mutually exclusive. On the contrary, success with pharmacological interventions involves many factors, only some of which are drug related. In general, the pharmacological evidence base is much better for younger patients. In particular, many clinical trials exclude older people, and this makes it difficult to extrapolate the findings to older people with mental illness. Older people may also be excluded because it is more difficult to control for confounding variables such as concurrent diseases and the medications needed to treat them. This must always be borne in mind when interpreting data from studies in younger people for use in older people. There is a need for more research on the use of psychotropic drugs in older people.

Pharmacological treatments

In the same way that it has proved difficult to classify mental disorders, so it has also proved difficult to classify psychotropic drugs, and a number of different classifications exist based on chemical structures, mechanisms of action or the main effects on brain function. The classification is complicated by the fact that many drugs overlap and do not fit neatly into discrete categories. In general, the broad categories include antidepressants and mood stabilisers, antipsychotics, anxiolytics and hypnotics and antidementia drugs (these are discussed in Chapters 8, 9, 10, 11 and 12). Sub-classification is usually on the basis of chemical structures (e.g. tricyclic antidepressants), principal mechanism of action (e.g. cholinesterase inhibitors), pharmacokinetic properties (e.g. short- and long-acting benzodiazepines) and specific properties (e.g. sedation). However, this classification, although useful, is very broad and has a number of limitations.

Assessment: general considerations

Older people should be interviewed in a quiet, distraction-free environment, and every effort must be made to put them at ease. In addition, they generally need more time than younger people and they should not be rushed. This is particularly important when assessing 'liaison' referrals on medical wards. Otherwise, any confusion will be compounded and a falsely pessimistic impression of function may result. Older patients may be very reluctant to discuss their personal feelings, so establishing a good rapport is essential. Some patients, especially those with dementia or communication difficulties, may not be able to give real consent. The doctor's ethical obligation is to act in the patient's best interest. This principle is particularly important when the patient's ability to exercise autonomy properly is diminished. Where necessary, consideration should be given to using appropriate mental health legislation. However, in England and Wales patients with dementia who lack capacity can be treated or admitted to hospital without the need to use mental health legislation, provided that the healthcare professionals involved and the patient's family agree that this is the most appropriate course of action and that the patient is not actively refusing medication or trying to leave hospital. A detailed assessment of the patient is important for a number of reasons.

- First, it enables an accurate *diagnosis* to be made, and this has implications for both the treatment and prognosis of the specific condition under consideration.
- Secondly, it is the beginning of the process of developing a *trusting relationship* with the patient that will be crucial for providing a sound basis for treating the patient and maintaining compliance.
- Thirdly, the assessment of the patient's past and current medical problems will indicate which drugs to avoid, and will highlight potential *drug interactions*.
- Finally, a knowledge of the patient's past psychiatric history might point to the most appropriate treatments.

Assessment is often undertaken over a period of time. It usually involves several different disciplines with different insights into the needs of older people. All relevant assessments must be taken into account. The care plan should be modified if necessary as new assessments are made. The self-discipline of good practice in record keeping and review can be improved by the practice of regular peer-group audit, which depends on careful record keeping. The use of standardised assessments can facilitate audit. Assessment of the patient is not a 'one-off' event. It should be repeated throughout treatment in order to evaluate progress and, if necessary, modify treatment and care plans. This creates a 'feedback loop' which should result in high-quality care matched to the patient's current needs.

Psychiatric assessment

History

The psychiatric history starts with the *presenting complaint* (or complaints), including how long it has been present and how it developed. Quite often the patient lacks insight and believes that nothing is wrong. In these circumstances, careful probing is appropriate. Sometimes, when it is difficult to obtain a clear history of the time course of an illness, the situation can be clarified by using 'time landmarks' such as the previous Christmas or some important personal anniversary. Often a proper history of the presenting complaint can only be obtained by talking to a friend or relative before or after seeing the patient. In other cases information may have to be pieced together from a variety of sources, such as home care staff, the social worker and the GP.

Usually it is best to follow the history of the presenting complaint with an account of the *personal history*. Most of us enjoy talking about ourselves, and it is quite easy to introduce the subject. A useful opening line is 'Tell me a bit about yourself – were you born in this area?'. Memory can be unobtrusively assessed while going through the history by reference to important dates (e.g. the date of birth, call-up to the forces and date of marriage). The *family history* and the *history of past and current physical health* can be woven into this brief account of the patient's lifetime, and an assessment can be made of the patient's personality and characteristic ways of dealing with stress.

Old people, like young people, respond well to those who have a genuine interest in them. It is essential to ensure that the patient can see and hear the interviewer. Courtesy is vital. Talking 'across' patients to other professionals or to relatives generates anxiety and resentment, as does lack of punctuality. It is also necessary to enquire about *past psychiatric illness* and any treatments.

Drug history

It is important to establish the name, dose, frequency, duration, reason for starting, efficacy and tolerability of any psychotropic drug currently or previously prescribed. Information should be sought about drug allergies, compliance and any practical problems (e.g. difficulty swallowing tablets). Some drugs may cause or exacerbate psychiatric illness, and some may cause side-effects that might exacerbate an underlying physical illness which might then cause further distress. Drugs may also interact with other drugs, so this needs to be considered and evaluated. Medication for physical illness should also be recorded.

Antihypertensives, digoxin and diuretics may be responsible for depressive symptoms, and all drugs with anti-cholinergic effects (including many antidepressants and antipsychotics) may produce confusion and constipation, among other side-effects. The list is constantly expanding, and the only safe advice is to assume that any medicine can potentially cause a wide range of unwanted effects. Postural hypotension induced by tricyclic antidepressants or antipsychotics and other drugs may be mistaken for histrionic behaviour, and may be dismissed as part of the symptoms of an underlying depressive illness. Benzodiazepines often have a 'hangover' effect, and may accumulate over many days to produce confusion and daytime drowsiness. Many drug interactions occur in older people, who are often on a number of different medications. When an older patient presents with a new symptom, current medication should always be considered as a possible source of the symptom before further drugs are added. Ask about gastrointestinal symptoms, especially if selective serotonin reuptake inhibitors (SSRIs) are likely to be prescribed, as there is some evidence that these can increase the risk of gastrointestinal bleeding, and the risk is similar to that associated with aspirin and non-steroidal anti-inflammatory drugs (NSAIDs). These should be used with caution in older people (> 80 years) and in patients taking aspirin or an NSAID.[1] It is therefore important to be aware of current medications (drugs for physical health, and psychotropic and over-the-counter drugs), previous drug sensitivities, response to treatment, side-effects and the potential for side-effects and drug interactions.

In summary, the content of the history will vary according to time and circumstance, but should generally include the following:

- the presenting complaint and its history
- personal and family history (including illnesses and longevity)
- past illnesses and operations
- previous personality
- alcohol and tobacco consumption
- current social circumstances and support
- drug history.

Mental State Examination

Level of awareness

At an early stage in the interview the patient's level of awareness should be assessed. The patient may be drowsy as a result of lack of sleep or because of physical illness or medication. A rapidly fluctuating level of awareness is seen in acute confusional states, and a level of awareness that fluctuates from day to day is one of the clues to the diagnosis of chronic subdural haematoma and/or dementia with Lewy bodies. Impaired awareness can lead to poor function on tests of cognition and memory, and if it is not recognised can lead to an underestimation of the patient's true abilities. It is especially important to consider this if the patient has a recent-onset physical problem. The patient's ability to concentrate and pay attention is closely related to their level of awareness, but may be affected by more mundane factors. For example, if the patient is in pain, it may be very hard for them to understand the relevance of giving an account of their mental state. Disturbance of mood and abnormal perceptual experiences can also impair attention and concentration.

Behaviour (and general appearance)

The patient's general appearance, behaviour, dress, personal hygiene and attitude to the interviewer can be observed directly, and behaviour can also be deduced indirectly from the state of their house. Incontinence can often be smelled (and occasionally felt). Mobility can be checked by asking the patient to walk a few steps. Especially if the patient lives alone, inconsistencies between appearance and behaviour and the state of cleanliness and organisation of the household indicate either that there is a good social support network or that the patient has deteriorated over a relatively short period of time.

Various schedules enable the systematic assessment of behavioural 'problems'. These are best seen as a function of the interaction between patient and environment and not as intrinsic characteristics of the patient. The behavioural subscale of the Clifton Assessment Procedure for the Elderly[2] and a shortened form of the Crighton Royal Behavioural Assessment Form[3] are useful examples. A scale has also been developed for the rating of behavioural symptoms by caregivers.[4]

Behavioural and activities of daily living (ADL) scales enable numerical values to be attached to a person's needs, abilities and problems in various important areas of behaviour. Such scales remind the assessor of important areas and enable discrepancies between different areas of performance to be highlighted. Potentially treatable problems are more easily seen and dealt with. Standardised scales also enable a rough comparison to be made between different patients and between different points in time for the same patient, even when the assessment is made by a different person. Finally, some scales give an overall rating of disability that can be used as a guide to the patient's future needs for care. There are many such scales[5] and they are all imperfect, but they do at least enable a quick and systematic approach to the assessment of behaviour and abilities. The numerical values ascribed to such scales are, of course, arbitrary. For example, a patient who is disturbed all night may not be manageable at home, despite that factor only contributing a small amount to the overall score. Scores must therefore be interpreted skilfully, taking into account the amount of support available and the peculiar impact of certain behaviours.

Affect (mood)

Mood in the technical sense used by psychiatrists is more than just how we feel. It has been described as 'a complex background state of the organism', and it affects not only how we feel but also how we think and even the functioning of our muscles and bowels. Older people are not always used to talking about their feelings, and it can sometimes be quite difficult to find the right words. This is particularly true for men, who may not have the words to describe feelings (alexothymia). Especially where there are communication difficulties, one may have to resort to direct questioning (e.g. 'Do you feel happy?').

Although patients should always be asked to give an account of their mood, this account cannot always be relied upon. Some older patients who are quite depressed do not confess to a depressed mood. This is often accompanied by somatisation – that is, the presentation of physical (hypochondriacal) complaints. It may also signify a more or less deliberate 'cover-up' due to fear of hospital admission. Anhedonia (loss of the ability to take pleasure in life) is a useful indicator of depression. Psychomotor retardation (the slowing of thought and action) can be so profound that the patient is unable to report their mood or may even say 'I feel nothing', although their facial expression, tears, sighs, slowed movement or agitation may reveal depression. Specific questions should be asked about guilt feelings, financial worries, and concerns about health.

Where there is depressed mood, careful enquiry should be made about suicidal feelings. This can be introduced in a non-threatening way by a question such as 'Have you ever felt that life was not worth living?'. If the patient responds positively to this, further probes can be made about present ideas of self-harm. If psychomotor retardation is present, the answer will take some time to come, and it is very easy to rush on to the next question before the patient has had time to respond to the previous one. Risk factors for suicide which should always be borne in mind include the following:

- male gender
- depression
- living alone

- bereavement
- long-standing physical illness or disability
- alcohol abuse.

Being aware of such risk factors complements but does not replace individual questioning and judgement.

One group of symptoms is often associated with severe 'biological' depression. This includes early-morning wakening, low mood worse in the morning (diurnal variation in mood), and profound appetite loss and weight loss. Some self-rating scales have been designed to avoid the confusion produced by the use of 'somatic' symptoms in other scales. They include the following:

- the Geriatric Depression Scale (GDS)[6]
- short forms of the GDS[7] and
- the brief assessment schedule depression cards (BASDEC)[8] and related even briefer assessment scale for depression (EBAS-DEP)[9]

These scales can provide indications of possible mood problems and, together with other scales (especially the Hospital Anxiety and Depression Scale [HAD]),[10] can be useful in measuring severity of depression, response to treatment and outcome. However, the frequent somatisation of depression in old age may cause 'false negatives' on such scales.

The opposite of depressed mood is elated mood, which is seen in mania and hypomania. In older patients, as in younger ones, decreased sleep, hyperactivity, excessive spending, flight of ideas, irritability and hypersexuality may be prominent symptoms.

Anxiety is also common in old age, sometimes in response to the stresses of ageing in our society. The patient may be so worried about falling that, in order to avoid anxiety, they restrict their life severely. Thus a patient who has had one or two falls may, instead of seeking medical help, restrict him- or herself to a downstairs room in the house and never go out. As long as the patient continues to restrict their life, they experience little anxiety. Whereas in a young person such behaviour would almost certainly immediately lead to the patient being defined as 'sick' and a call for medical attention, in older people this restriction is all too easily accepted as 'normal'. When assessing anxiety, attention should therefore be paid not only to how patients feel during the interview (which may in itself provoke anxiety!), but also to whether they can engage in the tasks of daily living without experiencing undue anxiety. Anxiety is an affect with physiological accompaniments – a racing pulse, 'palpitations', 'butterflies in the stomach', sweating and diarrhoea. Patients not infrequently use the term 'dizziness' to describe not true vertigo, but a feeling of unreality associated with severe anxiety. Sometimes the physiological changes induced by over-breathing, such as tingling in the arms and even spasm of the muscles of the hand and arm, may make matters worse. The anxiety subscale of the HAD[10] provides an easy patient-rated measure of the intensity of anxiety problems. Interestingly, anxiety and depression are often found together, and tend to improve together with treatment.

Panic attacks of rapidly mounting anxiety, usually with physiological symptoms, may occur as part of a phobic disorder, in isolation or, perhaps most commonly in old age, in the context of a depressive disorder.

Phobias occur when the patient is afraid of particular things or situations. Specific phobias (e.g. fear of spiders) are relatively uncommon in old age, but generalised phobias (e.g. fear of going out or of social situations) are relatively common and can be crippling.[11]

Thought (and talk)

The form, speed and content of thought should all be assessed. Formal thought disorder occurs in schizophrenia and includes thought-blocking (when the patient's thoughts come to an abrupt end), thought withdrawal (when thoughts are felt to be withdrawn from the patient's head), thought broadcast and thought insertion. For a fuller description of these phenomena, the reader is referred to a standard textbook of psychopathology.[12] Slowing of the stream of thought (thought retardation) is found in many depressive disorders. Slow thinking is also characteristic of some of the organic brain syndromes caused by metabolic deficiencies. Thought is speeded up in mania, often leading to 'flight of ideas', where one thought is built upon another in a way that is founded upon tenuous associations. In dementia, spontaneous thought is often diminished, so-called 'poverty of thought'. The patient with an acute confusional state experiences difficulty in maintaining a train of thought because of fluctuating levels of awareness. In dementias of metabolic origin and in some cases of multi-infarct dementia, slowing of thought processes may be accompanied by difficulty in assembling the necessary knowledge to solve particular problems. The observer gains the impression that the patient grasps that there is a problem but is frustrated in trying to cope with it.

Content of thought is influenced by the patient's mood. The depressed patient will often have gloomy thoughts, with ideas of poverty or physical illness. The anxious patient's thoughts may be preoccupied with how to avoid anxiety-provoking situations, and there may be unnecessary worries about all aspects of everyday living. The patient who feels persecuted may think of little else. Every noise or event will be fitted into the persecutory framework. Talk generally reflects the patient's thought, unless suspicion leads to concealment. Speech is also influenced by various motor functions. Slurred speech may be found in the patient who is drowsy or under the influence of drugs or alcohol. Sometimes it also results from specific neurological problems, such as a stroke. Patients with multiple sclerosis may produce so-called 'scanning' speech where words are produced without inflexion and with hesitation between words. Patients with severe parkinsonism may have difficulty in forming sounds at all (aphonia). Some difficulty in finding words and putting speech together is found in many patients with dementia, particularly those with Alzheimer's disease. This is one form of dysphasia. A stream of apparent nonsense (so-called fluent dysphasia) may occur in dementia but is also sometimes associated with a small stroke. The general behaviour of the patient, which is not 'demented', and the sudden onset of the dysphasia provide important diagnostic clues. Occasionally, fluent dysphasia, especially when it includes new words 'invented' by the patient (neologisms) may be mistaken for the so-called 'word salad' produced by some schizophrenic patients. The sudden onset and absence of other signs of schizophrenia aid in diagnosis. An assessment by a speech therapist experienced in this area may also help not only in diagnosis but also in suggesting management strategies that build upon the patient's residual (sometimes non-verbal) communication skills.

Hallucinations

These can be defined as perceptions without external objects. Visual hallucinations are usually found in patients with acute confusional states or dementia, although occasionally they occur in patients with poor eyesight without measurable organic brain damage, especially if the patient is living alone in a relatively under-stimulating environment. In dementia they are more often found in dementia with Lewy bodies, and their presence may correlate with neuropathological findings.[13] Auditory hallucinations (hearing 'voices' or sometimes music or simple sounds) occur in a variety of mental illnesses, especially schizophrenia (where they may consist of a voice repeating the patient's thoughts or of voices talking about the patient in the third person). They also occur in severe depressive illness and mania, when they are often in keeping with the patient's mood. Hallucinations of touch (tactile), smell (olfactory) and even taste (gustatory) also occur. Hallucinations of being touched, especially with sexual connotations, occur in schizophrenia, and hallucinations of smell, especially of the patient believing him- or herself to smell 'rotten', in severe depression. Experiences like hallucinations sometimes occur in bereavement. These vary from 'hearing the footsteps' of the lost person to complex phenomena occurring in more than one modality. People explain these in different ways. Some see them as spiritual and comforting, while others may be afraid they are 'going mad'.

Delusions

A delusion is a false unshakeable belief that is out of keeping with the patient's cultural background. Delusions occur in fragmentary forms in organic mental states, but well-developed delusions are usually found only in schizophrenia and in severe affective disorders, when ideas of poverty, guilt or illness may develop into absolute convictions. Ideas of persecution are also sometimes found in patients with depression of moderate severity, and these too can develop into full-blown delusions. Delusions of grandeur (e.g. that the patient has extraordinary powers of perception or is fabulously rich) are found in manic states. In paranoid schizophrenia, the delusional content is often very complicated and may involve persecutory activities by whole groups of people. These delusions may be supported by hallucinatory experiences.

Obsessions and compulsions

Obsessions occur when the patient feels compelled to repeat the same thought over and over again. They can be distinguished from schizophrenic phenomena such as thought insertion by the fact that obsessional patients recognise the thoughts as their own and try to resist them. Sometimes such thoughts may result in compulsive actions (e.g. returning many times to check that the door has been locked). Although they are characteristically a part of obsessive-compulsive disorder, obsessional symptoms also occur in depressed patients, and repetitive (not strictly compulsive) behaviour can also be a result of memory loss (e.g. when a patient repeatedly checks that the door is locked because they have forgotten that they have already done so).

Illusions

Illusions occur when a patient misinterprets a real perception. Some somatic (hypochondriacal) worries can be based on this. For example, many older people have various aches and pains, but sometimes patients may become over-concerned by these and may begin to worry that they indicate some physical illness. Such misinterpretations of internal perceptions are not usually described as illusions, although the term would be quite appropriate. Acute confusional states also produce illusions when the patient, seeing the doctor approaching them, misinterprets this as someone coming to do them harm and strikes out.

Cognition: orientation, memory, concentration and attention

These are considered together because they are so interdependent. Orientation with regard to time, place and person should be recorded in a systematic way. The degree of detail would depend upon the time available and the purpose of the examination. Orientation for time can easily be divided into gross orientation, such as the year or approximate time of day (morning, afternoon, evening or night), and finer orientation, such as the month, the day of the week and the hour of the day. Orientation with regard to person depends upon the familiarity of the person who is chosen as a point of reference. Orientation with regard to place also depends upon familiarity. A useful brief scale which includes some items of orientation as well as some items of memory is the Abbreviated Mental Test (AMT) score, developed by Hodkinson[14] from a longer scale which has previously been correlated with the degree of brain pathology in demented patients.[15] A slightly longer related scale has been developed for community use,[16] although many people 'adapt' the AMT (e.g. by asking for the patient's home address rather than the hospital name). Like most short scales, the AMT is not always well used.[17] It is also frequently overused, leading to false positives.

Orientation is to a large extent dependent upon memory, although it should never be forgotten that the patient may not know the name of the hospital they are in, simply because they have never been told. Memory for remote events can be assessed when taking the patient's history. This can be done by checking against known facts such as date of birth, checking with family members, and also by the internal consistency of the history. The ability to encode new material can be assessed by the capacity to remember a short address or to remember the interviewer's name when tested a few minutes later. Many patients with dementia will have great difficulty in encoding and storing new memories. Sometimes, especially in the metabolic dementias, one can form the impression that the patient is encoding and storing new material but that they are having great difficulty in retrieving the memory when asked to do so. This has been described as 'forgetfulness'.

Apraxia (demonstrated by the inability to copy simple drawings) and nominal aphasia (the inability to remember the names of common objects) can also be simply tested. A popular and relatively brief assessment of organic mental state is the Mini-Mental State Examination (MMSE)[18] which examines memory and a variety of other functions. However, the MMSE has been criticised because it is sensitive to educational attainment, its 'parallel' forms are not truly parallel, and it is not sufficiently sensitive to change. Longer scales such as the Cambridge cognitive examination (CAMCOG)[19] are probably too lengthy for routine clinical use. A variety of measures are used for evaluating outcomes in drug trials,[20] but these are generally too lengthy for routine use. A promising development is the construction of scales designed to elicit changes in the patient's memory from relatives and carers, such as the informant questionnaire on cognitive decline in the elderly (IQCODE).[21]

Another useful brief test which assesses a variety of cognitive functions is the 'clock test', where the assessor presents the patient with a circle and asks them to fill in the numbers as on a clock face and set the time to (for example) ten to two. This test is a useful screening tool for a broad range of cortical function.[22] In more severe dementia, where other tests are disabled by 'floor' effects, the Hierarchical Dementia Scale (HDS)[23] may be useful. More detailed descriptions of organic mental state examination can be found in Lishman's *Organic Psychiatry*.[24]

Insight and judgement

In severe psychiatric illness, insight (in the technical psychiatric sense) is often lost. Depressed patients may be unable to accept that they will get better, despite remembering previous episodes that have improved with treatment. Manic and paraphrenic patients may act on their delusions, with disastrous consequences. Patients with severe dementia often do not fully realise their plight, which is perhaps fortunate. Patients with milder dementia may have some insight, especially in the metabolic and vascular types of dementia where mood is, not surprisingly, also often depressed. Judgement is related to insight. This can be a particularly difficult question with a moderately demented patient who is living alone, or living with relatives but left alone for a substantial part of the day. Patients may leave gas taps on and be dangerous to themselves and others, but at the same time maintain that they are looking after themselves perfectly well and do not need any help, much less residential or nursing home care. They may have a mistaken image of the care that they are refusing. Common sense, professional judgement and multi-professional, inter-disciplinary working are needed to make decisions in these cases.

Physical assessment

Specialists in the psychiatry of old age need to work closely with their medical colleagues, particularly GPs and physicians for older people, because of the overlap and interactions between physical and psychiatric illness.[25]

No psychiatric examination, particularly in older people, is complete without a physical examination. Even in the patient's home a selective examination may be carried out, although it may be more appropriate to bring the patient to the clinic or the surgery for a more thorough examination. For a fuller account of assessment from the point of view of geriatric medicine, the reader is referred to *Assessing Elderly Patients*.[26] A joint psychiatric–geriatric clinic can facilitate the management of difficult cases. However, simple things can make a big difference to patients, such as improving vision and hearing, foot care and dentures, as well as suitable walking and other aids.

Sensory impairment

Diminished sensory input, one of the techniques used in 'brainwashing', is often inflicted on old people by our slowness in recognising and correcting defects of sight and hearing. Sensory deprivation may be instrumental in producing paranoid states and in precipitating or worsening confusion. Poor hearing is also associated with depression. An estimate of visual and auditory acuity is part of the examination of every older person. Wax in the ears is an easily remedied cause of poor hearing. Other forms of deafness may require a hearing-aid. A good deal of patience may be needed to learn to use an aid properly, especially if poor hearing has been present for some time. Look out for flat or dirty battery contacts in hearing-aids. For assessment purposes, more powerful portable amplifiers are useful. Even the inexpensive amplifiers linked to simple headphones that are advertised in popular magazines can be surprisingly effective. Visual defects range from those that are easily corrected by spectacles and other aids to those like cataract and glaucoma that require more complicated surgical or medical intervention.

Laboratory investigations

Further investigations may be planned in the light of findings from the history, mental state and physical examinations. Many doctors would confine themselves to haemoglobin, full blood count and film, urea and electrolytes, liver function tests and thyroid function tests, and some would routinely add serum vitamin B_{12} and folate and a serological test for syphilis. Although the necessity for the last is disputed, clinics that perform such tests still report unexpected positive findings. Other tests, such as chest X-ray, skull X-ray, electroencephalogram, computerised axial tomography (CAT), nuclear magnetic resonance (NMR) imaging and other forms of brain scan are at present only justified by specific indications. Hopes that CAT scans might provide an easy and definitive diagnosis of 'senile dementia' by demonstrating brain atrophy have not been realised due to wide overlaps in the picture between normal, functionally ill and demented patients, although occasionally a scan will reveal an unsuspected tumour or other problem. Newer scanning techniques such as NMR[27] or positron emission tomography (PET) may eventually be able to help in definitive diagnosis before death. In one fascinating study involving post-mortem verification, even SPECT scanning only had similar accuracy to rigorously applied diagnostic criteria (NINCDS-ADRDA), and a medial temporal lobe CT scan was not much better than the use of DSM-III-R criteria.[28] The Royal College of Psychiatrists *Consensus Statement* gives a reasonable account of what might be expected of the evaluation of dementia by a secondary service in the UK.[29]

Additional investigations

A number of additional investigations might need to be performed prior to starting treatment with a specific drug. The list below is not exhaustive, and the reader is referred to the latest *British National Formulary*, the Summary of Product Characteristics (SPC) produced for each drug by the drug manufacturer, and *The Maudsley Prescribing Guidelines*.[30]

Antipsychotics

A full blood count (FBC) should be done before initiating treatment with clozapine. An FBC should then be measured every week for 18 weeks, then every 2 weeks for 1 year, and thereafter every month.

Sudden unexplained death has been known for some time to be associated with antipsychotics, but the frequency has not been clearly defined. Some antipsychotics are associated with QTc-interval prolongation, which increases the risk of sudden death from the potentially fatal ventricular arrhythmia known as torsades de pointes, and thioridazine has been linked most frequently with this.[31] Drugs with a moderate effect on QTc interval include chlorpromazine and quetiapine, and those with a high risk include thioridazine and sertindole. The risk is increased in patients with cardiovascular disease (e.g. long QT syndrome, bradycardia and ischaemic heart disease), use of high doses, metabolic disorders (hypokalaemia, hypocalcaemia, hypomagnesaemia) and other factors such as stress/shock, female gender and increasing age. Patients at risk should have an ECG at baseline and thereafter every 6 months. Switching to a different drug is required if the QTc interval is >440 ms in men and >470 ms in women. Antipsychotics can also cause hyperglycaemia, so blood sugar levels should be monitored, especially with olanzapine.

Antidepressants and mood stabilisers

Most antidepressants, but especially SSRIs and venlafaxine, can lower the serum sodium concentration, so this is worth measuring before and after initiating treatment. Sodium levels of 1.25 mmol/l or lower require urgent advice and treatment from a physician. Lofepramine can cause abnormal liver function tests (LFTs) and not uncommonly frank jaundice, making LFT measurement advisable. Mirtazepine and mianserin (not often used now) can suppress the white cell count, so this should be measured before treatment and regularly thereafter. Patients who are being prescribed lithium should have a baseline ECG, thyroid function tests (TFTs) and urine and electrolytes (U&Es). The lithium level should be measured weekly until levels are in the therapeutic range and stable, and thereafter should be measured every 3 to 6 months. U&Es should then be measured every 3 months and TFTs every 6 months. Carbamazepine requires a baseline FBC to be repeated every 2 weeks for 2 months and thereafter every 3 to 6 months. Sodium valproate requires a baseline FBC, LFTs and U&Es to be repeated every 6 months.[30]

Antidementia drugs

The cholinesterase inhibitors may cause bradycardia, and many clinics routinely undertake ECGs before commencing treatment. Patients will normally be screened for a range of problems to exclude the treatable causes of dementia, and this would usually include LFTs. The latter are more important in patients taking donepezil or galantamine, as these drugs are metabolised by the liver.[32] A recent study with rivastigmine that specifically looked at cardiovascular effects found no effect on heart rate, QRS and QT interval compared with placebo.[33] Before initiating treatment with an antidementia drug, the diagnosis should be established. The laboratory tests recommended by the National Institute of Health[34] in the USA for a patient with suspected dementia include the following:

- complete blood count
- electrolyte and metabolic screen
- thyroid function
- vitamin B_{12} and folate levels

- syphilis serology
- urine analysis
- chest radiograph
- ECG
- head CT scan.

Home assessment

This is usually an integral part of the assessment, and most older patients referred for psychiatric assessment should preferably be seen initially in their own homes. This is also an ideal opportunity to undertake a social assessment, including a review of social networks, relationships and coping strategies used by family and friends. Home assessments have a number of advantages, including the following.

- The patient is seen in the situation with which he or she is familiar.
- The confusion, disorientation and distress which may be caused by a trip to hospital or consulting rooms are avoided.
- The environment can be assessed as well as the patient.
- The patient's function in his or her own environment and the level of social support can be assessed.
- Neighbours and relatives are often readily available to give a history of the illness and its impact on them.

Set against this are the disadvantages from the clinician's perspective, including time spent travelling, difficulties parking and problems performing physical examinations and tests in the patient's home. However, the home assessment allows a range of important areas to be assessed quickly which would not be apparent if the patient was seen in a clinic setting. Some examples are summarised in Box 4.1.

Box 4.1 The home assessment: what can be assessed? (modified from Curran and Wattis[35])

- *Local environment*: Location of shops and busy roads.
- *General state of the house*: General state of repair and cleanliness.
- *Cooker and fire*: Is the cooker being used? Is there any evidence of fire risk?
- *Fridge*: Is the fridge well stocked with fresh food? Is any of the food out of date or rotten?
- *Heating, lighting and ventilation*: Is the house cold? Is there adequate lighting?
- *Fire risks*: Cookers and fires are obvious examples. Is there any evidence of cigarette burns (e.g. in the bed area)?
- *Toilet and bathing facilities*: Are these being used appropriately?
- *Accident hazards*: Can the patient use the stairs safely? Are the floors cluttered?
- *Sleeping arrangements*: Is the patient getting enough sleep? Where is the patient sleeping? If the patient is sleeping downstairs, are the arrangements adequate?
- *Alcohol*: Is there any evidence of alcohol misuse (e.g. lost or empty bottles)?

- *Vulnerability*: Is the patient vulnerable (e.g. leaving doors unlocked, leaving large amounts of money in exposed places)?
- *Medication*: Are there any problems with the patient's medication? Can the medication be found? Is it the same as the prescribed medication? Is the patient taking the medication?

The patient's family and neighbours often have a key role to play in assessment and continuing management. Therefore a good relationship with them is very important. At the first interview, the patient and family will express many anxieties. Some of these may be founded upon their own ideas about the purpose of the assessment. Time is well spent listening to the problems as the patient and relatives see them. A still popular misconception is that the doctor, nurse or social worker has come to 'put away' the patient in the local institution. The elderly patient's idea of what institutional care involves may also be quite different from that of the assessor. Older people sometimes find it difficult to conceive that an admission to hospital or a residential home could be anything other than permanent. We need to take time to listen to these fears and to explain why we are visiting, and the scope and limitations of any help we can offer. Anxiety may impair the patient's and relatives' ability to grasp and remember what is being said. It may be necessary to repeat the same information several times and to ask questions to clarify whether explanations have really been understood. Although an assessment may be commonplace to us, for the patient and their relatives it is often taking place at a crisis point in their life. An empathetic manner, acknowledging the patient's and relatives' concerns, will help them to realise that their worries have been taken seriously. This will help to form a good relationship, which is the basis for further treatment.

The quality of relationships can be assessed both indirectly from the past history of the patient and the family, and more directly during a joint interview. It is worth trying to assess what each member of the family is aiming for and how open family members are in their communication with each other. Sometimes there is a pathological attachment between family members, resulting in a maladaptive pattern of caregiving.

The growing physical and psychological dependence of old people with progressive illnesses such as Parkinson's disease and Alzheimer's dementia can put extraordinary stress on family relationships that will reveal previously carefully disguised 'fault lines'. Because services are sometimes only made available when a crisis has occurred and members of the family are at the end of their tether, we do see relatives who may be labelled as 'rejecting'. This happens less frequently than it used to, as the development of more effective services has led to earlier intervention before a crisis has occurred. Even when a crisis has occurred, it may be possible to manage it in such a way that the relatives realise that they can continue to cope if they have the help of appropriate services. In addition, carers now have a statutory right to have their own care needs assessed by the social services.

Making allies of the family

An important factor here is a prompt response, usually in the form of a home visit. This is the first step in impressing upon the family the fact that help is available. Carers are relieved to find someone who has time and is willing to listen to the problems they are facing and provide practical help. This can cause family members to re-evaluate their attitudes and avoid premature decisions to put an elderly relative into a care home. The understanding and assessment of a situation by family members may be quite different from the professional viewpoint, and must be 'heard' and respected by the team that is planning help. The appropriate use of short-term care home or hospital admission, day care, family care and home care services to relieve perceived strains can enable the family to cope. Although the medical members of the team should include social and support needs in their initial assessment, where these are complicated, further expert assessment by another team member is justified, whether by a social worker, an occupational therapist or a community psychiatric nurse.

The need for 24-hour care

When an older person lives alone and suffers from moderate or severe dementia, it may be impossible to provide adequate supervision without admitting them to a long-stay care facility. This should not be viewed as a 'failure' to keep the person 'in the community', but as the appropriate use of one of a range of options for providing care. Management depends upon psychiatric and medical diagnosis as well as the family and social situation, and the skill of the psychogeriatric team lies in understanding the various components of the situation and how they interact in order to produce the best possible management plan.

Problem formulation and management: 'care planning'

Each patient needs a 'tailor-made' care plan of medical, psychological, nursing and social management. This will often need to be agreed on a multi-disciplinary basis after assessments have been made by several different members of the team. Some teams insist that the initial assessment is made by a senior member of the medical staff, as physical and severe psychiatric illness usually needs to take precedence in any management plan. Another member of the team may attend either with the doctor or later. The alternative pattern of using specially trained and supervised nursing staff, for example, may become increasingly common in the face of rising demand and limited resources. In any case, it is essential that the initial assessment includes an overall view of medical, psychological and support needs and social factors, and that the family is given some idea of the likely management and the help available at that first assessment. This includes at least an outline knowledge of local home care, day care, voluntary groups, financial allowances and other relevant sources of help. The care plan will usually evolve and develop as the patient's condition and circumstances change.

The care planning procedures[36] provided an official framework for this process in the UK. They introduced a more carefully monitored procedure to replace the informal approach that previously prevailed. The advantages of a more formal procedure are that all stakeholders are more likely to have a 'say' in producing the plans, and that there is less likelihood of poor communication leading to failure. The disadvantages are that the new procedures can be time-consuming and impose a bureaucratic burden on overworked clinicians. This in turn can lead to a slower and less flexible team response where the central purpose of caring for the patient is obscured by the necessity of filling in forms. Ideally a synthesis of the personal clinical approach and methodical documentation and process can be achieved, but not without supporting clerical resources and information technology. Case management is a related philosophy which is used by social services departments in the UK and elsewhere. This approach potentially allows a more flexible deployment of resources, although there is also a danger that it will simply become a crude mechanism to control costs and transfer blame. A review of research into care management suggests that approaches in which the care manager is a clinician actively involved with the patient work better than those in which the care manager is a 'broker' who is not directly involved with the patient.[37]

A medical, psychosocial and nursing 'diagnosis' is only the beginning of patient management. Because of the multiplicity of problems faced by patients, a haphazard approach to management is time-wasting, inefficient and potentially dangerous. For example, arranging long-term home care support for people who are suffering from undiagnosed and untreated depressive episodes may 'keep them going' in the community, but it does not permit them to have the best possible quality of life, and it may lead to a treatment-resistant depressive illness or even to suicide. Arranging nursing home care for people whose confusion is due to an undiagnosed medical condition denies them proper treatment, reduces their independence, wastes resources and may also have fatal consequences. On the other hand, a narrowly medical approach to people's problems will also reduce their prospects of independent living.

Teamwork is therefore essential, and it is most important that case management and care planning procedures do not detract from the tradition of multi-disciplinary teamwork that has been built up in many psychogeriatric services. The traditional psychiatric formulation of a patient's problems has always included not only the psychiatric diagnosis but also all relevant medical, psychological and social factors. Care plans achieve the same thing by listing the patient's needs, planning interventions to meet those needs, and agreeing responsibility between professionals and agencies for different components of the plan. Although these plans are ideally agreed at a meeting of the patient, caregiver(s), health service and social services staff, in practice we have found this too time-consuming to be accommodated within the available resources. We now reserve full meetings for difficult cases, and we use an abbreviated (although still firmly multi-disciplinary) procedure for the majority of cases. Community team members review patients regularly in a multi-disciplinary forum, but only arrange formal meetings as and when circumstances demand.

Starting drug treatments

Lader and Herrington[38] have suggested that 'unless there is intense distress there is no need to proceed with haste'. There are a number of important reasons for delaying treatment.

- The additional time allows for more detailed assessment, which will make the eventual treatment more informed.
- Psychotropic drugs can be harmful, and older people are often very sensitive to their side-effects, so they should not be given unnecessarily.
- Some patients improve after the initial assessment/admission, rendering psychotropic drugs unnecessary. For example, in general practice patients with minor disorders often improve after simple discussion, and drugs may reinforce the patient's view that they have a 'serious illness'.[39] Admission to hospital may be associated with a significant improvement in symptoms. However, this is not always sustained.
- Other reasons include the increased risk of drug interactions and the financial implications.

Where possible, older people should be on as few drugs as possible. However, if a decision is made to prescribe a particular drug, then choosing the most appropriate medication can be a complex process. Response to previous treatments is not always a good guide,[38] but this needs to be considered. In general, drugs should be introduced gradually (unless there is a single dose) and stopped gradually. Sometimes small, apparently 'subtherapeutic' doses can be useful for people who are intolerant of psychoactive drugs (e.g. the patient can be given half or a quarter of the normal dose). However, some patients will require standard doses of drugs, and antidepressants in particular should not generally be abandoned without a trial of an adequate dose for an adequate period of time. There is also variation in response depending on the illness and comorbid clinical factors such as personality factors.[40] Age itself is an important determinant of response to treatment, due to reduced drug clearance, increased side-effects, reductions in receptor density and increased risk of interactions with other drugs. Physical illness can also impair the response to treatment through a variety of mechanisms. Reduced diet can also have an impact through changes in the proportion of body fat, reduced plasma proteins, reductions in the levels of amino acids and vitamins, with consequences for enzyme function,[41] and changes in receptor density.

In general, it is better to know a few drugs in detail so that one becomes familiar with their doses, side-effects and interactions with other drugs. Confusion is also reduced if the generic name is used whenever possible. Complex drug regimes should be avoided, and in general it is not usually necessary to use two or more drugs from the same class of drugs (e.g. two or more antipsychotic drugs). Drugs should be commenced cautiously. Similarly, drugs should be stopped cautiously and over a few days or weeks, particularly if the patient is on high doses and/or has been taking the drug for extended periods of time. This will depend in part on the individual patient, the drug in question, the dose and the duration of treatment. There is a range of factors that have to be considered before prescribing drugs in older people. One of the possibilities that should always be considered is the advantage of prescribing nothing.[38]

Consent is another important issue. In order to consent to treatment, the patient should have a broad understanding of the treatment, including the risks and benefits, the consequences of not taking the treatment, and the alternatives currently available (with their risks and benefits). Patients who lack capacity to give consent should normally be treated under the Mental Health Act 1983, but patients with dementia who lack capacity are frequently treated without this legal framework. This has generated considerable medical and legal debate.[42] The current legal position in England and Wales is that patients with dementia who lack capacity can be treated or admitted to hospital without the need to use mental health legislation, provided that the healthcare professionals involved and the patient's family agree that this is the most appropriate course of action, and that the patient is not actively refusing medication or trying to leave hospital.

Thus some of the factors that need to be considered before commencing treatment include the diagnosis, the likelihood of safe compliance, and the response to previous treatments, including tolerability and patient preferences. The efficacy and tolerability of the drug for a particular patient need to be considered. Does the drug have a licence for the indication for which it is being used? Is the patient aware of this? Are there any age-specific considerations? What are the likely side-effects based on the patient's physical health? Are there likely to be any drug interactions? Has the patient been given adequate information? Some of these questions will now be explored in slightly more detail.

Age-related changes

Older people are more sensitive to the side-effects of drugs and experience these more frequently than younger patients.[43] Pharmacodynamic and pharmaco-kinetic changes with increasing age both play a part in explaining increased drug sensitivity.[44] Pharmacodynamic changes include increased receptor sensitivity and a reduction in total receptor numbers with increasing age. Changes in drug distribution, metabolism and excretion are the main pharmacokinetic factors involved. A shift in body composition with a relative reduction in total body water compared with fat alters the distribution of lipid-soluble drugs in particular. As a result, the half-life of many lipid-soluble psychotropic drugs is prolonged. Hepatic metabolism of psychotropic drugs is reduced because of decreased hepatic blood flow and slowed enzyme metabolism. The glomerular filtration rate declines by 50% between young adulthood and the age of 70 years,[44] which is of particular importance in explaining the increased risk of lithium toxicity in older patients. In summary, some of the important pharmaco-kinetic and dynamic changes that occur with increasing age include the following:

- increased risk of side-effects and drug interactions
- increased receptor sensitivity
- decreased receptor numbers
- prolonged half-life of lipid-soluble drugs
- increased blood levels of water-soluble drugs
- decreased plasma albumin levels
- decreased gastric acid production and emptying
- reduced hepatic metabolism
- decreased glomerular filtration rate.[45]

Large variations in plasma concentrations of tricyclic antidepressants occur after similar doses, and this variation is greater in older people, particularly with amitriptyline, nortriptyline and imipramine. Reduced clearance and increased half-lives are also observed. The clearance of trazodone is also reduced in older people, and there is an increased half-life. Age-related increases in plasma concentrations have been reported with citalopram, paroxetine, fluoxetine and sertraline. Lithium clearance is reduced in older people, so smaller doses are needed to achieve the same therapeutic benefit. Benzodiazepines tend to have an increased half-life in older people, especially diazepam. There has been very little research with regard to antipsychotics, but in general smaller doses are needed to achieve a therapeutic outcome.

Side-effects of psychotropic drugs in older people

Mental illness is common in older people, especially the very old, and psychotropic drugs are commonly prescribed. Older people are more likely to have a range of physical illnesses, and psychotropic drugs may exacerbate these. These conditions include cardiovascular (e.g. arrhythmias and hypertension), endocrine (e.g. diabetes), gastrointestinal (e.g. constipation, malnutrition), urological (e.g. prostatic hypertrophy), central nervous system (e.g. dementia, seizure disorders) and ophthalmic (e.g. glaucoma) conditions.[46] These disorders can cause particular risks for older patients treated with psychotropic drugs, but an awareness of them can lead to more focused prescribing.

The side-effects of psychotropic drugs can be categorised according to their effects on neurotransmitter systems. These include anticholinergic (e.g. reduced salivation, sweating and gastric acid production, increased intraocular pressure, blurred vision, urinary retention, tachycardia, impotence and delirium), antidopaminergic (extrapyramidal side-effects, galactorrhoea, gynaecomastia and pigmentation), antihistaminic (sedation, hypotension, weight gain) and anti-α_1-adrenergic (tachycardia, arrhythmia, angina, insomnia and tremor) effects.[46] Knowledge of the mechanism of action of particular psychotropic drugs will enable the prescriber to predict the likely side-effects in older people with specific physical illnesses, and thus avoid them. In addition, a knowledge of drug interactions should reduce side-effects through more focused prescribing.

Drug interactions

Older people will often be taking a wide range of psychotropic drugs as well as drugs for physical health problems. Hurwitz[47] reported a higher level of drug interactions in inpatients, and studies in outpatients have reported similar findings.[48] There is therefore an increased risk of drug interactions. Older people are more sensitive to these and the consequences can be serious, and are a common cause of poor efficacy with psychotropic drugs. Some of the common and/or important drug interactions are summarised in Tables 4.1 and 4.2.

Table 4.1 Common adverse drug reactions and interactions: antidepressants and mood stabilisers (modified from Curran and Wattis[45])

Drug	Comments
Antidepressants	• *Tricyclic antidepressants (TCAs)*: Increased drowsiness with sedative drugs; enhanced anticholinergic effects with anticholinergic drugs; increased levels with haloperidol; reduced levels with high-fibre diet; reduced metabolism with cimetidine; increased metabolism of imipramine, doxepin and amitriptyline by carbamazepine; raised phenytoin levels with imipramine
	• *Citalopram*: Increased risk of hyponatraemia and serotonin syndrome with buspirone
	• *Fluoxetine*: Carbamazepine levels increased; cardiac arrhythmias with cisapride; increased risk of serotonin syndrome with lithium; increased phenytoin levels; increased risk of cardiotoxicity with terfenadine
	• *Paroxetine*: Reduced bioavailability with cimetidine and phenytoin
	• *Sertraline*: Possible cardiac arrhythmias with cisapride; raised phenytoin levels
	• *Mirtazepine*: Increased sedation with benzodiazepines
	• *Moclobemide*: Increased half-life with cimetidine
	• *Reboxetine*: Increased risks of hypokalaemia with diuretics; avoid using with erythromycin and flecainide
	• *Venlafaxine*: Increased diazepam clearance; reduced clearance with cimetidine. Serious adverse reaction with selegiline
Mood stabilisers	• *Lithium*: These are extensive. Reduced excretion caused by ACE inhibitors and NSAIDs and increased excretion caused by sodium bicarbonate, acetazolamide, loop diuretics, thiazides and theophylline. Lithium toxicity reported with SSRIs. Increased risk of neurotoxicity with carbamazepine and phenytoin, diltiazem and verapamil and methyl-dopa. Increased risk of EPS with clozapine, haloperidol and phenothiazines. Enhanced effect of muscle relaxants
	• *Sodium valproate*: Enhanced effect of aspirin. Decreased metabolism caused by erythromycin and cimetidine. Increased effect of warfarin. Increased risk of neutropenia when combined with olanzapine
	• *Carbamazepine*: These are extensive, and only a brief summary is provided here. Increased level of carbamazepine with erythromycin and isoniazid. Reduced anticoagulant effect with warfarin. Increased plasma concentrations of fluoxetine and fluvoxamine. Metabolism of mianserin and TCAs is accelerated. Avoid with MAOIs. Plasma concentrations of mirtazepine and paroxetine are decreased. Decreased metabolism with cimetidine. Metabolism of clozapine, haloperidol, olanzapine, quetiapine and risperidone is increased

Table 4.2 Common adverse drug reactions and interactions: benzodiazepines, antipsychotics and antidementia drugs (modified from Curran and Wattis[45])

Drug	Comments
Benzodiazepines	• Increased drowsiness with sedative drugs (e.g. alcohol, antihistamines, TCAs, phenothiazines)
	• Absorption reduced by antacids and anticholinergic drugs
	• Clearance of diazepam reduced by propranolol
	• Cimetidine inhibits the metabolism of long-acting benzodiazepines
	• Levels of diazepam increased by fluoxetine
	• Potentiation of phenytoin by diazepam and chlordiazepoxide
	• Clearance increased by smoking (nicotine)
	• Antagonism of levodopa by diazepam, nitrazepam and chlordiazepoxide
Antidementia drugs	• *General*: Antagonism by and of anticholinergic medication; exacerbation of succinylcholine-type muscle relaxation during anaesthesia. Enhance the effect of suxamethonium and antagonise the effect of non-depolarising muscle relaxants
	• *Galantamine*: Plasma levels increased by paroxetine; clearance reduced by paroxetine and fluoxetine
	• *Memantine*: Risk of CNS toxicity increased with ketamine and dextromethorphan. Enhances the effect of antimuscarinics and possibly decreases the effect of antipsychotics. Avoid with dopaminergics because of the increased risk of CNS toxicity
Antipsychotics	• *General*: Increased drowsiness with sedative drugs; enhanced anticholinergic effects with anticholinergic drugs
	• *Chlorpromazine*: Enhanced hypotensive effect with hypotensives; reduced absorption with antacids; reduced levels with cimetidine; reduced metabolism of sodium valproate
	• *Haloperidol*: Absorption reduced by antacids; levels decreased by rifampicin
	• *Risperidone*: Clearance increased by carbamazepine
	• *Olanzapine*: Clearance increased by carbamazepine
	• *Quetiapine*: Levels reduced with carbamazepine; raised levels with erythromycin; slightly raised lithium levels; levels reduced by phenytoin

Information for patients

Psychotropic drugs are powerful agents and they can sometimes have serious consequences. Before starting treatment, patients should be given adequate information and time to make an informed choice. Unfortunately, because of limited time as well as clinical pressures this is often a neglected part of the process. The *Drug and Therapeutics Bulletin*[49] has recommended that patients should be given the following information before starting treatment:

- the name of the drug
- the aim of the treatment (relief of symptoms, cure, prevention of relapse or prophylaxis)
- how the patient will know if the drug is or is not working
- when and how to take the medication
- what to do if a dose is missed
- how long to take the drug
- side-effects
- effects on performance (e.g. driving ability)
- interactions with other drugs.

There are few who would disagree with these recommendations, but unfortunately this is a very time-consuming process and it can sometimes be difficult to determine how much choice and information should be given. Some years ago a patient with bipolar affective disorder stormed out of SC's clinic in a very angry mood. She later contacted SC to explain that the reason she had left was because she had been given a choice – 'You are the doctor, I expect you to decide'. She was not well enough to make a decision. Another example is that of a carer who complained that her husband had had a heart attack from his chlorpromazine because the list of side-effects for the drug had increased his anxiety so much that this had precipitated the heart attack. This can be a difficult balance to achieve. Patient information leaflets such as those available from the Royal College of Psychiatrists (www.rcpsych.ac.uk) and the Alzheimer's Society (www.alzheimer.org.uk) have been specifically written for patients and carers, and they strike a balance between providing sufficient information to enable the patient to make an informed choice, and not scaring the patient and preventing them from benefiting from what can be life-saving treatments.

Assessing response to treatment

Evaluation of the response to treatment is intricately linked with assessment and initiation of treatment. Response should be evaluated fairly frequently after commencing treatment, but there are no universally accepted guidelines, and practice depends in part upon clinical judgement (see below). It is usual for contact to be maintained with the patient for as long as the patient remains on psychoactive drugs, although again there are no guidelines. In any event there should be clear discussion with the GP and the team if formal contact comes to an end. It is also important to determine the aim of treatment (e.g. relief of acute symptoms, prevention of relapse or prophylaxis).

Stopping drugs

Drugs also need to be stopped carefully and in a planned manner. Many drugs, if stopped quickly, especially if they have been given at high doses for long period of time, can cause withdrawal symptoms. In general, drugs with longer half-lives cause fewer problems. For example, the withdrawal symptoms frequently associated with SSRI withdrawal include dizziness, lethargy, nausea, vivid dreams and irritability. These were significantly more common in patients stopping paroxetine (17.2%) than in those stopping fluoxetine (1.5%) – fluoxetine has a much longer half-life.[50]

Yellow Card system

In the UK the Yellow Card scheme was introduced in 1964 after the thalidomide tragedy, to allow for the spontaneous reporting of suspected adverse drug reactions. Since then more than 400 000 reports have been submitted to the Committee on Safety of Medicines on a voluntary basis by doctors, dentists, pharmacists, coroners and nurses, and by pharmaceutical companies under statutory obligations. Forms are available in issues of the *British National Formulary*. An electronic version became available in 2002 and is easy to use. More information is available at the Medicines and Healthcare Products Regulatory Agency website (http://medicines.mhra.govuk).

Measuring outcome

The emphasis on accountability and, in the UK, the emphasis on clinical governance adds a new imperative to the need to measure outcomes.[51] Ideally, outcomes should be assessed from a variety of perspectives (e.g. those of the patient, carer, provider and commissioner), and measures should be found which will reflect a broad consensus on 'good' and 'bad' outcomes between different viewpoints. A distinction should also be made between overall measures of outcome such as the HoNOS 65+, individualised measures focused on each patient, and specific measures designed for use in particular diagnostic groups. The HoNOS 65+ belongs to the HoNOS family (Health of the Nation Outcome Scales), the usefulness of which as tools in routine practice has been questioned.[52] In one small study of outcomes on an acute psychiatric ward for old people, the HAD completed by the patient emerged as a good overall measure for the outcome of depression, and correlated well with a variety of 'viewpoints'.[53] Measures such as this, which can 'summarise' outcomes in specific disorders and settings, ideally need to be combined with the less sensitive but more global measures. Building such measures into care pathways would enable routine audit of performance. This could produce feedback to the clinical team and enable comparisons of performance both between teams and within teams over time. As well as increasing accountability, this kind of measure should encourage reflective practice and improve clinical quality. The snag is that researching *and applying* such measures requires time and money. The time needed can be reduced by increasing efficiency through good information technology, but this also requires investment.

Key points

- Psychotropic drugs have an important role to play in the treatment of mental disorders in older people.
- A detailed assessment before starting treatment is essential in order to achieve the best therapeutic outcome with minimal side-effects and good compliance.

> * Patients should be given adequate information and time to make an informed choice before starting treatment.
> * Once initiated, treatments should be properly monitored for clinical benefit and tolerability and, when appropriate, cautiously discontinued.
> * More research is needed that specifically focuses on the use of psychotropic drugs in older people.

References

1 Drug and Therapeutics Bulletin (2004) Do SSRIs cause gastrointestinal bleeding? *Drug Ther Bull.* **42**: 17–18.

2 Pattie A and Gilleard C (1979) *Manual of the Clifton Assessment Procedure for the Elderly (CAPE).* Hodder and Stoughton Educational, Sevenoaks.

3 Cole MG (1989) Inter-rater reliability of the Crichton Geriatric Behaviour Rating Scale. *Age Ageing.* **18**: 57–60.

4 Rabins PV (1994) The validity of a caregiver-rated brief Behaviour Symptom Rating Scale (BSRS) for use in the cognitively impaired. *Int J Geriatr Psychiatry.* **9**: 205–10.

5 Burns A, Lawlor B and Craig S (1999) *Assessment Scales in Old Age Psychiatry.* Martin Dunitz, London.

6 Yesavage J, Brink T, Rose T *et al.* (1983) Development and validation of a geriatric depression screening scale: a preliminary report. *J Psychiatr Res.* **17**, 37–49.

7 Yesavage J (1986) Geriatric Depression Scale (GDS): recent evidence and development of a shorter version. *Clin Gerontol.* **9**: 165–73.

8 Adshead F, Day CD and Pitt B (1992) BASDEC: a novel screening instrument for depression in elderly medical inpatients. *BMJ.* **305**: 397.

9 Allen N, Ames D, Ashby D, Bennetts K, Tuckwell V and West C (1994) A brief sensitive screening instrument for depression in late life. *Age Ageing.* **23**: 213–18.

10 Zigmond A and Snaith P (1983) The Hospital Anxiety and Depression (HAD) Scale. *Acta Psychiatr Scand.* **67**: 361–70.

11 Lindesay J (1991) Phobic disorders in the elderly. *Br J Psychiatry.* **159**: 531–41.

12 Sims AC (1988) *Symptoms in the Mind: an introduction to descriptive psychopathology* (2e). WB Saunders, London.

13 Forstl H, Burns A, Levy R and Cairns N (1994) Neuropathological correlates of psychotic phenomena in confirmed Alzheimer's disease. *Br J Psychiatry.* **165**: 53–9.

14 Hodkinson HM (1972) Evaluation of a mental test score for assessment of mental impairment in the elderly. *Age Ageing.* **1**, 233–8.

15 Blessed G, Tomlinson BE and Roth M (1968) The association between quantitative measures of dementia and senile change in the grey matter of elderly people. *Br J Psychiatry.* **144**: 797–811.

16 Kay DW, Black SE, Blessed G, Jachuck SJ and Sahgal A (1972) The prevalence of dementia in a general practice sample: upward revision of reported rate after follow-up and reassessment. *Int J Geriatr Psychiatry.* **5**: 179–86.

17 Holmes J and Gilbody S (1996) Differences in use of abbreviated mental test score by geriatricians and psychiatrists. *BMJ.* **313**: 465.

18 Folstein MF, Folstein SE and McHugh PR (1975) 'Mini-Mental State'. A practical method for grading the cognitive state of patients for the clinician. *J Psychiatr Res.* **12**: 189–98.

19 Greifenhagen A, Kurz A, Wiseman M, Haupt M and Zimmer R (1994) Cognitive assessment in Alzheimer's disease: what does the CAMCOG assess? *Int J Geriatr Psychiatry.* **9**: 743–50.

20 Curran S and Wattis J (1997) Measuring the effects of antidementia drugs in patients with Alzheimer's disease. *Hum Psychopharmacol.* **12**: 347–59.
21 Christensen H and Jorm AJ (1992) The effect of premorbid intelligence on the Mini-Mental State and IQCODE. *Int J Geriatr Psychiatry.* **7**: 159–60.
22 Shulman KI, Gold DP, Cohen CA and Zucchero CA (1993) Clock-drawing and dementia in the community: a longitudinal study. *Int J Geriatr Psychiatry.* **8**: 487–96.
23 Ronnberg L and Ericsson K (1994) Reliability and validity of the hierarchic dementia scale. *Int Psychogeriatr.* **6**: 87–94.
24 Lishman WA (1987) *Organic Psychiatry: the psychological consequences of cerebral disorder.* Blackwell Scientific Publications, Oxford.
25 Wattis JP and Curran S (2003) Physical complaints and psychiatric disorders. *Geriatr Med.* **23**: 33–9.
26 Philp I and Ebrahim S (1994) *Assessing Elderly Patients.* Farrand Press, Nottingham.
27 O'Brien JT (1995) Is hippocampal atrophy on magnetic resonance imaging a marker for Alzheimer's disease? *Int J Geriatr Psychiatry.* **10**: 431–5.
28 Jobst KA, Barnetson LP and Shepstone BJ (1998) Accurate prediction of histologically confirmed Alzheimer's disease and the differential diagnosis of dementia: the use of NINCDS-ADRDA and DSM-III-R criteria, SPECT, X-ray CT and Apo E4 in medial temporal lobe dementias. *Int Psychogeriatr.* **10**: 271–302.
29 Royal College of Psychiatrists (1995) *Consensus Statement on the Assessment and Investigation of an Elderly Person with Suspected Cognitive Impairment by a Specialist Old Age Psychiatry Service.* Royal College of Psychiatrists, London.
30 Taylor D, Paton C and Kerwin R (2003) *The Maudsley Prescribing Guidelines* (7e). Martin Dunitz, London.
31 Reilly JG, Thomas HL and Ferrier IN (2002) Recent studies on ECG changes, antipsychotic use and sudden death in psychiatric patients. *Psychiatr Bull.* **26**: 110–12.
32 Inglis F (2002) The tolerability and safety of cholinesterase inhibitors in the treatment of dementia. *Int J Clin Pract.* **127(Suppl. 1)**: 45–63.
33 Morganroth J, Graham S, Hartman R and Anand R (2002) Electrocardiographic effects of rivastigmine. *J Clin Pharmacol.* **42**: 558–68.
34 Arnold SE and Kumar A (1993) Reversible dementias. *Med Clin North Am.* **77**: 215–30.
35 Curran S and Wattis JP (2001) *Practical Psychiatry of Old Age* (3e). Radcliffe Medical Press, Oxford.
36 Department of Health (1990) *Caring for People: the Care Programme Approach for people with a mental illness referred to the specialist psychiatric services. Joint Health/Social Services Circular. Health and Social Services Development.* Department of Health Publications Unit, London.
37 Burns T (1997) Case management, care management and care programming. *Br J Psychiatry.* **170**: 393–5.
38 Lader M and Herrington R (1990) *Biological Treatments in Psychiatry.* Oxford Medical Publications, Oxford.
39 Thomas KB (1978) The consultation and the therapeutic illusion. *BMJ.* **1**: 1327–8.
40 Young MA, Keller MB, Lavori PW *et al.* (1987) Lack of stability of the RDC endogenous subtype in consecutive episodes of major depression. *J Affect Disord.* **12**: 139–43.
41 Williams RT (1978) Nutrients in drug detoxification reactions. In: JN Hathcock and J Coon (eds) *Nutrition and Drug Interactions.* Academic Press, New York.
42 Livingston G, Hollins S, Katona C *et al.* (1998) Treatment of patients who lack capacity. *Psychiatr Bull.* **22**: 402–4.
43 Ray WA, Fought RL and Decker MD (1992) Psychoactive drugs and risk of injurious motor vehicle crashes in elderly drivers. *Am J Epidemiol.* **136**: 873–83.
44 Lader M (1994) Neuropharmacology and pharmacokinetics of psychotropic drugs in old age. In: J Copeland, M Abou-Saleh and D Blazer (eds) *Principles and Practice of Geriatric Psychiatry.* John Wiley and Sons, Chichester.

45 Curran S and Wattis JP (2004) Psychopharmacology in the elderly. In: DJ King (ed.) *Seminars in Clinical Psychopharmacology* (2e). Gaskell, London.

46 Smith D (1998) Side-effects of psychotropic drugs. In: D Wheatley and D Smith (eds) *Psychopharmacology of Cognitive and Psychiatric Disorders in the Elderly*. Chapman and Hall Medical, London.

47 Hurwitz N (1969) Predisposing factors in adverse reactions to drugs. *BMJ.* 1: 536–40.

48 Learoyd BM (1972) Psychotropic drugs and the elderly patient. *Med J Aust.* 1: 1131–3.

49 Drug and Therapeutics Bulletin (1981) What should we tell patients about their medicines? *Drug Ther Bull.* 19: 73–4.

50 Coupland NJ, Bell CJ and Potokar JP (1996) Serotonin reuptake inhibitor withdrawal. *J Clin Psychopharmacol.* 16: 356–62.

51 Charlwood P, Mason A, Goldacre M, Cleary R and Eilkinson E (1999) *Health Outcome Indicators: severe mental illness. Report of a working group to the Department of Health.* National Centre for Health Outcomes Development, Oxford.

52 Stein GS (1999) Usefulness of the Health of the Nation Outcome Scales. *Br J Psychiatry.* 174: 375–7.

53 Wattis JP, Butler A, Martin C and Sumner T (1994) Outcome of admission to an acute psychiatric facility for older people: a pluralistic evaluation. *Int J Geriatr Psychiatry.* 9: 835–40.

Chapter 5

Old age psychopharmacology: the pharmacist's perspective

Paul Hardy and Mary Crabb

Introduction

This chapter will discuss the role of the pharmacist in the care of the older mentally ill person. In the first part it will describe specific medicines which may require special care due to the physiological changes that occur with increasing age, and it will then go on to discuss medicines management using the example of a patient journey.

Pharmacokinetic changes in old age

As people get older their use of medicines tends to increase. Four in five people aged over 75 years take at least one prescribed medicine, with 36% taking four or more medicines.[1] These changes, together with polypharmacy (taking multiple medicines for multiple medical conditions), mean that the elderly are more prone to adverse drug reactions (ADRs). Adverse drug interactions are an important cause of morbidity, and even mortality, in older people. There is a threefold greater incidence of drug-induced morbidity in patients over the age of 60 years compared with those under 30 years. ADRs have been reported to be solely or partly the cause of 10–16% of admissions of elderly people to acute geriatric wards.[2]

Pharmacokinetic changes

Pharmacokinetics can be defined as 'how the body handles a drug', whereas pharmacodynamics is described as 'what a drug does to a patient'. Pharmacokinetic parameters of drug handling (absorption, distribution, metabolism and elimination) may be significantly altered in the elderly (*see* Table 5.1).

Table 5.1 Pharmacokinetic changes with
increasing age

Absorption	Increased gastric pH
	Decreased intestinal blood flow
	Decreased surface area for absorption
	Decreased gastrointestinal motility
	Decreased gastric emptying
	Decreased gastric acid secretion
Distribution	Increased total fat content
	Decreased total body water
	Decreased lean body mass
	Decreased serum albumin
Metabolism	Decreased liver mass
	Decreased liver blood flow
	Decreased liver enzyme activity
Elimination	Decreased glomerular filtration
	Decreased renal tubular filtration

Absorption

Difficulties with swallowing are relatively common among elderly patients with psychiatric disorders, especially those that are associated with neurodegenerative or cerebrovascular conditions. Factors such as an increase in gastric pH and a reduction in absorptive surface area and mesenteric blood flow may contribute to a reduced rate of drug absorption. This slowing can be compounded by drugs that cause anticholinergic effects, the administration of antacids and the ingestion of food.[3]

Distribution

The distribution of drugs may be significantly altered because of age-related changes in body fat, total body water, lean body mass and plasma albumin levels. Total body fat increases between the ages of 18 and 35 years from 18% to 36% in males and from 33% to 48% in females.[4] This increase in body fat results in an increase in the volume of distribution of lipid-soluble drugs such as diazepam, and can result in a prolonged elimination half-life leading to accumulation. A decrease in lean body mass reduces the volume of distribution of water-soluble drugs such as digoxin and lithium that bind to muscle in older adults. Therefore smaller doses may be required in elderly people. Factors which may affect binding and that have special applicability in older people include protein concentration, disease states, co-administration of other drugs, and nutritional status.[4]

Following absorption into the bloodstream, most medication binds to plasma proteins, albumin and α1-acid glycoprotein. Acidic drugs tend to bind to plasma albumin, whereas basic drugs bind to α1-acid glycoprotein. Only an unbound drug is able to cross the blood–brain barrier and interact with the intended target in the brain. In the elderly, plasma albumin levels fall resulting in higher levels of protein-bound drugs (e.g. diazepam, phenytoin and warfarin), which may have an increased free concentration and therefore an enhanced effect. Plasma α1-acid glycoprotein levels may remain unchanged or may rise slightly with ageing.

Total body water may decrease by 15%, reducing the volume of distribution of water-soluble drugs such as lithium and leading to higher plasma concentrations. Concomitant administration of diuretics may exacerbate this problem.

Metabolism

Hepatic metabolism is decreased in the elderly due to a loss of liver mass and a decrease in liver blood flow. Other disease states such as heart failure will further decrease liver blood flow.

First-pass metabolism of drugs with a higher extraction ratio, such as barbiturates and propranolol, are blood flow dependent and are impaired, resulting in increased drug levels. Liver metabolism of drugs by phase 1 reactions (e.g. oxidation) decreases with age, and this leads to age-related reductions in clearance for drugs such as diazepam, chlordiazepoxide and nortriptyline. Phase 2 reactions (e.g. conjugation) show few or no age-related changes.[2] Note that in the elderly, normal liver function tests (LFTs) do not imply normal metabolism of drugs. The cytochrome P450 group of isoenzymes is responsible for the metabolism of most commonly used drugs. The CYP1, CYP2 and CYP3 families are responsible for the majority of drug metabolism in humans.[5] Antidepressants such as selective serotonin reuptake inhibitors, mirtazepine and venlafaxine are all primarily eliminated by oxidative metabolism via the cytochrome P450 enzymes.[6] Antipsychotic drugs are also metabolised by this pathway, and caution is advised as these drugs may have reduced clearance in the elderly.

Elimination

This is the most important age-related change, and disease states such as diabetes and heart failure can worsen renal function, as can an acute illness which leads to dehydration, such as a chest infection.[7] Renal function deteriorates with increasing age. The glomerular filtration rate decreases by 1% per year after the age of 40 years. A decrease in renal excretion of cleared medicines may lead to an increase in serum concentration, resulting in accumulation and toxicity. Drugs that are removed by renal excretion include allopurinol, atenolol, digoxin and spironolactone. Lithium is dependent on renal function for elimination. Serum levels of lithium above the therapeutic range may result in nephrogenic diabetes insipidus. In older adults, toxicity may occur at levels that would be considered therapeutic in younger adults. Signs of toxicity include increased tremor, confusion and ataxia. Creatinine clearance can be estimated from serum creatinine levels using the Cockcroft–Gault equation:[8]

$$\text{Creatinine clearance} = \frac{F \times (140 - \text{age}) \times \text{body weight (kg)}}{\text{serum creatinine concentration } (\mu\text{mol/l})}$$

where $F = 1.03$ for females and 1.23 for males. In obese patients, ideal body weight should be used, as total body weight will overestimate renal function. Renal impairment is often missed in the elderly, especially as a decrease in muscle mass may prevent an increase in plasma creatinine levels. One way to grade renal impairment is summarised in Table 5.2.

Table **5.2** Glomerular filtration rate and degree of
renal impairment

Degree of renal impairment	Glomerular filtration rate (ml/min)
Mild	20–50
Moderate	10–20
Severe	< 10

Pharmacodynamic changes

Pharmacodynamic changes may be defined as 'what a drug does to the patient'.
The most important changes seen in older people are summarised in Table 5.3.

Table **5.3** Pharmacodynamic changes
observed in older people

Increased sensitivity to some drugs

Decreased drug receptor population

Decreased cholinergic transmission

Decreased thermoregulatory mechanisms

Decreased orthostatic circulatory responses

Increased postural instability

Pharmacodynamic changes with age have not been studied to the same extent as
pharmacokinetic changes, but it is evident that some systems in the body become
increasingly sensitive to drugs that act on them. There is an increased sensitivity
to central nervous system drugs, such as benzodiazepines. These may cause
sedation, confusion, disorientation, memory impairment and delirium. Reduced
cholinergic transmission in the brain with increasing age may explain why the
elderly are more prone to drug-induced cognitive disorder. Drugs which may
cause cognitive impairment include anticholinergics (benzhexol, orphenadrine
and procyclidine), benzodiazepines, opioids and tricyclic antidepressants. The
selective serotonin reuptake inhibitors (SSRIs) and reversible inhibitors of
monoamine oxidase A have not been shown to have negative effects on
cognition.

The elderly are more susceptible to anticholinergic side-effects, and many
medication classes, including tricyclic antidepressants, antipsychotics, antihistamines and anti-arrhythmics, have anticholinergic properties.[9] Anticholinergic
side-effects include dry mouth, blurred vision, constipation, confusion and
urinary retention.

Thermoregulatory mechanisms are often impaired in the elderly, and hypo-
thermia may occur. Commonly implicated drugs include phenothiazines, tricyclic
antidepressants, benzodiazepines, opioids and alcohol. Older people are more
prone to drug-induced hypotension because of an impaired reflex tachycardia

response. Medicines responsible for orthostatic effects include tricyclic antidepressants, phenothiazines and levodopa. It is appropriate to assume that there is an impaired baroreflex function in elderly people,[10] and to monitor these medicines carefully.

Other effects of psychotropic medicines in the older person include agitation, mood and perceptual disturbances, headache, sweating, sexual dysfunction, gastrointestinal disturbances (nausea, anorexia, changes in weight or bowel habits) and hyponatraemia.[3]

Medication and falls in the older person

About 30% of older people over 65 years of age fall at least once a year, often resulting in fractures.[11] The aetiology of falls is complex, and medicines are seldom the sole cause, but they do make a major contribution to the problem.

Medication may cause falls by various mechanisms, including the following:

- increased sedation
- reduced balance
- reduced reaction time
- postural hypotension
- drug-induced parkinsonism
- confusion
- hypoglycaemia
- postural instability – this increases with age and drugs that increase postural sway may precipitate falls.

Tinetti[12] has shown the strongest link to an increased risk of falling to be with selective serotonin reuptake inhibitors, tricyclic antidepressants, neuroleptic agents, benzodiazepines, anticonvulsants and class IA anti-arrhythmic medications. One-third of prescriptions given to older patients admitted to hospital could be stopped without detriment to the patient, either because the drugs are unnecessary or because they are absolutely contraindicated. Despite this, many drugs are still prescribed unnecessarily.[13]

Pharmaceutical care of older people with mental illness

Pharmaceutical care has been defined as 'the responsible provision of drug therapy for the purpose of achieving definite outcomes which improve the patient's quality of life.'[14] Philosophically, it may be seen as the latest stage in a process of moving the focus of pharmacists' activity from a supply-oriented role to a patient-oriented one. Typically a series of pharmaceutical care needs will be identified for a patient (*see* Table 5.4) to guide the pharmacist in devising that patient's care plan.

Table 5.4 Pharmaceutical care planning: examples of some of the key issues (adapted with permission from Shaw et al.[15])

Adherence problems

Administration problems

Side-effects/adverse drug reactions

Medication review

Therapeutic drug monitoring (TDM)

Special monitoring requirements

Drug interactions

Polypharmacy

Other medications (non-prescribed remedies, illicit drug use)

In the area of old age psychiatry there are relatively few examples of pharmaceutical care initiatives directed towards the elderly mentally ill which have been shown to have positive outcomes for patients. Examples of programmes designed for the elderly[25,28–9] or for the mentally ill, which can give pointers to the types of service which might be developed in the future, are included in this book.

To demonstrate the range of activity in this area, we shall follow a hypothetical patient journey through secondary and primary care and highlight some of the programmes which have been developed at each stage on the journey. Note that the programmes discussed are largely pilot schemes and not available in all areas.

Hospital admission

When a patient is admitted to hospital, it can often be their drug therapy which has precipitated the admission. It has been estimated that 10–20% of hospital admissions are caused by adverse drug reactions. Mannesse et al.[16] examined admissions of patients over 70 years of age to general medical wards. A severe adverse drug reaction was present in 24 of cases, and 12% of admissions were classified as probably caused by an adverse drug reaction. Badcott et al.,[17] in a 10-day audit of admissions via Accident and Emergency, identified 90 patients (45%) in whom drug-related problems were a likely causative factor with regard to their admission.

Following admission to hospital, the patient is prescribed medication for inpatient use which is usually intended to replicate the drug regime taken by the patient immediately prior to admission. For a variety of reasons this may not always be accurate. Drewett[18] studied admissions to a general hospital in order to quantify these discrepancies on their medication charts. In total, 34% of patients were found to have errors. As well as mis-transcriptions of dose and frequency, patients had medicines omitted in many instances.

Pharmacist-conducted drug histories on admission have been used to avoid some of these problems. The pharmacist's greater familiarity with the range of products available commercially can help to improve the accuracy of the medication history. However, the scope for pharmacy intervention in this area is limited. It is not clear whether the information gleaned is more helpful than careful checks with practice records or with medication records in community pharmacies. Also, patients admitted to psychiatric settings may be unable to provide the pharmacist with an adequate medication history for various reasons, and the introduction of another health professional to the patient at this early stage of treatment can be counter-productive.

Many pharmacies now implement strategies of reusing patients' own drugs, or the 'one-stop' dispensing system, as advocated in the National Service Framework for Older People.[19] Reuse of patients' own drugs has been associated with a reduction in medication errors.[20] One-stop dispensing reduces the risk of transcription errors when inpatient medication is rewritten for discharge, and provides the opportunity for patients to retain responsibility for their medication before discharge. However, this approach may not suit patients in mental health environments. Generally, inpatient stay for psychiatric conditions tends to be of a longer duration, which requires the resupply of medication that one-stop dispensing is designed to avoid. In addition, small supplies of medication are still required for short periods of home leave.

The inpatient stay

Pharmacist involvement with prescription monitoring at ward level, and attendance at multi-disciplinary ward rounds, is now an established practice in many UK hospitals. In addition, many pharmacists have developed other services to help to meet the needs of their patients. Longitudinal drug histories are one example. Paton[21] reviewed the drug history request service provided at their hospital (an acute adult mental health unit). A longitudinal history for a long-stay patient could take an experienced pharmacist up to a full day to prepare, and on the basis of its findings would conclude by providing some suggestions for future pharmacological management to be considered for the patient. A questionnaire was circulated among users (medical and nursing staff) to assess whether this service offered good value. Respondents indicated an overall high level of satisfaction with the service. Of ten patients studied for 6 months following the drug history, nine had changes to their treatment plan as a result of the recommendations made, and the majority of these led to improvements in the patient's mental state.

The use of computerised pharmacy records has assisted this process at Rampton Hospital.[22] The 'PPS' database presents a patient 'timeline', with medication record, blood histories and other patient data and events co-ordinated on the timeline. The relationship between onset of drug therapy and progression of disease has become easier to observe, and has added a layer of objective observational data to the assessment of whether or not psychiatric drugs are working.

Increasingly as evidence-based and protocol-driven practice takes hold in patient management, more objective criteria for directing pharmacist activity will be needed. Beers et al.[23] have attempted to devise a list of medication deemed inappropriate for use in the elderly. Using an expert panel, a review of the literature resulted in a list of 33 medications or categories of medications considered less suitable or unsuitable for use in elderly patients. The list was later revised[24] to keep abreast of developments in the field of pharmacotherapy, and is now an important assessment tool in studies of prescribing practice.

Similarly, Osborne *et al.*[25] attempted to devise an indicator for appropriate neuroleptic prescribing in nursing homes in the UK. Developing an indicator based on US consensus criteria, the authors examined neuroleptic prescribing in 934 residents in 22 nursing homes in the South Thames region. In total, 45% of prescriptions for antipsychotics in this cohort were initiated prior to admission to the nursing home. Only 17.8% of prescriptions fulfilled the criteria for appropriate prescribing.

Hospital discharge: the secondary/primary care interface

The risk of readmission during the first 6 months after discharge is very high for psychiatric patients.[26] Therefore, as our patient moves towards hospital discharge, continuity of care across the interface becomes a major concern. A number of studies have looked at improving communication between primary and secondary care pharmacists by means of pharmacy discharge information.

In a study of general medical patients,[27] discharge prescription details were passed on to community pharmacists in an active group, and not in a comparison group. The number of unintentional discrepancies in subsequent community-based supply of medication was lower for the intervention group than for the comparison group, and the number of discrepancies judged to have a definite adverse effect was also lower. The authors calculated that giving such information to 19 patients would prevent one patient from being exposed to one unintentional discrepancy with a definite adverse effect.

In another study on pharmacy discharge planning in adult patients from a large psychiatric hospital,[15] 97 patients were randomly assigned to either an intervention group or a control group. Intervention took the form of pharmaceutical needs assessment, provision of medication information and sending discharge planning information to the patient's community pharmacy. Patient knowledge did not differ between the two groups. Medication problems post-discharge (supply, administration and storage/handling issues, and therapeutic problems) were greater for the control group than for the intervention group. There was a trend in the control group for lower readmission rates in the 3 months following discharge, but this did not reach the level of clinical significance.

However, the overall benefits of discharge pharmaceutical care planning may be limited. Nazareth *et al.*[28] studied the effectiveness of a pharmacy discharge plan in 362 older medical patients. The primary outcome measure of readmission rates at 3 and 6 months did not differ between the intervention and control groups. Secondary outcomes of the number of deaths, hospital outpatient or general practice appointments, and the number of days in hospital during the follow-up period also did not differ.

This finding contrasts with the positive assessment of discharge planning seen in the other studies. It is theoretically possible that mental health patients would gain greater benefit from this type of intervention than medical patients, precisely because of the high risk for readmission during this period, but this cannot be confirmed on the basis of the present data.

Community-based interventions

As our patient becomes reintegrated in their domestic environment, ongoing pharmaceutical care can continue to offer health benefits. Specialisation in mental health pharmacy has been almost exclusively a secondary care phenomenon in the past. Community pharmacists who have supported patients with mental health problems in the community have had no formal structures to support or recognise their contribution. However, the study programmes available from the Centre for Postgraduate Pharmacy Education and the United Kingdom Psychiatric Pharmacy Group are beginning to improve this situation.

Bernsten *et al.*[29] studied community pharmacy-based care for elderly patients with a variety of medical and/or psychiatric problems in seven European countries. A harmonised, structured pharmaceutical care programme was provided by community pharmacists who received training. A general decline in health for the whole study cohort was seen over the course of the 18-month study. However, significant improvements were seen in the intervention group compared with the control group. Patients in the intervention group reported better control of their medical conditions as a result of the survey. The authors noted that the chief beneficial outcomes of the study seemed to be in the humanistic aspects, such as satisfaction with treatment and sign and symptom control, and (perhaps surprisingly) less impact was seen on drug therapy, drug knowledge and adherence.

One of the most well-regarded community-based schemes of recent years has been the work conducted in South Derbyshire by Harris.[30] In this project, 24 community pharmacists were recruited to work alongside other health professionals in providing advice, support and information, visiting patients in their own homes, and rationalising treatment regimes and supporting patient adherence. The pharmacist provides a pharmaceutical care plan to the patient or carer. This scheme has proved popular with other health workers and with carers.

Following the success of this project, Harris was commissioned by the Mental Health Foundation to investigate the level of provision of community-based pharmaceutical care for the elderly mentally ill throughout the UK. This work has recently been updated.[31] Respondents reported that the main perceived medication difficulties for this patient group included obtaining information about medicines, understanding the instructions for taking medicines, removing medicines from the container, and taking medicines as prescribed. Only a third of respondents considered that routine support for elderly mentally ill patients was available. Provision of support for community teams or home-based services was inconsistent, and the level of continuity of care between hospital and the community was low. Funding problems were commonly seen as a barrier to provision of services.

Key points

- This chapter has discussed the impact on patient care made by pharmacists at all stages of the patient journey. The model schemes that have been highlighted demonstrate the untapped potential of pharmacists to make significant contributions to medicines management.
- In time it is hoped that provision of these value-added services will be able to make improvements to the lot of greater numbers of elderly patients with mental health problems.

References

1 Erens B and Primatesta P (eds) (1999) *The Health Survey for England in 1998: cardiovascular disease.* The Stationery Office, London.
2 Denham MJ and Barnett NL (1998) Drug therapy and the older person – role of the pharmacist. *Drug Safety.* **4**: 243–50.
3 Zubenko GS and Sunderland T (2000) Geriatric psychopharmacology: why does age matter? *Harvard Rev Psychiatry.* **7**: 311–33.
4 Young LY and Koda-Kimble MA (eds) (1995) *Applied Therapeutics: the clinical use of drugs* (6e). Lippincott Williams & Wilkins, Philadelphia, PA.
5 Adams P (1998) Drug interactions that matter: mechanism and management. *Pharm J.* **261**: 618–21.
6 Devane CL and Pollock BG (1999) Pharmacokinetic considerations of antidepressant use in the elderly. *J Clin Psychiatry.* **60 (Suppl. 20)**: 38–44.
7 Phillips PA, Johnston CI and Gray L (1993) Disturbed fluid and electrolyte homoeostasis following dehydration in elderly people. *Age Aging.* **22**: S26–33.
8 Kuczynska J and Evans H (2000) Prescribing drugs for patients with renal failure. *Prescriber.* **11**(5): 115–23.
9 Gray SL, Lai KV and Larson EB (1999) Drug-induced cognition disorders in the elderly: incidence, prevention and management. *Drug Safety.* **2**: 101–22.
10 Mets TF (1995) Drug-induced orthostatic hypotension in older patients. *Drugs Aging.* **6**: 219–28.
11 Anon (2000) Managing falls in older people. *Drug Ther Bull.* **38**: 68–72.
12 Tinetti M (2003) Preventing falls in elderly persons. *NEJM.* **348**: 42–9.
13 Royal College of Physicians (1997) *Medication for Older People* (2e). Royal College of Physicians, London.
14 Hepler CD and Strand LM (1990) Opportunities and responsibilities in pharmaceutical care. *Am J Hosp Pharm.* **47**: 533–43.
15 Shaw H, Mackie CA and Sharkie I (2000) Evaluation of effect of pharmacy discharge planning on medication problems experienced by discharged acute admission mental health patients. *Int J Pharm Pract.* **8**: 144–53.
16 Mannesse CK, Derxx FHM, De Ridder MAJ *et al.* (2000) Contribution of adverse drug reactions to hospital admission of older patients. *Age Aging.* **29**: 35–9.
17 Badcott S, Fernandes R, Hargreaves D and Freij R (1999) Target drug-related admissions. *Pharm Pract.* **9**: 358–61.
18 Drewett NM (1998) Stop regular medicine errors. *Pharm Pract.* **8**: 193–6.
19 Department of Health (2001) *National Service Framework for Older People.* The Stationery Office, London.
20 Nicholls M (2000) Medicines: peace in a POD. *Health Serv J.* **111**: 35.
21 Paton C (2000) Are we clinically effective? *Pharm Pract.* **8**: 198–200.

22 Anon. (2002) Innovative database gives pharmacists passport into clinical team. *Med Manag.* **1**: 7–8.
23 Beers M, Ouslander JG, Rollingher I *et al.* (1991) Explicit criteria for determining inappropriate medication use in nursing home residents. *Arch Intern Med.* **151**: 1825–32.
24 Beers M (1997) Explicit criteria for determining inappropriate medication use by the elderly: an update. *Arch Intern Med.* **157**: 1531–6.
25 Osborne CA, Hooper R, Li KC *et al.* (2002) An indicator of appropriate neuroleptic prescribing in nursing homes. *Age Ageing.* **31**: 435–9.
26 Walker SA and Eagles JM (2002) Discharging psychiatric patients from hospital. *Psychiatr Bull.* **26**: 241–2.
27 Duggan C, Feldman R, Hough J and Bates I (1998) Reducing adverse prescribing discrepancies following hospital discharge. *Int J Pharm Pract.* **6**: 77–82.
28 Nazareth I, Burton A, Shulman S, Smith P, Haines A and Timberall H (2001) A pharmacy discharge plan for hospitalised elderly patients – a randomised controlled trial. *Age Aging.* **30**: 33–40.
29 Bernsten C, Björkman I, Caramona M *et al.* (2001) Improving the well-being of elderly patients via community pharmacy-based provision of pharmaceutical care. *Drugs Aging.* **18**: 63–77.
30 Harris D (1999) Helping elderly people with mental health problems. *Pharm J.* **263**: 23–4.
31 Milne A and Lingard J (2001) *Medicines and Good Health in Later Life. The Mental Health Foundation Updates. Volume 3, Issue 8*; http://www.mentalhealth.org.uk/html/content/Updatev03i08.pdf

Chapter 6

The role of the nurse in the assessment, diagnosis and treatment of older people with psychotropic drugs

Richard J Clibbens

Introduction

For many older people with mental health needs, nurses are the healthcare professionals with whom they are likely to have most frequent contact. The nurse may also be the main link and information source for the person's family and carers. Where the Care Programme Approach or social care management packages are in place for the older person, this may be a formalised arrangement, where the nurse acts as the communication hub for all agencies and professionals involved in the person's package of care. With regard to psychotropic medication, the nurse's role in working with older people requires a special awareness and knowledge of the potential effects of ageing on how psychotropic drugs are metabolised and excreted, and the nature and prevalence of potential adverse effects of these drugs. Psychotropic medications are those intended to have an effect on mental functioning, such as antidepressants, anxiolytics, hypnotics, antipsychotics and antidementia drugs. These drugs are frequently prescribed for older people experiencing mood disorder, sleep disorder, delerium, dementia, and thought or behavioural disturbance.

The potential benefits of prescribing any drug must be weighed against the possible risks. The nurse must be skilled in identifying when a prescription is not the best first option for treatment or intervention. He or she must be familiar with the range of methods available for the administration of drug treatments and the appropriate use of measured delivery systems, especially in community settings, such as 'blister packs' and other measured 'daily' systems designed to enable the older person to take their medicines independently and safely.

The nurse must always consider issues of concordance. Will the person take the drug as prescribed? Do they want to take this drug? Do they understand what it is for and how it should be taken? What will they do if they experience side-effects? The nurse working with older people with mental health problems and their families and carers has a vital role in providing appropriate information and education to enable an effective partnership approach with the older person. From initial assessment and diagnosis to treatment with and monitoring of psychotropic medication, nurses have an essential role to play in ensuring that best prescribing practice is enabled in true partnership with the older person.

Assessment

All nurses caring for older people must be alert to the importance of screening for and assessment of mental health needs, whatever the setting. Early detection of mental health needs in older people enables appropriate intervention to minimise further distress or deterioration.[1] Where drug treatments for mental health problems are being considered, comprehensive nursing assessment will provide key information to enable accurate diagnosis and appropriate prescribing practice that is tailored to the patient's individual needs.

Assessment information gathered by the nurse may form part of a global health screening assessment such as the 'EASY-Care' tool,[2] which contains specific brief questions to identify possible depression or cognitive impairment. Nurses in contact with older people in the community or acute general hospital environment will often have sustained contact with the person, which enables the identification of possible mental health needs through their privileged knowledge of the individual. Nurses in these environments can utilise screening tools[3] and thoughtful day-to-day practice with older people, to ensure that conditions such as depression are not missed in cases where there is a primary focus on physical health or social care interventions. This information may inform multi-disciplinary discussion and decision making on appropriate interventions and treatment, or prompt referral for a more detailed specialist mental health assessment.

Nurses working within mental health roles may complete a more detailed specialist mental health assessment, including the completion of screening instruments such as the Geriatric Depression Scale[4] or the Mini-Mental State Examination.[5] Completion of a comprehensive mental health assessment with the older person will enable the nurse to identify any problems or needs that require intervention. The nurse may use this information to form a treatment plan with the person for relevant psychological or psychosocial interventions, or to inform an accurate diagnosis to enable appropriate drug treatment prescribing by the GP or psychiatrist.

Effective comprehensive assessment will ensure that the nurse provides key information to enable appropriate and effective prescribing. A knowledge of the person's previous and current medication, physical health and social history and situation will enable the nurse to provide the prescriber with key information to enable the best treatment decision. The nurse's knowledge of the person's previous experience of medication and preferences for any particular interventions and therapies will all inform individually tailored prescribing decisions which increase the likelihood of concordance with the person receiving the prescription.

Nurses are often well placed to obtain key assessment information to enable the multi-disciplinary team to weigh up the potential benefits and risks of drug treatment for the older person with mental health problems. Other interventions such as facilitating increased social contact and activity in depression, for example, or the use of cognitive behavioural therapy (see Box 6.1), may be more appropriate first-line interventions to be implemented and evaluated prior to considering the suitability of drug treatments. The nurse has a responsibility to ensure that other non-pharmacological interventions are appropriately considered either as an alternative to or in conjunction with any pharmacological treatments. Clear communication with and the provision of timely information to the older person at all stages of assessment and diagnosis will ensure a partnership approach whereby individual preferences are recognised and considered.

Box 6.1 Conditions that can be helped by cognitive behavioural therapy

- Phobias
- Certain anxiety disorders, including panic attacks and panic disorder
- Depression
- Eating disorders
- Obsessive-compulsive disorder
- Anger
- Post-traumatic stress disorder
- Sexual and relationship problems
- Drug or alcohol abuse
- Some sleep problems

Adapted from Prodigy.[6]

Nurses working with older people in specialist roles may have a key function in ensuring the appropriate prescribing and administration of psychotropic medication. For example, specialist liaison nurses may be requested to provide information and advice on appropriate prescribing for older people's mental health in general hospital wards or in the care home sector. Where the older person is identified as demonstrating difficult or 'challenging' behaviour, the liaison nurse can work with the care or treatment team to ensure that appropriate assessment information is gathered, alternatives to drug treatment are considered and, if appropriate, that prescribing follows national or local good practice guidelines or protocols.[7,8]

Diagnosis

Increasingly, nurses working with older people with mental health problems are formally establishing a nursing diagnosis for conditions such as depression or anxiety, from which a treatment plan is identified which may include social interventions (such as reducing isolation) and psychological interventions (such as cognitive behavioural therapy).[9] Mental health nurses may utilise the diagnostic criteria outlined in the DSM-IV[10] or ICD-10[11] classification systems to assist them in reaching an effective nursing diagnosis and to ensure a compatible approach with medical colleagues who may also be involved in the person's care, particularly where prescribing of a psychotropic medication is appropriate.

Nurses will often be well placed to offer advice or interventions directly to the older person before a psychotropic medication is prescribed. For example, if the older person is experiencing sleep disturbance, management strategies should be the first intervention before consideration of the prescribing of a hypnotic medication (*see* Box 6.2):

Hypnotics and anxiolytics should be avoided where possible and reserved for short courses to alleviate conditions after causal factors have been established.[12]

Box 6.2 General tips to help with sleep

- Body rhythm – get up at the same time each day and never sleep during the day.
- Routines – are useful before bedtime (e.g. a warm drink, hot bath and reading).
- Bedroom – should be free of noise and not used for watching television, eating or work.
- Stimulants – such as alcohol, caffeine and smoking should be avoided in the evening.
- Exercise – regularly earlier in the day, but not within a few hours of bedtime.
- Eat – only a light snack before bedtime and not a large meal.
- Relaxation – may be improved by a relaxation tape.

Adapted from Prodigy.[12]

Locally agreed protocols for the detection and treatment of specific conditions such as depression increasingly provide a framework for the diagnosis of and interventions for common mental health needs such as dementia and depression. These protocols indicate diagnostic steps with appropriate intervention strategies, including pharmacological intervention where appropriate. Such agreed protocols provide evidence-based practice guidelines which the nurse can utilise both to inform their own individual care and treatment of the older person with mental health needs and to guide appropriate interventions in discussion with the wider multi-disciplinary team.[13]

Increasingly in the care of older people with mental health needs, nurses are completing initial comprehensive assessments and formal psychometric tests which directly inform medical colleagues with regard to the provision of appropriate prescribing decisions. This partnership approach with medical colleagues reduces unnecessary repetition of diagnostic assessment and enhances nurse-led, community-focused care for older people with mental health needs.

Treatment

When administering any psychotropic drug the nurse must ensure that they adhere to the Nursing and Midwifery Council (NMC) guidelines for the administration of medicines[14] (*see* Box 6.3). It is good practice to enable the self-administration of medicines by the patient or carers where appropriate, particularly for hospital patients approaching discharge.[14,15] However, effective policies and procedures must be in place to ensure safe practice, and for some older people with mental health problems the potential risks and benefits of this approach must be carefully considered. Where a concordance aid such as a monitored-dose container or daily/weekly dosing aid is proposed, this should ideally be dispensed, labelled and sealed by a pharmacist. The nurse will need to ensure both the ongoing appropriateness of any such aid and that the patient or their carer has sufficient information and understanding to use this equipment safely.[14]

Box 6.3 Principles for the administration of medicines

When exercising your professional accountability in the best interests of your patients you must:

- know the therapeutic uses of the medicine to be administered, its normal dosage, side-effects, precautions and contraindications
- be certain of the identity of the patient to whom the medicine is to be administered
- be aware of the patient's care plan
- check that the prescription, or the label on medicine dispensed by a pharmacist, is clearly written and unambiguous
- have considered the dosage, method of administration, route and timing of the administration in the context of the condition of the patient and coexisting therapies.

During the administration of medicines to older people, or monitoring of treatment concordance, the nurse will need to evaluate whether any prescribed drug is prescribed in the most appropriate form for the individual. Alternatives to tablets, such as liquids or solubles, may be available and more comfortable or suitable for some older people with mental health needs.

Nurses have an essential role in effective medication management, and may find it helpful to review local trust policies and work with local pharmacists, clinical governance committees and prescribing committees to achieve a systematic approach to ensuring that appropriate prescribing and monitoring of psychotropic medication is a reality for patients in their care. Nurses are required to maintain their professional competence in relation to the administration of medicines, and will need to ensure that they participate in effective continuing professional development linked to their role, job description and identified competencies. Formally identifying and meeting ongoing competency and training needs through annual appraisal and training plans is an essential part of ensuring effective medications management. An increasing range of electronic resources are available to guide and support nursing practice, such as the electronic *BNF*[15] and Prodigy[6] internet sites.

When administering drug treatments for older people with mental health problems, nurses must take account of the physiology of ageing and the potential consequences of this for those in their care. Trounce[16] has identified that older people may be more at risk of altered distribution, metabolism and excretion of drugs. An older person with reduced blood albumin levels may experience greater pharmacological effects than a younger person at the same drug dose, due to reduced protein binding with the drug. The enzymes which break down many drugs in order to metabolise them may be less active with increased age, and the blood supply to the liver may also be reduced. This can potentially lead to an over-accumulation of the drug and symptoms of overdose. Renal function in an

80-year-old may be half that of someone aged 40 years, and the resultant reduced excretion of drugs may cause potential accumulation. Some body organs and systems may also be more sensitive to drug treatment in older patients, with a higher incidence of disturbance of blood pressure, for example, in an older population. Adverse drug reactions may be two to three times more common in older people, due to a range of potential factors including the number of drugs taken, the presence of severe illness and reduced elimination of drugs from the body.[16,17]

Management of behavioural disturbance

In 2004, important concerns were identified regarding the use of specific atypical antipsychotics for behavioural and psychological symptoms in dementia.[8] This report produced expert guidance to the effect that when behavioural and psychiatric symptoms are identified in people with dementia, assessment of the person's needs must consider the following:

> Any changes in environment, relationships or physical health?
> To whom is the symptom a problem and why?
> Do family carers and care staff need additional training to improve therapeutic interactions?[8]

In considering the use of drug treatment for behavioural and psychiatric symptoms, the Royal College of General Practitioners recommends that psychosocial, behavioural and environmental interventions are tried first, with additional consideration of the appropriate use of aromatherapy. The Nursing and Midwifery Council guidelines[14] suggest that nurses who practise complementary and alternative therapies must have successfully undertaken training and be competent in this area. It is essential to have considered the appropriateness of any such therapy to both the condition of the patient and any coexisting treatments. It is also essential that the patient is aware of the therapy and gives their informed consent.

Nurses are often in key roles of responsibility with regard to planning and delivering the care and treatment of people who are experiencing dementia. Nurses must ensure that appropriate assessment and education have taken place with the person with dementia and their family, carers and care staff in cases where there is distressing behaviour or psychiatric symptoms. Nurses will often be able to lead the way in providing non-pharmacological interventions, working creatively with the person with dementia to identify individual solutions that are acceptable to that person and their carers.[18]

Within busy and stressful roles with demanding workloads, medication can often be viewed as a 'quick fix' for behaviour that presents challenges or difficulties. A more individualised approach, focused on the individual with dementia and their unique needs, will often be more time-consuming, but is ultimately often more rewarding as the nurse works creatively to identify person-centred solutions. Many nurses in this situation may be required to adopt a clear stance and demonstrate leadership both in trying alternative individual approaches, and in resisting any inappropriate pressure for a drug to be prescribed before other options have been implemented and evaluated. This approach will require clear communication with all members of the multi-disciplinary or multi-agency team, as well as crucially with the person him- or herself and his or her family. This nursing role can be a challenging one, particularly if carers or care staff show resistance to exploring the impact of their own behaviour and response to the person with dementia. However, persistence in finding individual solutions will bring benefits as those who are being introduced to this more creative way of responding to difficult behaviour recognise their successes and become more familiar and comfortable with this approach.

Use of shared care guidelines

Nurses working with older people with mental health problems have played a key role in the development and implementation of shared care protocols for conditions such as dementia and depression, with target dates for the implementation of these protocols previously identified within the National Service Framework for Older People[1] (*see* Box 6.4).

Box 6.4 An example of a shared care protocol for antidementia drug treatments

In South West Yorkshire Mental Health NHS Trust, local shared care protocols have been implemented for the prescribing of antidementia drugs. Memory service nurses respond to initial referrals, completing home-based assessments and liaising with psychiatrist colleagues in diagnosis and the monitoring and titration of prescribed antidementia medication, prior to the GP taking over prescribing responsibility. The memory services remain involved in monitoring the person with dementia at agreed intervals and informing the GP of their progress and the suitability of continuation of treatment. This role has provided the memory service nurses with the opportunity to develop improved information and support for people with dementia and their carers, both pre- and post-diagnosis.

A comparison study of two locality memory services for people with dementia has highlighted the value that both the person with dementia and their carers place on the opportunity to have consistent access to the same nurse, who visits them at home at a convenient time and provides pre-diagnostic support and information, diagnostic and monitoring assessments and follow-up monitoring and support.[19] This approach, which has been developed in response to the availability of antidementia drugs, demonstrates that in addition to the availability of the drug itself, it is the communication, information and support that this brings with it from the memory service nurse that is of significant value to the person with dementia and their family. A valid concern may be whether people with dementia who are not identified as suitable for antidementia drug treatment receive equal access to these benefits from local health and social care providers.

Seeking the consent of the older person is an essential component of all aspects of the provision of nursing care and treatment. When prescribing or administering psychotropic medication, as with any intervention, for a person's consent to treatment to be valid they must be:

- capable of taking that particular decision
- acting voluntarily
- provided with enough information to enable them to make the decision.[20]

It is the right of any older person to refuse medicines. If prescribed drugs are refused, the nurse should record the reason for refusal and identify an opportunity to review this with the prescriber and other relevant members of the multidisciplinary team. When someone refuses offered prescribed medication (e.g. in a hospital ward), every effort should be made to identify the reasons for this refusal. Does the person have any safety concerns about the drug? Has it made them feel unwell? Have the purpose and anticipated benefits of the drug been clearly explained? Do they require any written information about the drug or an opportunity to discuss the treatment with their doctor? If the tablets are difficult for the person to swallow, or have an unpleasant taste, are there any alternatives available? It will often be useful to discuss this with a pharmacist in order to obtain advice and information on alternatives.

Any nurse who identifies the potential need for the covert administration of medicines to older people with mental health problems will need to follow the guidelines set out in the *UKCC Position Statement on the Covert Administration of Medicines*,[21] endorsed by the Nursing and Midwifery Council. However, this practice is best avoided if at all possible, and should only be considered in exceptional circumstances. It is the right of an individual to refuse any treatment, and every adult is assumed to have the capacity to consent to or refuse a treatment until the contrary is proven. This includes people with severe dementia, as no older person should be assumed to lack capacity in any situation unless this has been formally assessed and identified. Assessments of capacity to make a particular decision will only relate to that decision at that particular time, and must not be generalised to any other situation or intervention.

When adults lack capacity and this has been formally determined, it is possible to lawfully provide treatment and care, but this must be in the person's 'best interests'. Any determination of the person's best interests must include information from those who know the person well, and also identification of previously expressed wishes and preferences. In addition to the person's 'medical' or health need, attention must be given to the impact of any treatment on their psychological, social and spiritual well-being. No one can give consent on behalf of another adult. The healthcare professional responsible for the person's care is legally accountable for deciding whether the treatment is in the person's best interests, but ideally decisions will reflect agreement between professionals and those 'close to the older person'.[20]

Efficacy and safety

The National Service Framework for Older People[1] identifies the need for regular medication reviews for older people to minimise the risk and harm of polypharmacy. Once an older person has been prescribed a psychotropic drug, nurses are often best placed to monitor the effects of the drug, in terms of its benefit and any possible experienced adverse effects. This requires a working knowledge of the drug, its anticipated treatment benefits and possible side-effects. The nurse can consider this information in the context of the individual patient's lifestyle and health history, to ensure that appropriate dose titration, medication review, consideration of alternatives or discontinuation of treatment all occur when appropriate.

Polypharmacy in older people has been identified as a significant risk factor for falls.[1] Medication review and monitoring of possible side-effects of prescribed drugs, such as hypotension, can play an important role in falls prevention. The prescribing of antipsychotic medications for patients in nursing and residential homes has been identified as a particularly significant concern:[17]

> Such medicines used to treat behavioural complications of dementia may hasten cognitive decline.[17]

Nurses have a clear role in ensuring that any behavioural disturbance is fully and appropriately assessed, and that the prescribing of medication is viewed as a last resort once other interventions have been appropriately implemented.

The provision of timely, appropriate and understandable information on drug treatments, anticipated benefits and possible side-effects is likely to improve the patient's concordance and provide him or her with an opportunity to raise any concerns prior to treatment. If the patient has a communicative, trusting relationship with the nurse, a more open discussion of prescribed medication is likely to occur, minimising the risk of prescriptions that are not dispensed or unused stockpiles of tablets in the patient's medicine chest.

Reporting adverse events

The Yellow Card scheme is available to enable nurses to report any suspected adverse drug reactions. It is available in a paper version at the back of the *Nurse Prescribers Formulary (NPF)*[22] and the *British National Formulary (BNF)*.[15] The Committee on Safety of Medicines (CSM) and the Medicines Control Agency (MCA)[23] recommend that nurses use the electronic version of the Yellow Card, which is available at: www.mca.gov.uk/yellowcard. The CSM/MCA identify an adverse drug reaction as follows:

> an unwanted or harmful reaction experienced following the administration of a drug or combination of drugs under normal conditions of use and suspected to be related to the medicine.[23]

All adverse reactions, including non-serious ones, should be reported for black triangle medicines (which indicates intensive monitoring of that product by the CSM/MCA). For established medicines or vaccines, all serious suspected adverse reactions should be reported, including those that are:

> fatal – life-threatening – disabling – incapacitating – congenital abnormality – involve hospitalisation – and/or medically significant.[23]

Nurse prescribing

Nurses have a key role in the assessment, diagnosis and treatment of older people with psychotropic drugs. Historically, nurses have supported medical prescribing practice, providing timely accurate information to enable appropriate prescribing decisions by medical staff. Registered mental nurses working with older people in community or inpatient settings have for many years prompted timely appropriate prescribing and advised non-mental-health prescribers (e.g. in primary care settings) on suitable and appropriate drug treatments in the field of older people's mental health. More recently, national procedures and validated training programmes have been established to enable nurses to achieve a registrable qualification in independent, extended independent and supplementary prescribing, where autonomous appropriate prescribing is undertaken directly by mental health nurses, rather than 'through the back door' by advising medical colleagues.

The role of experienced mental health nurses in advising doctors on appropriate prescribing for mental health needs has been recognised for many years.[24] In this context the development of extended roles for nurses, enabling them to supplement the medical workforce in mental health prescribing, is a natural development. However, concern has been expressed that in undertaking formal prescribing roles, nurses may become less focused on care and concentrate more on medical treatment, at a time when a much greater emphasis on psychosocial approaches, talking therapies and health promotion is required in older people's mental health nursing. De-facto prescribing by community mental health nurses has been identified,[25] where nurses have described influencing and advising doctors on prescribing decisions.

User views on mental health nurse prescribing have been identified as including concerns about the appropriateness of prescribing by nurses rather than doctors,[26] and currently any psychotropic drugs prescribed by a nurse as a supplementary prescriber require that the agreement of the patient to this form of prescribing is documented.

Mental health nurses have been described as having a mixed level of existing knowledge of pharmacology, and concern has been raised about potential underestimation of the level of knowledge and experience needed to prescribe psychotropic medication.[27,28] This may be addressed by the development of a nurse prescribing training curriculum to include additional content on psychotropic pharmacology for nurses working in the field of mental health.[29]

Since 2003 the opportunity has been available for nurses to undertake training to become *extended independent and supplementary prescribers*. At the time of writing, psychotropic medications for older people's mental health problems are not included within the list of approved medicines that registered nurse prescribers can prescribe independently. However, qualification as a supplementary prescriber does enable the prescription of psychotropic medications by the nurse, within strict specific parameters.[30] The supplementary prescribing role is described as follows:

> A voluntary prescribing partnership between the independent prescriber (a doctor or dentist) and a supplementary prescriber, to implement an agreed patient-specific Clinical Management Plan.[30]

The independent prescriber (IP) is responsible for diagnosis and the parameters of the clinical management plan. The supplementary prescriber (SP) has discretion with regard to the dosage, frequency and product, within the limits of the clinical management plan. Once a clinical management plan has been completed, this must be reviewed by the IP at least annually if not more frequently. The IP and SP must share access to a common patient record. Agreement to the clinical management plan must be recorded by the independent prescriber and supplementary prescriber before prescribing can begin.[30]

Clearly the supplementary prescriber should not prescribe any medicine that they do not feel competent to prescribe. The independent prescriber can choose not to implement a clinical management plan where there is concern for any reason that supplementary prescribing may not be appropriate. The independent prescriber can also resume full direct responsibility for prescribing at any time if required. An example of supplementary nurse prescribing for antidementia drug treatments is given in Box 6.5.

Box 6.5 Supplementary prescribing of antidementia medication in a memory service

Community memory clinic nurse completes comprehensive home assessment

↓

Patient attends memory clinic for completion of baseline psychometric tests and diagnostic interview with medical and nursing team. Information is provided on diagnosis and available drug treatments

↓

Patient is in agreement with supplementary prescribing by the nurse

↓

Clinical management plan for named patient is signed by doctor (independent prescriber) and nurse (supplementary prescriber)

↓

Nurse provides ongoing monthly prescriptions, including dose titration, in accordance with NICE guidance[31] and locally approved shared care guidelines for antidementia medication

↓

At 4 to 6 months from initial prescription, GP takes over prescribing in accordance with the shared care guidelines

---

There is no legal restriction on the clinical conditions that the supplementary prescriber may treat. It is anticipated that supplementary prescribing may be most useful in the treatment of some long-term conditions. All prescription-only medicines can be prescribed except controlled drugs.[30]

A scoping study conducted by the National Prescribing Centre for the Department of Health identified that clinical management plans need to be relatively simple and quick to complete in order to be worthwhile, and should not include a lot of information that is already available within the shared record. The clinical management plan should make reference to appropriate reputable guidelines or agreed protocols for the treatment of specific conditions.[32]

Registered nurses are personally accountable for their prescribing practice, and must work to the same standard or competence that applies to all other prescribers.[30] Nurse prescribers are also accountable to the Nursing and Midwifery Council and must act in accordance with its code of professional conduct. All nurse prescribers should have professional indemnity. The National Prescribing

Centre has produced a framework document to enable nurses to maintain ongoing competency in their prescribing.[33]

Key points

- Nurses have contact with older people in many different settings, and have significant opportunities to enhance the appropriate detection, assessment and treatment of mental health problems for these people.
- Knowledge of psychotropic medications for older people, including when and how these should be prescribed, monitored and evaluated, together with a knowledge of alternative or complementary non-pharmacological interventions, is essential for all nurses involved in the care of older people.

References

1 Department of Health (2001) *National Service Framework for Older People*. Department of Health, London.
2 Sheffield Institute for Studies on Ageing (1999) *EASY-Care Elderly Assessment System*. Sheffield Institute for Studies on Ageing, University of Sheffield, Sheffield.
3 Royal College of Nursing (1997) *Guidelines for Assessing Mental Health Needs in Old Age*. Royal College of Nursing, London.
4 Van-Marwijk H, Wallace P, de-Boc G *et al.* (1995) Evaluation of the feasibility, reliability and diagnostic value of shortened versions of the Geriatric Depression Scale. *Acta Psychiatr Scand.* **67**: 361–70.
5 Folstein M, Folstein S and McHugh P (1975) 'Mini-Mental State': a practical method for grading the cognitive state of patients for the clinician. *J Psychiatr Records.* **12**: 189–98.
6 Prodigy (2004) *What is Cognitive Behaviour Therapy (CBT)?* www.prodigy.nhs.uk
7 Royal Pharmaceutical Society of Great Britain (2003) *The Administration and Control of Medicines in Care Homes and Children's Services*. Royal Pharmaceutical Society of Great Britain, London.
8 Royal College of General Practitioners (2004) *Guidance for the Management of Behavioural and Psychiatric Symptoms of Dementia and the Treatment of Psychosis in People with a History of Stroke/TIA*. Royal College of General Practitioners, London.
9 Woods R (1999) *Psychological Problems of Ageing: assessment, treatment and care*. John Wiley and Sons, Chichester.
10 American Psychiatric Association (1994) *Diagnostic and Statistical Manual of Mental Disorders* (4e). American Psychiatric Association, Washington, DC.
11 World Health Organization (1992) *The ICD-10 Classification of Mental and Behavioural Disorders: clinical descriptions and diagnostic guidelines*. World Health Organization, Geneva.
12 Prodigy (2003) *Guidance: hypnotic or anxiolytic dependence*; www.prodigy.nhs.uk
13 Alzheimer's Society (accessed 2004) *Dementia: diagnosis and management in primary care. An evidence-based educational package about dementia for primary care teams in CD-ROM format*; www.alzheimer's.org.uk
14 Nursing and Midwifery Council (2002) *Guidelines for the Administration of Medicines*. Nursing and Midwifery Council, London.
15 The Pharmaceutical Press (2003) *Nurse Prescribers' Formulary 2003–2005*. The Pharmaceutical Press, London.

16 Trounce J (2000) *Clinical Pharmacology for Nurses* (16e). Churchill-Livingstone, Edinburgh.

17 Department of Health (2001) *Medicines and Older People: implementing medicines-related aspects of the NSF for Older People*. Department of Health, London.

18 Clibbens RJ and Lewis D (2004) The role of the nurse in the assessment, diagnosis and management of patients with dementia. In: S Curran and J Wattis (eds) *Practical Management of Dementia: a multi-professional approach*. Radcliffe Publishing Ltd, Oxford.

19 Timlin A, Gibson G, Curran S and Watttis JP (2005) *Memory Matters: A report exploring issues around the delivery of anti-dementia medication*. University of Huddersfield, Huddersfield.

20 Department of Health (2001) *Seeking Consent: working with older people*. Department of Health, London.

21 Nursing and Midwifery Council (2002) *UKCC Position Statement on the Covert Administration of Medicines*. Nursing and Midwifery Council, London.

22 The Pharmacutical Press (2003) *The British National Formulary*. The Pharmaceutical Press, London; www.bnf.org/

23 Committee on Safety of Medicines and the Medicines Control Agency (2002) *Extension of the Yellow Card Scheme to Nurse Reporters*. Medicines Control Agency, London.

24 Gournay K and Barker P (2002) Prescribing: the great debate. *Nurs. Standard.* 17: 22–3.

25 Ramcharan P, Hemmingway S and Flowers K (2001) A client-centred base for nurse prescribing. *Ment Health Nurs.* 21: 6–11.

26 Harrison A (2003) Mental health service users' views of nurse prescribing. *Nurse Prescrib.* 1: 78–85.

27 McCann TV and Baker H (2002) Community mental health nurses and authority to prescribe medications: the way forward? *J Psychiatr Ment Health Nurs.* 9: 175–82.

28 Davis J and Hemmingway S (2003) Supplementary prescribing in mental health nursing. *Nurs Times.* 99: 28–30.

29 Department of Health (2004) *Nurse Prescribing Training and Preparation: extended formulary nurse prescribing and supplementary prescribing*. Department of Health, London.

30 Department of Health (2004) *Supplementary Prescribing: key principles*. Department of Health, London.

31 Department of Health (2001) *Guidance on the Use of Donepezil, Rivastigmine and Galantamine for the Treatment of Alzheimer's Disease*. NICE Technology Appraisal guidance No. 19, Department of Health, London.

32 Department of Health (2004) *Scoping Study of Supplementary Prescribing*. Department of Health, London.

33 National Prescribing Centre (2001) *Maintaining Competency in Prescribing: an outline framework to help nurse prescribers*. National Prescribing Centre, London.

Chapter 7

The GP and 'medicines management' for older people with mental health problems in primary care

Owen P Dempsey

Introduction

The general practitioner (GP) in the UK has a pivotal gate-keeping role with unique opportunities for the early detection of memory or behavioural problems and mental illness in older people. However, the early recognition of problems such as dementia and depression can be very difficult in the hurly-burly of everyday practice, and unfortunately GPs do not always have the time, the motivation or the skills required.[1] In older people in particular, depression and dementia can be very difficult to recognise, but despite the large and increasing prevalence of these problems, less than 40% of GPs have received any specialist training in gerontology, and even less will have received training in old age psychiatry.[1,2] A report from the Audit Commission has recommended that mental health experts provide more training for primary care health workers.[1]

As well as the early recognition of mental health problems, GPs also have clinical and legal responsibility for the vast majority of prescribing for older people who have already been established on psychotropic medication. This is a huge and important problem. Four out of five people over 75 years of age take at least one prescribed medicine, with 36% taking four or more medicines, and almost half of the NHS drugs bill is spent on medicines for older people.[3,4] Care homes are a special case. Residents receive up to four times as many prescription items as older people living in their own homes, and up to 53% of care home residents receive at least one inappropriate prescription[5,6] (*see* Case study 7.2). Understandably, GPs struggle to cope. Zermansky found that 72% of repeat prescriptions sampled in 50 practices had not been reviewed in the past 15 months.[7]

In order to address this issue, the National Service Framework for Older People (www.nelh.nhs.uk/nsf/older_people/default.htm) has emphasised the need for GPs to perform regular face-to-face clinical medication reviews and to consider flexible ways of managing this issue, such as collaborative working with pharmacists or nurse specialists/practitioners.[8]

For those who are interested, there is an excellent pack produced by the University of Leeds on behalf of the Task Force on Medicines Management Partnership. This is available online to support medication reviews (www.medicines-partnership.org/medication-review/toolkit).

Depression

Special considerations and epidemiology

Depression is common in older people, with perhaps 10–15% of the over-65s experiencing significant depressive symptoms. It is often 'masked'. The patient may have predominantly anxiety symptoms masking an underlying depression, or they may have a multitude of physical problems causing anxiety about potential illness, and may feel that physical complaints are more 'acceptable' than emotional ones. Depression is under-recognised, is associated with twice the suicide rate for younger people, and is strongly associated with physical illness.[9,10] It is associated with a poorer prognosis than physical illness, even allowing for illness severity.[10] Milder depressive symptoms may be recognised by GPs but are often not treated, perhaps because of uncertainty about the effectiveness of treatment.

Diagnosis

GPs should be alert for the early warning signs and prepared to ask specifically about anhedonia (lack of pleasure in life), poor appetite, weight loss and suicidal ideas (*see* Boxes 7.1 and 7.2). If in doubt, the Geriatric Depression Scale (GDS) or its shorter version (GDS-15) can be used. It contains 30 questions with a yes/no response, and concentrates mainly on cognitive rather than physical symptoms.[11] A score of >11 suggests depression.[12]

Box 7.1 Early warning symptoms of depression[13]

- Sleep disturbance
- Fatigue
- Failure to care for oneself
- Withdrawal from social life
- Unexplainable somatic symptoms
- Hopelessness about a coexisting physical disorder

Box 7.2 People at increased risk of depression and/or suicide[10]

- Living in an institution
- Older white men
- Living alone
- Multiple physical illness
- Sleep disturbance
- Recent bereavement
- Previous suicide attempt
- Other loss (income, children moving away)
- Alcohol or drug abuse

Assessment

Possible medical causes or drug-related causes should be evaluated. The list of drugs associated with depression is long, and the medications are common and not always easily reduced or stopped (*see* Box 7.3). The GP should consider reduction of the drugs listed in Box 7.3 if depression is diagnosed.[14]

Box 7.3 Common drugs associated with depression

- Benzodiazepines and buspirone
- Anticonvulsants
- Anti-parkinsonian drugs (e.g. anticholinergics and L-dopa)
- Cardiovascular system drugs (e.g. beta-blockers, enalapril, methyl-dopa)
- Gastrointestinal drugs (e.g rantidine/cimetidine)
- Non-steroidal anti-inflammatory drugs
- Aminophylline
- Steroids

The patient should be examined with particular reference to signs of conditions associated with depression, including appearance (unkempt, parkinsonian facies, oedema of myxoedema, pallor of anaemia), blood pressure (may affect choice of treatment), pulse (myxoedema), weight (useful baseline), fundi (raised intracranial pressure – brain tumours) and central nervous system, particularly rigidity, tremor, cog-wheeling and ataxia (Parkinson's disease or multiple sclerosis).

Consider, as a minimum, blood tests for the following:

- thyroid function tests – hypothyroidism
- calcium/phosphate – hypercalcaemia (malignancy)
- full blood count, ferritin, vitamin B_{12}/folate – iron, vitamin B_{12}/folate deficiency (anaemia)
- random plasma glucose – diabetes
- electrolytes and creatinine – renal failure.

Consider formally testing for cognitive impairment with the Mini-Mental State Examination (MMSE) (see section on dementia) to check for early dementia and ask (both the patient and the carer if possible) about the four domains of functioning that are commonly affected in dementia, namely:

- use of transport
- managing a budget
- using a telephone
- managing medication.

Treatment

The GP and the primary healthcare team can provide important 'general support' and encouragement, including attention to practical issues, access to social services, bereavement counselling, and a sharing with the patient of the problem, its nature, possible causes, effective treatments, the likely length of the illness and its possible consequences. There are two useful leaflets that the GP can provide:

- *Depression in the Elderly* (www.rcpsych.ac.uk/public.help/depeld/depeld.html)
- *Bereavement* (www.rcpsych.ac.uk/public/help/bereav/bereavem.html).

Drugs

The first-line treatment for older people should be a selective serotonin reuptake inhibitor (SSRI). The National Service Framework on Mental Health[15] (www.doh.gov.uk/pub/docs/doh/mhmain.pdf) recommends that tricyclic anti-depressants (TCAs) should not be prescribed for depression in patients over 70 years of age. Even though older people are particularly susceptible to the adverse effects of the older TCAs, analysis of prescribing shows that elderly patients are more likely to be prescribed an older TCA and less likely to be prescribed an SSRI than younger patients.[16] In a prescribing analysis study using appropriate doses for primary care, only 43% of those over 65 years of age received an adequate dose in cases where a TCA was prescribed.[16]

The response takes longer in older people, and may take up to 12 weeks. Treatment should be continued for 6 to 12 months, and lifelong treatment may be indicated in recurrent or severe depression.

GPs need to be aware of potential side-effects and interactions. Reduction in or cessation of treatment should be gradual. The side-effects include anticholinergic (urinary retention, constipation and glaucoma), antihistaminic (sedation) and α_1-adrenergic-blocking (postural hypotension) effects (*see* Table 7.1).

Table 7.1 Side-effects of common antidepressants[17]

	Anticholinergic	Antihistaminic	α_1-adrenergic blocking
TCAs			
Amitriptyline	++++	++++	++++
Dothiepin	+++	++	++
Lofepramine	+	+	+
SSRIs			
Paroxetine	0/+	0	0
Citalopram			
Atypical			
Trazodone	0	+++	+

Referral to secondary care

This should be considered in cases where there is a high risk of self-harm (e.g. serious suicidal thoughts, previous suicide attempts), self-neglect, failure to respond to treatment after 12 weeks on a therapeutic dosage, or significant carer stress (*see* Case study 7.1).

Case study 7.1

Mr A lived with his 'young-for-her-age', active and busy 67-year-old wife who continued to work as a seamstress/dressmaker from home. At the age of 72 years he presented at the surgery with low back and left leg pain and a left-sided foot drop and absent left-sided ankle jerk. His wife was with him and she did most of the talking for him. He had always had an introspective personality, had had no hobbies or interests since retirement, and for months had spent all day on the sofa, and was reluctant to mix with others. He presented a very flat expressionless affect, denied feeling depressed but kept referring back to the awful pain in his leg that was preventing him from sleeping. His wife said that he made 'a big thing' of keeping the blankets off his leg at night with a home-made cradle. He was anxious about the possibility of spinal cancer. He was given opiate analgesics (tramadol). His wife did everything for him, and seemed exasperated. He was referred to the orthopaedic surgeons. Investigations of the spine revealed a prolapsed disc, but surgery was decided against because of the chronicity of the symptoms. Blood tests, including bone screen and plasma viscosity, were all normal. The surgeons suggested amitriptyline for relief of the neuralgia. This (and the strong opiate analgesia) led to a home visit because of acute urinary retention and Mr A was admitted and eventually had a transurethral resection of the prostate. He remained tormented and obsessed by the pain in his foot, was apathetic and became forgetful. An MMSE revealed a score of 13/20. He was started on fluoxetine, with little noticeable benefit. He was referred to the community psychiatric nurse for the elderly, and much to his discomfort (and his wife's guilt) started on day care 3 days a week to provide respite for his wife. During this time his wife became ill, with faints and weakness of no apparent cause, and was admitted acutely from her home. All her investigations were negative and her own depressive symptoms, heavily overlaid with anxiety, eventually became apparent. She responded well to a combination of counselling and paroxetine.

Mr A's mood has proved resistant to treatment with a range of antidepressants, and he remains on citalopram and tramadol. His deteriorating cognitive impairment has made attempts to reduce his anxiety about cancer by attempts to link his fears to his mood very difficult. He asks repetitive questions of his wife and becomes extremely anxious if he can't see her. He attends surgery regularly with his wife, who is adapting to her circumstances.

Dementia

Special considerations and epidemiology

Based on the *Morbidity Statistics in General Practice*,[18] it is possible to estimate the incidence, prevalence and workload for patients with dementia. The figures in Table 7.2 are based on an assumed list size of 2000 patients per GP principal.

Table 7.2 Incidence, prevalence and workload for patients with dementia[18]

Classification category	Incidence	Prevalence	Workload
	New patients per general practitioner per year	Patients consulting per general practitioner per year	Condition-related consultations per general practitioner per year
Early- and late-onset organic psychotic conditions	1.6	3.6	7.4

About 5% of people aged 65 years or over have some form of dementia, with the prevalence rising to about 20% by 80 years, and one in three by 90 years.[19] In care homes, 70–80% of residents will have functional impairment due to dementia.

There are guidelines for the primary care management of dementia from the North of England Evidence-based Guidelines Development Group.[20] These are helpful if used in conjunction with local guidelines (e.g for referring to a memory monitoring nursing service for assessment for suitability for an acetylcholinesterase inhibitor).

Diagnosis

There is evidence that GPs lack the skills and knowledge to diagnose and manage dementia effectively, and increased training has been recommended.[1] With the emerging new treatments recommended for use within the NHS for mild to moderate dementia[21] (www.nice.org.uk), there is a renewed emphasis on early diagnosis. However, early diagnosis is difficult and the GP needs to be alert for early signs (see Table 7.3). The diagnosis should be suspected if the patient has difficulty with one or more of the following four domains of daily activity, and questions about these should be directed to the carer as well as the patient:

- managing medication
- managing use of the telephone
- managing a budget
- managing public transport.

Note that problems with these domains of functioning may appear before obvious memory loss, especially in patients with vascular dementia.

Table 7.3 Features of dementia at different points in its path (adapted from Iliffe and Drennan[19])

	Early changes	*Later changes*
Emotional changes	Shallowness of mood Lack of emotional responsiveness and consideration of others	Irritability and hostility Aggression
Cognitive changes	Memory deficits Perseveration and repetitive speech Getting lost	Receptive and expressive dysphasia Thought processes fragmented Psychotic features in 30–40% (paranoid delusions) Auditory and visual hallucinations
Behavioural changes	Social withdrawal Self-neglect Disorientation	Wandering Evening and nocturnal restlessness prominent Turning night into day Aggression and violence
Physical changes	Usually later in the disease process	Weight loss Incontinence Rigidity Seizures (late)

Once the diagnosis is suspected it is recommended that general practitioners or a member of their team use a cognitive function test, such as the Mini-Mental State Examination (MMSE).[11] This gives a score out of 30 and takes about ten minutes to complete, so is not easy to incorporate into an ordinary consultation. It would probably be best to set up a separate consultation specifically to perform this test, as it is easy to perform it inaccurately. It is also probably best to become familiar with one test. In Huddersfield the guidelines for referral to the memory monitoring service (for consideration for treatment with an acetylcholinesterase inhibitor) include the criterion of an MMSE score of >12.

Assessment

A physical examination is required, with the same level of detail as for depression (see above). The patient should be examined with particular reference to signs of conditions associated with memory problems or depression, including appearance (unkempt, parkinsonian facies, oedema of myxoedema, pallor of anaemia), blood pressure (may affect choice of treatment), pulse (myxoedema), weight (useful baseline), fundi (raised intracranial pressure – brain tumours) and the central nervous system, particularly rigidity, tremor, cog-wheeling and ataxia (Parkinson's disease or multiple sclerosis).

For vascular dementia, which is characterised by a step-wise deterioration in cognitive function, it is worth assessing for additional risk factors for athero-sclerosis, such as blood pressure, carotid bruits, body mass index (BMI), lipids (if under 75 years of age) and smoking status. However, there is increased recognition of the overlap between Alzheimer's disease (AD) and vascular dementia, and vascular risk factors also increase the risk of AD. Consider using the Geriatric Depression Scale (GDS) to exclude depression, which is more common with dementia and can also cause cognitive impairment.[11]

Other problems may contribute to cognitive impairment (e.g. infections, drug toxicity, alcohol, and pain and its underlying causes) (see Case study 7.2).

Blood tests are as described for depression above, namely:

- thyroid function tests – hypothyroidism
- calcium/phosphate – hypercalcaemia
- full blood count, ferritin, vitamin B_{12}/folate – iron, vitamin B_{12}/folate deficiency
- random plasma glucose
- electrolytes and creatinine.

There are a number of rarer and potentially reversible causes of dementia, such as normal-pressure hydrocephalus (classical triad of dementia, ataxia and incontinence).

The GP should also take time to discuss with the patient and their carer the diagnosis of early cognitive impairment. There is evidence that people value information, although GPs often shy away from a full discussion.[22] Discussion of how memory impairment and dementia affect people (especially in terms of emotional or behavioural changes), what causes these conditions, what can be done to help (both the illness and in terms of support), and the possible time course and consequences can be achieved over a number of consultations. This process can also be supported by referral to the old age psychiatry service, which can co-ordinate further assessments, consider the treatment options and provide support for the carer.

Case study 7.2

Mr P was a new patient at the practice, admitted to a local residential home for older people. He was 87 years old, and had been bereaved 3 years previously. He had had dementia for about 3 years, and was no longer able to cope on his own. He had one daughter who visited him regularly. The GPs at his new practice were alerted to his presence when a repeat prescription request came through which included aspirin, ramipril, metformin, frusemide 80 mg per day, oxpentifylline, atorvastatin, amitriptyline 50 mg at night, and temazepam 20 mg at night.

The GP visited the patient, whose old notes had not yet come through from the previous practice. He was pleasantly confused, sitting most of the time in a chair dozing, well-mannered when woken, and obese. He had marked peripheral oedema but no other abnormalities on examination. His blood sugars were around 10 mmol/l. His blood pressure was 130/80 mmHg, his pulse rate was regular, and he was a little unsteady on his feet. He was not causing the staff any problems. He was disorientated with regard to season, place and time, and appeared cheerful. The GP decided to reduce the temazepam and the amitriptyline by half, and to stop the atorvastatin (it has unproven benefit at this age and can cause gastrointestinal upset) and oxpentifylline (limited value), to check Mr P's electrolytes, full blood count and thyroid function tests, and to await the records, arranging to review the patient in 2 weeks time. The notes revealed that he had been on amitriptyline for several years for dysaesthesiae affecting his legs and thought to be due to amiodarone that had been discontinued a few years previously. There was no history of depression, and he was thought to have congestive cardiac failure. The GP visited again, and the electrolytes, full blood count and thyroid function tests were normal. In himself Mr P was much the same. Although he had peripheral oedema, his lungs were clear and there was no breathlessness or tachycardia. He remained unsteady. The GP stopped the temazepam and the amitriptyline completely, and reduced the frusemide to 40 mg per day, and arranged a follow-up visit in a month's time. The home was attempting a weight-reducing diet, and was also monitoring sugars. Two weeks later Mr P's daughter rang the GP to ask why the tablets had been stopped. She said her father was anxious as he was used to taking his sleeping tablets, and he had not been sleeping well. The GP explained the rationale for the changes, and promised to review Mr P soon. He rang the home, who said that Mr P was not sleeping well at night, tending to wander, and became anxious at bedtime without his sleeping tablet, but was much more alert during the day, less confused, and taking part in some of the activities to a limited extent during the day. He was also less unsteady in his gait. The GP planned to review the patient with a view to further reduction of medication if clinically possible. The daughter agreed that the home could offer her father a paracetamol tablet at night.

A week later the home rang the GP to report that Mr P was unsettled at night, getting up and getting dressed, and he was upset about not having his sleeping tablets. The GP agreed to restarting the temazepam, and arranged to review Mr P in 1 month's time.

Issues raised by the above case study include the following.

- This patient's medication had clearly not been adequately reviewed for some time.
- Should the psychotropic medication have been withdrawn more slowly?
- Should the GP have discussed the changes in medication with the patient and the daughter before initiating them?
- Is it ethical to offer a paracetamol tablet at night to allay such a patient's anxieties about missing his sleeping tablets?
- Should the patient remain on temazepam indefinitely?

Special considerations in dementia

These include the following:

- use of the newer antidementia drug
- management of behavioural and psychiatric problems.

Use of the newer antidementia drugs: the acetylcholinesterase inhibitors

The National Institute for Clinical Excellence (NICE) has recommended that these drugs should be made available on the NHS, but only according to strict guidelines.[21] However, one major study on effectiveness has demonstrated that approximately seven (95% CI, 4–16) people would have to be treated with donepezil for one person to benefit in terms of an outcome based on a clinical impression of impairment and a carer rating.[23]

- The patient must have mild to moderate Alzheimer's disease, with an MMSE score of >12.
- The drug must be prescribed by a specialist.
- The patient must be carefully monitored after commencing treatment by the specialist services.
- If there is no improvement after 3 months (e.g. on the MMSE score or the activities of daily living score), the drug should be discontinued.
- The GP should only take over prescribing with an agreed shared care protocol with clear end points.

Use of antipsychotics

This is a particularly thorny issue and deserves special attention. Up to 60% of residents in care homes are on psychotropic medication, and up to 30% are on antipsychotics. The drugs prescribed have the potential to cause serious side-effects, and there is good evidence that this level of prescribing is excessive and causing harm, and that it can be reduced without causing significant problems.[24–29]

In our own survey of 200 residents in 20 nursing homes (all non-'Elderly Mentally Infirm' care homes) and residential homes across Huddersfield, 56% of residents were taking a regular psychotropic medication (60% in nursing homes and 51% in residential homes), and of these 31% were taking antipsychotics, 21% were taking benzodiazepines, and 22% were taking antidepressants (13% TCAs vs. 63% SSRIs).[30] There was significant cognitive impairment in approximately 80% of residents in both nursing and residential homes, as measured by capacity to provide informed consent.

The antipsychotic drug bill is also rising. Between 1999 and 2000 there was a 70% increase in the use of atypical antipsychotic drugs for people aged 60 years or over in the UK. Some of this increase was due to the discontinuation of thioridazine and the introduction of more expensive atypical antipsychotics, but nevertheless overall prescribing of all antipsychotic drugs rose by 6%. In the year 2000–01, antipsychotic prescribing costs rose by £39 million (32%), compared with statins which rose by £103 million (33%).[8]

In the UK there are guidelines available such as *Interventions in the Management of Behavioural and Psychological Aspects of Dementia* issued by the Scottish Intercollegiate Guidelines Network (SIGN) (www.sign.ac.uk),[31] and the North of England Group guidelines on the primary care management of dementia.[20]

When to prescribe and when not to

It is very common for GPs to be presented with behavioural problems of patients, particularly in care homes. Sometimes this is manifested as agitation of some form (see below), and sometimes it is a poor sleep pattern. It is also common for GPs to have several older residents on repeat prescriptions for antipsychotic medication (up to 30% of residents in care homes). There is often pressure for the GP to prescribe (*see* Case studies 7.3 and 7.4).

Case study 7.3

In the office at the practice the GP was given a prescription to sign for Mrs Z, a resident in a local nursing home. It was for zopiclone, lansoprazole, co-codamol lactulose and ferrous sulphate, none of which was on the patient's list of repeat prescriptions. The GP had a look at Mrs Z's electronic record. She had last been seen 13 months previously for a chest infection, when she had been prescribed some antibiotics. Her paper notes were found. They were very thin indeed, with a few scribbled entries from many years previously. The GP rang the matron at the home. It transpired that Mrs Z, a thin, normally quiet 74-year-old, had had a fall one Saturday about a month ago and fractured her femur. She had been discharged to the home 2 weeks ago, on zopiclone from the hospital. She was glad that the GP had telephoned, because Mrs Z seemed confused at times, she had lost weight, she was not eating, she was shouting out at people who weren't there, and had been trying to hit out at other residents and staff who walked near her. The matron had been thinking of asking for a visit. In the office at the practice the GP found a discharge 'flimsy' that had not yet been filed, with illegible writing on it relating to the recent admission. The GP visited, and Mrs Z's medications had all been started during her recent hospital admission. She was frail, dozing and difficult to rouse. The scar from the internal fixation was well healed, but movement at the hip joint provoked grimacing and an angry aggressive attempt to push the GP away. Her abdomen was distended and tender with a suspicion of an epigastric mass, and rectal examination revealed a rectum loaded with hard faeces. Her chest was clear. She would not respond to any commands and did not say anything. The matron said that Mrs Z had become increasingly tetchy and withdrawn prior to her admission, with a tendency to wander at night. The GP contacted the hospital. Her haemoglobin level had been 9.5 post-operatively and she had been started on iron and lactulose. She had been disturbed at night and had also been prescribed zopiclone. Her post-operative electrolytes and sugar levels were normal. The GP arranged for a repeat full blood count, plasma viscosity, ferritin, vitamin B_{12} and folate, random plasma glucose, electrolytes, calcium and thyroid function tests. The nurse performed an enema with good results. The co-codamol was changed to paracetamol, and the zopiclone, lansoprazole and ferrous sulphate were stopped. Her haemoglobin level was 10.2, plasma viscosity was 1.9 (<1.72 normal range), ferritin was 22 (15–150), vitamin B_{12} was 185 (200–1100), urea was elevated consistent with dehydration, and glucose, calcium and thyroid function tests were normal. She remained agitated and restless with what seemed to be visual hallucinations, and was striking out at staff while being dressed, fed or bathed. The GP discussed with the relatives their expectations and concerns. They just wanted their mother to be comfortable, and they appreciated that she was seriously ill. The GP explained that he thought that Mrs Z probably had an underlying malignancy, possibly of the stomach, that she was suffering from dementia which was causing distressing hallucinations (probably accelerated by her recent operation), that she was too frail to move (and this would probably cause more distress than benefit), and that the aim was to reduce her distress. She was started on a small dose of risperidone, and her bowels were monitored. Fluids were encouraged, together with a light diet. She became less agitated, started to eat and started to mobilise. She developed some rigidity and tremor, but no akathisia or tardive dyskinesia. Over the next 3 months she remained comfortable and less agitated, but she slowly continued to lose weight.

Case study 7.4

Mrs N was discharged from hospital following a hip operation after a fall, back to her nursing home. She was 90 years old, physically quite strong and on no medication apart from paracetamol. She had severe cognitive impairment, and the GP was asked to visit because of worsening agitation, with verbal aggression and physical violence towards other residents and staff, who she accused of taking her things. Examination and blood tests were normal. The agitation and violence were most troublesome when Mrs N was being dressed and undressed. She had some day–night reversal, with a tendency to wander into other residents' rooms. After discussion with relatives she was started on haloperidol, which did calm her agitation, but during the next 4 weeks she became increasingly immobile and restless at rest, persistently tapping her feet and moving in her seat. On examination she was found to have become quite rigid with a parkinsonian tremor and she exhibited akathisia. She was started on procyclidine, an anticholinergic, but this led to worsening confusion and a dry mouth. The local psycho-geriatrician was asked for advice. The haloperidol and procyclidine were stopped, and he explained that anticholinergics should always be avoided in patients with dementia, and that the newer antipsychotics had fewer side-effects, and Mrs N was started on a small dose of risperidone. He suggested that she should be given more time when dressing and undres-sing, and allowed to do as much as she could by herself. The akathisia and parkinsonian symptoms abated, she remained calmer, and after 2 months the risperidone was reduced and stopped with no ill effects.

The introduction to this chapter included a discussion of the evidence for excessive prescribing of antipsychotics to older people (i.e. when there is no valid indication for their use), especially in care homes. Faced with agitated behaviours (agitation can cover a range of issues, including hallucinations, delusions, sleeplessness, excitement, hostility, belligerence or emotional instability) it is important to exclude underlying, often reversible causes. Iliffe and Drennan have described a useful mnemonic, namely **PAID** (Physical, Activity related, Intrinsic to dementia, Depression or delusion) for underlying causes (*see* Table 7.4).

Table 7.4 The causes of behavioural problems (after Iliffe and Drennan[19])

Physical	Pain (e.g. from osteoarthritis) causing aggression or wandering, or infection (e.g urinary tract infection); also consider retention of urine, and constipation
Activity related	For example, when a carer is helping with an intimate task such as dressing or bathing; also in response to a lack of activity or company
Intrinsic to dementia	Wandering, repetitive stroking of another person, uncontrollable laughter or crying (sometimes seen in vascular dementia)
Depression or delusions	Hallucinations or delusions with paranoia; treat the psychosis itself but be careful with medication (see below)

When presented with a behavioural problem the GP should:

- exclude other causes as described above
- obtain a clear description
- identify contributory factors
- identify others involved and what they were doing
- consider coming back to review the problem after a diary has been kept by the home for a short time period.

Not all agitation requires an antipsychotic drug, and some behavioural problems may be ameliorated by the use of skilful approaches that avoid confrontation. These include the following:

- calmness
- approaching the patient in their line of vision
- doing things at the patient's pace
- using non-verbal cues (e.g. smiling)
- providing reassurance.

A small dose of an antipsychotic may be indicated for some of the 30–40% of patients with dementia who develop psychosis in terms of paranoid delusions or hallucinations associated with aggression and violence. Before medication is considered the GP should establish that these behaviours are actually causing a significant problem, as they do not always do so. Systematic reviews have suggested that the antipsychotic drugs can have a modest beneficial effect on 'agitation' in dementia. The effect is on the behaviours, and the studies did not measure the effects on the patient's overall well-being or any adverse effects. The trials also show a large placebo effect.

The antipsychotic drugs include the traditional dopamine antagonists thioridazine (now withdrawn), haloperidol and chlorpromazine, as well as the newer atypical drugs such as olanzapine, sulpiride and risperidone, which have an additional therapeutic serotonin-blocking action. The newer drugs cause fewer extrapyramidal (parkinsonian) side-effects, although they may still cause confusion, sedation and postural hypotension, and there is little evidence for their effectiveness in dementia even though they are widely and increasingly being prescribed to the older population (see introduction to this chapter).

The drugs take up to 1 week to have an effect on psychotic behaviours and, given the number needed to treat to benefit (NNT) of 5 (i.e. five patients would need to be prescribed the drug for one to benefit from it), for the majority there will be no beneficial effect.[32] This means that consideration should be given to stopping the drug after a 4 to 6-week trial. There are no easy-to-use, reliable and objective measures of behavioural problems, although a simple diary kept by care staff might be useful.

Guidelines for the use and monitoring of antipsychotic drugs[33]

- The atypical antipsychotics have a better side-effect profile.
- Start with the smallest dose prescribable.
- Make increases slowly, with careful monitoring for emergent side-effects.
- You may need to wait several weeks for the full effects to occur.
- Only continue if there is demonstrable evidence of efficacy (this is not easy to obtain; you could consider asking the home to monitor it with one of the behavioural scales, such as the 'Nursing Home Behavior Problem Scale'[34]).
- Care should be taken to identify Lewy body dementia (see below).
- Avoid the use of anticholinergics.
- Review continued need for treatment every 3 months.
- Encourage trials of drug-free periods to test whether treatment is still needed.
- Careful monitoring of emergent side-effects should take place *at least fortnightly* (this requires the patient to be seen and examined). Such side-effects include:
  - confusion
  - a worsening of cognitive impairment over time
  - falls
  - tardive dyskinesia (orofacial or buccolingual movements, or athetoid movements of limbs – due to a rebound dopamine hypersensitivity; 15% prevalence; may worsen if the drug is withdrawn too quickly; no effective treatments)
  - parkinsonian features (tremor and rigidity)
  - akathisia (restlessness).

Sleep problems

About a quarter of patients with dementia develop sleep problems. These can range from interrupted sleep to a complete night–day reversal. The GP needs to take the following steps:

1 Establish whether there really is a problem.
   - Does the care home have unrealistic expectations, putting the patient to bed at 9pm only for him or her to wake 6 hours later at 3am, well rested and fully awake?
   - Is the resident him- or herself adversely affected by the change in sleeping pattern? If not, then the home may be able to work round the problem, being up with the resident, keeping them occupied and then trying them

back to bed in half an hour, rather than trying to keep them in bed throughout the night. However, for lone carers this would be difficult.

2   Check for any factors that may disturb sleep, including the following:
   * pain
   * urinary frequency (nocturnal dose of diuretic)
   * disturbance by others
   * psychotic symptoms
   * depressed mood.

If there is a persistent problem with sleep without psychotic symptoms, a short course of a short-acting hypnotic can be tried.

Lewy body dementia

Patients with Lewy body dementia are excessively sensitive to antipsychotics. These drugs should therefore be avoided and, if necessary, specialist help sought. The features suggestive of Lewy body dementia are as follows:

* intermittent clouding of consciousness
* visual hallucinations
* parkinsonian features
* falls.

Schizophrenia and other psychoses

The antipsychotics have an important role to play in the management of schizophrenia and other forms of psychosis not related to dementia, and usually in these situations a specialist has initiated the drug. Once the GP takes over prescribing responsibility, they must be careful not to stop or reduce the medication injudiciously.

Key points

* Organise a system for the regular face-to-face medication review of older patients in care homes.
* Be aware of and seek out the early warning signs of dementia and depression (think **T**ransport, **M**edication, **P**hone, **B**udget).
* Avoid using tricyclic antidepressants in older people.
* Avoid using antipsychotics for older people. They are rarely indicated and rarely work, and they cause side-effects. If they are used, consider a short course only.
* Seek out the underlying causes of agitation before trying medication (think **P**hysical, **A**ctivity, **I**ntrinsic to dementia, **D**epression).

References

1 Audit Commission (2000) *Forget Me Not: mental health services for older people.* Audit Commission Publications, London.

2 Millard P et al. (1999) Nursing Home Placements of Older People in England and Wales: a National Audit 1995–1998. Department of Geriatric Medicine, St George's Hospital Medical School, London.

3 Department of Health (2000) Prescriptions Dispensed in the Community. Statistics for 1989 to 1999: England, Bulletin 2000/02. Department of Health, London.

4 UK Data Archive (1998) Health Survey for England: findings. www.data-archive.ac.uk

5 Walley T and Scott A (1995) Prescribing in the elderly. Postgrad Med J. **71**: 466–71.

6 Lunn J, Chan K and Donohughe J (2003) A study of the appropriateness of prescribing in nursing homes. Int J Pharm Pract. **5**: 6–10.

7 Zermansky A (1996) Who controls repeats? Br J Gen Pract. **46**: 643–7.

8 Department of Health (2001) Medicines and Older People. Supplement to the NSF for Older People. Department of Health, London.

9 Iliffe S and Drennan V (2000) Depression, anxiety and dementia. In: Primary Care for Older People. Oxford University Press, Oxford.

10 Katona C (1989) The epidemiology and natural history of depression in old age. In: K Ghose (ed.) Antidepressants for Elderly People. Chapman and Hall, London.

11 Burns A, Lawlor B and Craig S (1999) Assessment Scales in Old Age Psychiatry. Martin Dunitz, London.

12 Yesavage J, Brink T and Rose T (2003) Development and validation of the Geriatric Depression Screening Scale: a preliminary report. J Psychiatr Res. **17**: 37–49.

13 World Health Organization (1992) The ICD-10 Classification of Mental and Behavioural Disorders. World Health Organization, Geneva.

14 Dhondt T, Derksen P, Hooijer C et al. (2003) Depressogenic medication as an aetiological factor in major depression: an analysis in a population of depressed elderly people. Int J Geriatr Psychiatry **14**: 875–81.

15 Department of Health (1999) A National Service Framework for Mental Health. Department of Health, London.

16 Donoghue J, Katona C and Tyle A (1998) The treatment of depression: antidepressant prescribing for elderly patients in primary care. Pharm J. **260**: 500–2.

17 Katona C and Livingstone G (2004) Drug Treatment in Old Age Psychiatry. Martin Dunitz, London.

18 McCormick A, Fleming D and Charlton J (1995) Morbidity Statistics in General Practice: fourth national study 1991–1992. HMSO, London.

19 Iliffe S and Drennan V (2001) Primary Care and Dementia. Jessica Kingsley Publishers, London.

20 Eccles M, Clarke J, Livingstone M, Freemantle N and Mason J (1998) North of England Evidence-based Guidelines Development Project: guidelines for the primary care management of dementia. BMJ. **317**: 802–8.

21 National Institute for Clinical Excellence (2003) Guidance on the Use of Donepezil, Rivastigmine and Galantamine for the Treatment of Alzheimer's Disease. National Institute for Clinical Excellence, London.

22 Maguire C, Kirby M, Coen R et al. (2003) Family members' attitudes towards telling the patient with Alzheimer's disease their diagnosis. BMJ. **313**: 529–30.

23 Rogers S, Farlow M, Doody R et al. (2003) A 24-week double-blind, placebo-controlled trial of donepezil in patients with Alzheimer's disease. Neurology. **35**: 136–45.

24 Waxman H, Klein M and Carner E (1985) Drug misuse in nursing homes: an institutional addiction? Hosp Commun Psychiatry. **36**: 886–7.

25 McGrath AM and Jackson GA (1996) Survey of neuroleptic prescribing in residents of nursing homes in Glasgow. BMJ. **312**: 611–12.

26 Ruths S, Straand J and Nygaard HA (2001) Psychotropic drug use in nursing homes – diagnostic indications and variations between institutions. Eur J Clin Pharmacol. **57**: 523–8.

27 Furniss L, Burns A and Craig S (2000) Effects of a pharmacist's medication review in nursing homes. Randomised controlled trial. *Br J Psychiatry*. **176**: 563–7.

28 Thapa PB, Meador KG, Gideon P, Fought RL and Ray WA (1994) Effects of anti-psychotic withdrawal in elderly nursing home residents. *J Am Geriatr Soc*. **44**: 280–6.

29 Hopker S (2003) *Drug Treatments and Dementia*. Jessica Kingsley Publishers, London.

30 Dempsey OP, Moore H and Mulligan E (2003) *A survey of psychotropic prescribing and behavioural problems in residential and nursing homes*. Unpublished paper.

31 Scottish Intercollegiate Guidelines Network (1998) *Interventions in the Management of Behavioural and Psychological Aaspects of Dementia*. Scottish Intercollegiate Guidelines Network, Edinburgh.

32 Schneider LS, Pollock V and Lyness S (1994) A meta-analysis of controlled trials of neuroleptic treatment in dementia. *J Am Geriatr Soc*. **38**: 553–63.

33 Howard R, Ballard C, O'Brien J *et al*. (2001) Guidelines for the management of agitation in dementia. *Int J Geriatr Psychiatry*. **16**: 714–17.

34 Ray WA, Taylor JA, Lichtenstein MJ and Meador KG (1992) The Nursing Home Behavior Problem Scale. *J Gerontol*. **24**: M9–16.

Chapter 8

Management of geriatric mood disorders

Naila Jawaid and Robert C Baldwin

Unipolar depression

Introduction

Despite its prevalence and seriousness, depressive disorder in older people remains under-treated.[1,2] Knowledge of the efficacy of antidepressant treatment in the elderly has been restricted by the exclusion from most antidepressant drug trials of the very old, and those who are frail and/or with cognitive impairment, which are the majority of those seen in the routine practice of old age psychiatry.

The optimal treatment of depression in later life is crucial, and requires appreciation of several age-related factors such as comorbidity, polypharmacy, altered drug kinetics,[3] variable treatment response and increased predisposition to side-effects.[4,5]

This chapter reviews the development and use of antidepressants in older depressed patients. The relevant literature on neurochemistry, kinetics, dosing, efficacy and differential side-effect profiles of various classes of drugs will be reviewed, with special emphasis on geriatric data.

Subtypes of depression and treatment modalities

There is insufficient space to discuss the nosology of mood disorders in older people. However, there is some relationship between different types of depressive disorder and treatment options, summarised in Table 8.1.[6] In dysthymia there are the same symptoms as for major depression, but fewer of them and with a duration of at least 2 years. Dysthymia in older people is often associated with poor health. 'Minor' depression is still an experimental category, but it seems to be especially common in older people and is certainly not a trivial condition. It is defined in the same way as dysthymia, but with a much shorter duration and often with additional symptoms such as anergia, poor motivation and poor cognition. The only evidence that pharmacological treatment works comes from a study in which symptoms were present for at least 4 weeks and were associated with functional decline.[7]

Table 8.1 Summary of evidence: treatment modality and type of depression[6]

Type of depression	Treatment modality
Psychotic depression	Combined antidepressant/antipsychotic or electroconvulsive therapy (ECT)
Severe (non-psychotic) depression	Combined antidepressant and psychological therapy (e.g. cognitive behavioural therapy, problem-solving, interpersonal therapy or brief psychodynamic psychotherapy)
Moderate depressive episode	Antidepressant *or* psychological therapy (as above)
Dysthymia	Consider an antidepressant
Recent onset sub-threshold (minor) depression (1–4 weeks)	Watchful waiting
Persistent sub-threshold (minor) depression with functional impairment (>4 weeks)	Consider an antidepressant

Assessment

This includes a detailed history from both patient and informant covering aspects such as recent change in mood state, physical illness, drug and alcohol use, adverse life events and available support systems. A mental state examination with emphasis on suicidal ideation and plans, delusional phenomena and cognitive impairment (wherever possible using a standardised test such as the Mini-Mental State Examination, MMSE[8]) is an essential component of the assessment process along with relevant physical examination and laboratory investigations. An issue of particular importance is the assessment of suicidal risk. Any deliberate self-harm in an older person should be taken very seriously, as depressive disorder often underlies it.

Measuring depression in older people

Screening for depressive disorder in older people can be achieved with the Geriatric Depression Scale (GDS),[9] which has been validated and widely used in elderly subjects. It is quick to administer and exists in several versions (ranging from 4 to 30 items). It has been translated into a number of languages and further information can be obtained from its public-domain website (http://stanford.edu/~yesavage/GDS.html).

The severity of a diagnosed case of depression can be assessed with the Montgomery-Asberg Depression Rating Scale (MADRS)[10] or the Hamilton Rating Scale for Depression (HRSD).[11] Both have been validated in elderly depressed subjects,[12] although some clinicians find that the MADRS has greater face validity in patients with comorbid medical conditions. Both are useful in assessing response to treatment.

Principles of drug treatment

The first challenge is to break down the barriers which prevent treatment from being instituted in the first place. All treatment options available to depression earlier in life remain effective in old age and, as with younger people, therapy in more than one modality may be more effective and appropriate than one modality alone.[13,14]

Education about depressive disorder and its treatments is vital in building a trusting and therapeutic relationship with the patient. It may cover the following:

- counselling the patient that depression is a treatable disorder
- explaining that antidepressants are non-addictive
- discussing the importance of compliance (taking tablets regularly, not missing tablets, no sudden discontinuation)
- emphasising to the patient that they must not stop treatment when recovery has occurred
- explaining that acute treatment in older people may typically last for 6–8 weeks at the minimum.

Pharmacotherapy

There are now many antidepressants available, so it is imperative to operate within some general guidelines. The choice of antidepressant should be guided by factors such as type and severity of depression, tolerability, side-effects and contraindications to the drug. Antidepressants available in the UK can be classified as shown in Box 8.1.

Box 8.1 Classification of antidepressants

Tricyclics
Secondary amines (nortriptyline, desipramine)
Tertiary amines (imipramine, amitriptyline, dosulepin, clomipramine)
Newer tricyclics (lofepramine)

Monoamine oxidase inhibitors
Irreversible (phenelzine)
Reversible (moclobemide)

Selective serotonin reuptake inhibitors (SSRIs)
(fluvoxamine, fluoxetine, paroxetine, sertraline, citalopram, escitalopram)

Serotonin/noradrenaline reuptake inhibitors (SNRIs)
(venlafaxine, duloxetine)

Noradrenaline reuptake inhibitors (NARIs)
(reboxetine)

Noradrenaline and specific serotonin enhancers (NASSs)
(mirtazepine)

Atypical antidepressants
(trazodone, minaserin)

Others
(L-tryptophan) (licensed use only)

Table 8.2 lists antidepressants according to their main mode of action, side-effects, starting doses and average daily dosages. Altered pharmacokinetics (see below) in older people mean that for the tricyclics (but not for SSRIs and many of the newer drugs) there is considerable inter-individual variation in how these drugs are handled, and therefore predicting the final dose can be difficult. Furthermore, a dose-titration period is necessary, which will lengthen treatment trials compared with newer antidepressants.

Table 8.2 Side-effect profiles and dosages of the main antidepressants (Baldwin et al.[6])

Drug	Main mode of action	Anti-cholinergic	Anti-histaminic	$\alpha 1$-adrenergic blocking	Starting dosage (mg)	Average daily dose (mg)
Amitriptyline	NE++ 5HT+	++++	++++	++++	25–50	75–100
Imipramine	NE++ 5HT+	+++	++	+++	25	75–100
Nortriptyline	NE++ 5HT+	+++	++	++	10–30	75–100
Dothiepin (Dosulepin)	NE++ 5HT+	+++	++	++	50–75	75–150
Mianserin	α_2	0/+	+++	0/+	30	30–90
Lofepramine	NE++ 5HT+	+	+	+	70–140	70–210
Trazodone	$5HT_2$	0	+++	+	100	300
Fluvoxamine	5HT	0/+	0/+	0	25–100	100–200
Sertraline	5HT	0/+	0	0	25–50	50–100
Fluoxetine	5HT	0/+	0	0	10	20
Paroxetine	5HT	0/+	0	0	10–20	20–30
Citalopram	5HT	0/+	0	0	10–20	20–30
Escitalopram	5HT	0	0	0	5–10	0–20
Phenelzine	MAO-I (non-reversible)	0/+	0	++	15	30–45 (divided dosages)
Moclobemide	RIMA	0/+	0	0	300	300–400
Venlafaxine XR	NE+ 5HT++	0/+	0	0/+	25–75	75–200
Mirtazapine	α_2 $5HT_2$	0	++	0	7.5–15	15–30

5HT, serotonin reuptake inhibitor; NE, norepinephrine (noradrenaline) reuptake inhibitor; DA, dopamine reuptake inhibition; RIMA, reversible inhibitor of monoamine oxidase ihibitor α_2 antagonism at the presynaptic α_2 receptor. α_2 +/++ indicates magnitude of effect from small (+) to marked (++++).

Tricyclic antidepressants

The majority of tricyclic antidepressants have three rings in the molecule, with two benzene rings fused to a central seven-membered carboxylic or heterocyclic ring. In attempts to avoid some of the side-effects, compounds with differing ring structures, ranging from monocyclic to tetracyclic, were synthesised. All of these compounds are inhibitors of noradrenaline uptake, with a variable potency of inhibition of 5-hydroxytryptamine (5-HT) uptake as well. Tricyclics are sometimes subdivided into secondary and tertiary amines (*see* Box 8.1). Secondary amines are predominantly noradrenaline reuptake inhibitors and have a more benign side-effect profile.

Pharmacokinetics and pharmacodynamics

Tricyclic antidepressants are by and large well absorbed orally. They are lipophilic and widely distributed in the body, being strongly bound to plasma proteins and tissue constituents. They are metabolised in the liver to a variety of metabolites, some of which are active antidepressant compounds. The major route of elimination is via renal excretion. Minor amounts enter the bile and are then excreted in the faeces. The lower rates of both hepatic metabolism and renal clearance in this age group need to be taken into account when dosing, otherwise considerably higher than expected steady-state plasma levels may develop in older patients. For this reason, some clinicians have recommended plasma level monitoring for tricyclic antidepressants in elderly patients. The newer tricyclic, *lofepramine*, has minimal anticholinergic properties and cardiac toxicity in older patients compared with older drugs. Inter-individual differences usually account for the majority of the variance in kinetic parameters, rather than the effect of ageing *per se*.[15]

Side-effects (see Table 8.2)

Drugs with tertiary amine structure tend to produce more antagonism of α_1-adrenergic receptors with subsequent hypotension, blockage of histamine receptors (leading to sedation) and blockage of cholinergic receptors (causing dry mouth, blurred vision, urinary retention, dizziness, tachycardia, memory impairment and, at high and toxic doses, delirium). The tendency to produce orthostatic hypotension is a serious side-effect in the elderly that leads to an increased risk of falls and limb fracture.

Monoamine oxidase inhibitors (MAOIs)

Traditional MAOIs bind non-selectively, either irreversibly or almost so, to both type A and type B monoamine oxidase enzymes to prevent monoamine destruction. Because they lack selectivity, traditional MAOIs can lead to serious side-effects when food rich in tyramine or other amines is ingested. In addition, these drugs show strong interactions with other drugs that seriously limit their use compared with other antidepressants. They may have a place in the treatment of resistant depression,[16] but they are hardly ever used as first-line drugs nowadays and will therefore not be discussed further here.

Reversible MAOIs, represented by moclobemide, have considerably fewer dietary constraints and problematic drug interactions. Moclobemide achieves this by reversibly inhibiting largely monoamine type A enzyme. The MAOIs are all rapidly absorbed. The reversible ones have shorter half-lives and require multiple daily doses. A period of 2 weeks must elapse when irreversible MAOIs are stopped before starting other drugs that may interact with the MAOIs and with SSRIs.

Selective serotonin reuptake inhibitors (SSRIs)

SSRIs are third-generation antidepressants with a specific effect on serotonin reuptake, making them less likely to cause the side-effects encountered with the use of tricyclics. The main class members are represented by fluvoxamine, fluoxetine, paroxetine, sertraline, citalopram and escitalopram. The latter is the active s-enantiomer of rs-citalopram. The r-enantiomer is essentially pharmacologically inactive. Escitalopram has been demonstrated to show greater efficacy and to provide a more rapid response than citalopram.[17]

Pharmacokinetics and pharmacodynamics

SSRIs are rapidly absorbed from the gut and metabolised to several metabolites (often with antidepressant activity), each with a different drug half-life. All SSRIs are extensively protein-bound and have a large volume of distribution. For example, the plasma half-lives of fluvoxamine and fluoxetine are relatively unaffected by age, whereas the steady-state plasma concentrations of paroxetine, sertraline and citalopram are higher in the elderly and the elimination half-life is longer than for the same dose in adult patients.[18] Paroxetine also has a notable affinity for muscarinic cholinergic receptors, thus making it the most sedative of the SSRIs. Administration of all SSRIs can augment TCA activity, as well as the activity of other drugs metabolised by the hepatic cytochrome P450 system. SSRI interactions with the P450 system appear to be dose dependent and are important in elderly people, who are much more likely to be on concurrent medication.

Side-effects

The most commonly reported side-effects of SSRIs include nausea, agitation, anxiety, headache, sleep disturbance and tremor. Less frequently there are changes in appetite and weight, dry mouth, sweating, weight loss and sexual dysfunction, especially anorgasmia. The SSRIs have a major advantage in that they lack the cardiotoxicity and major cholinergic and adrenergic side-effects of tricyclics. Withdrawal reactions with some SSRIs can be severe and prolonged.[19–21] They are usually characterised by rebound anxiety, dysphoria, insomnia and parasthesiae, but are relatively short-lived. Most problems arise with SSRIs that have short half-lives.

Table 8.3 Cytochrome P450 isozymes inhibited by SSRI antidepressants (*in vitro*)

Drug	1A2	2C9	2C19	2D6	3A4
Fluoxetine	+	++	+	+++	++
Sertraline	+	+	+	+	+
Paroxetine	+	+	+	+++	+
Citalopram	+				
Escitalopram					
Fluvoxamine	+++	++	+++	+	++

For more details see Greenblatt *et al.*[22] and von Moltke *et al.*[23]

SSRIs such as paroxetine and fluoxetine are inhibitors of P450 isoenzymes (CYP 2D6), which can considerably influence the metabolism of tricyclic anti-depressants and other medication (see Table 8.3).

Other antidepressants

Venlafaxine selectively inhibits the uptake of serotonin and noradrenaline, and in contrast to tricyclics shows no affinity for other neuroreceptors. No dosage adjustments are recommended for older people. Compared with SSRIs, venlafax-ine affects the cytochrome P450 enzyme system relatively little. The most common side-effects are nausea, headache, dry mouth, dizziness, constipation and hypertension, although postural hypotension can be a problem in older people. To minimise the risk of discontinuation symptoms, the dose of vena-flaxine should be gradually tapered over a period of a few weeks. The possibility of serotonergic syndrome should be taken into account when venlafaxine is co-administered with other serotonergic drugs.[24] SSRIs and venlafaxine are also associated with hyponatraemia in elderly inpatients.[25] Duloxetine is a newer SNRI which may have a safer cardiovascular profile than venlaxafine but data on older patients are awaited.

Mianserin and *mirtazapine* both have potent effects on antagonising α_2-adrenergic auto- and heteroreceptors. This leads to an increase in noradrenaline release. These drugs have a low affinity for muscarinic, cholinergic and dopamine receptors, and this in turn is related to reduced side-effects. Mirtazapine has effects on both the noradrenergic and serotonergic systems. It enhances central noradrenergic and $5HT_1$-receptor-mediated serotonergic neurotransmission. It is an antagonist at α_2-adrenergic presynaptic autoreceptors, and it also blocks $5HT_2$ and $5HT_3$ receptors. This results in increased noradrenergic release. Differences in pharmacokinetics with age are considered to be minor.[26] Mianserin has fallen out of favour because of the small risk of agranulocytosis necessitating blood monitoring. The main adverse effects of mirtazapine are sedation and weight gain.

Reboxetine is a specific noradrenaline reuptake inhibitor. It has not been recommended for use in older people in the UK because there are insufficient efficacy data for the elderly. There have been some uncontrolled efficacy studies, and it appears to be well tolerated and safe in this patient group.[27]

Efficacy of antidepressants

There have been a limited number of double-blind, placebo-controlled trials of antidepressants involving elderly people, and most of these are of tricyclics. Most of the efficacy data involving double-blind, placebo-controlled trials is for tricyclic drugs.[28,29] Newer drugs usually involve head-to-head comparisons with estab-lished drugs. In all age groups the use of tricyclic drugs to treat depression has been declining in favour of SSRIs, although views differ as to whether SSRIs should be used as first-line treatment in depression.[30]

The assessment of efficacy has been made easier by the publication of two recent systematic reviews of antidepressants in older people, namely a Cochrane Review[29] and a systematic review of number needed to treat (NNT) by Katona and Livingston.[31] The NNT is the number of patients who need to be given the treatment in question compared with another treatment or placebo in order for one further patient to gain benefit. The lower the NNT, the more efficacious the drug. In the Cochrane Review by Wilson et al.,[29] the NNT for tricyclics was 4 (a figure as good as many other treatments in medicine), and for SSRIs it was 7, although only two trials met the criteria for the analysis (both of fluoxetine). In the study by Katona and Livingston,[31] most antidepressant trials showed efficacy, but this was less clear for moclobemide and fluoxetine. In head-to-head comparisons between antidepressants there was a trend for the superiority of SSRIs and venlafaxine over tricyclics, but most of the trials were under-powered statistically.

There is some evidence that in melancholic depressive disorder the tricyclics are superior to SSRIs, but there are no data specific to older patients.[32]

Efficacy in special patient groups

Depression associated with systemic disease
A meta-analysis by Gill and Hatcher[33] has shown that antidepressants are effective in the management of depression complicating a variety of systemic illnesses. The NNT was the same as for tricyclic antidepressants in the meta-analysis of older patients conducted by Wilson et al.[29] SSRIs are preferred because of their favourable side-effect profile in depression that is comorbid with medical disorder. Cole et al.[34] calculated that 38–87% of elderly medically ill inpatients have contraindications to the use of older heterocyclic antidepressants, but only 4% have contraindications to SSRIs.

Dementia
Studies show a high rate of spontaneous recovery in mild to moderate depression complicating dementia. Current advice suggests providing support to the patient and caregiver with a review in 2 to 4 weeks, rather than initiating antidepressants.[6]

For moderate to severe cases of depression complicating dementia there is evidence of antidepressant efficacy. For example, citalopram was found to improve a variety of emotional symptoms, including depression in dementia,[35,36] while moclobemide significantly improved depressive symptoms in those with dementia.[37] Fluoxetine treatment was shown to be effective in patients with severe physical illness.[38] In an open-label study by Zimmer[39] involving 18 geriatric patients with concurrent cardiovascular and cerebrovascular illness, depression was successfully and cost-effectively treated (78% of patients responded) with venlafaxine at dosages of 50–262.5 mg/day. The logistic problems inherent in such studies mean that large placebo-controlled studies of such patients are unlikely to be feasible.

Stroke
In a review of antidepressants in stroke, Gustafson et al.[40] do not recommend the use of the older tricyclic antidepressants because of the high rate of contra-indications and side-effects, including delirium. As with dementia, there is a high rate of spontaneous recovery, but this diminishes rapidly after 6 weeks.[41] Citalopram[42] and fluoxetine have been shown to be more effective than placebo.[43]

Nursing home residents
Few studies have been conducted on this population. This represents an important gap in knowledge, as these patients are likely to encompass the most difficult to treat, namely the very old and the very frail. Tricyclic antidepressants have

been shown to be effective but associated with unacceptably low tolerability.[13] In an open study of SSRIs by Trappler and Cohen,[44] the response rate was poor if the patient had associated dementia, but otherwise it was good. Likewise, in an open pilot study of sertraline in patients with minor (sub-threshold) depression, outcome and tolerability were good.[45]

Current best practice suggests that the patient should be treated with an SSRI or moclobemide, starting with a low dose and titrating upwards. An alternative is to deploy psychosocial interventions. In one study a socialisation programme was associated with short-term benefit.[46]

Treatment of major depressive episode

The pharmacological management of depressive disorder is divided into three phases, namely acute treatment, continuation therapy and maintenance treatment. These will be discussed in turn.

Acute treatment phase

Antidepressants are usually the first-line treatment in patients with moderate and severe depressive episode. In general, no antidepressant drug is clearly more effective than another, but rather antidepressants should be tailored to the patient, taking account of the likely side-effects and tolerability. Older antidepressants should be avoided in patients at risk of suicide.

Therapeutic response may occur within 2 weeks. Likewise, if there has been no response within 4 weeks recovery is unlikely.[47] Once recovery has started it may take up to 12 weeks for a full response (i.e. longer than in younger patients).

Continuation phase

Continuation drug therapy reduces the risk of relapse after remission. It is not a fixed period, but in older people a 12-month period of continuation with antidepressants is recommended, in contrast to a 6-month period for younger patients.[6] However, patients with recurrent depression can be treated for 2 years.[6] For patients with delusional depression on antipsychotic medication, it is recommended that this be continued for 6 months before being tailed off.

Maintenance phase

Major depression often follows a recurrent course, and older people benefit from maintenance therapy even after a first episode of depression. Evidence comes from several studies. A placebo-controlled trial of dothiepin (dosulepin) showed that over a 2-year period the relapse rate was reduced by a factor of 2.5 in the actively treated group.[48] In another study, by Reynolds et al.,[14] most protection was conferred by a combination of nortriptyline, a secondary amine tricyclic, and interpersonal therapy. Patients who received placebo and usual care had a very high rate of relapse/recurrence.

Citalopram, an SSRI, prevented recurrence over a period of 1–2 years, suggesting that a protection effect is not confined to tricyclic antidepressants.[49] Extrapolating from studies of younger patients, the risk of relapse is increased if there are residual symptoms or if chronic life stresses exist.[50] Wilson et al.[29] did not find any benefit from sertraline in prophylaxis. Possibly the dose used was too small, otherwise this study cautions against assuming that all antidepressants are equally effective in prevention.

The case for long-term antidepressant treatment needs to be balanced against adverse effects, which for the older antidepressants can include troublesome weight gain, tooth decay and cardiovascular disturbance.

Resistant depression

At least a third of patients fail to respond to first-line antidepressant therapy.[51] In such patients it is important to first review the diagnosis, rule out undetected systemic disease or dementia, ensure treatment adequacy in terms of duration and compliance, and attend to the possibility of psychosocial reinforcers. This has been described as a *stepped care approach*, meaning that each step of treatment follows a logical sequence rather than a chaotic mishmash.[52] This has been reinforced in a study by Flint and Rifat,[53] in which over 80% of patients recovered if a logical process was adopted – for example, starting with a trial of anti-depressant monotherapy and eventually moving up to electroconvulsive therapy (ECT).

The various strategies for treating resistant depression include the following.

- *Increasing the dose.* This may be beneficial for TCAs and venlafaxine, but there is little evidence that increasing the dose significantly alters the outcome in the case of SSRIs.[54]
- *Prolonging the length of treatment.* Here the therapeutic trial is continued beyond what is usually considered to be an 'adequate' period of time. There is evidence that an extension to 9 weeks or even longer may improve recovery from a depressive episode in older patients,[16] but not if there has been no improve-ment in the first 4 weeks.[47]
- *Switching antidepressant class.* Switching between classes of antidepressants has been shown to have a modest benefit, although there has been little systematic evaluation of this. The most popular strategy is a change from one antide-pressant to another from a different class (e.g. from a TCA to an SSRI, or vice versa).[55] Use of the traditional MAOIs has been mentioned. Venlafaxine shows some promise in resistant depression, but evaluation is mostly confined to clinical experience[56] or open trials.[57] It has been estimated that the overall success rate for class switching is about 50%.[54]
- *Augmentation.* Most of the evidence is for lithium augmentation.[54] Austin *et al.* conducted a meta-analysis of five small double-blind trials and found that 18 out of 50 of patients augmented with lithium responded, compared with 6 out of 49 of those who were given a placebo.[58] In another study,[59] venlafaxine and lithium augmentation was studied in an open trial in outpatients aged 18–70 years. At the end of the 7-week study, 35% of the patients showed more than a 50% reduction in depressive symptoms, and the combination was well tolerated. Other augmentation approaches include the use of neuroleptics, anti-epileptics, thyroid hormone and L-tryptophan, but the evidence base is too small to allow recommendations to be made.

Prevention

Depression in old age frequently follows a chronic and relapsing course. As endorsed by the US National Institute of Health,[60] a major goal of the treatment is to prevent relapse, recurrence and chronicity. Antidepressant pharmacotherapy is the mainstay of this therapeutic goal. Studies published to date have established the maintenance efficacy of TCAs and some SSRIs, as discussed above.

Bipolar affective disorders

Introduction

Bipolar disorder affects approximately 0.1% of individuals over the age of 65 years, compared with 0.4% of those aged 45–64 years, and 1.4% of those aged 18–44 years.[61] Little is known about the course of illness in elderly patients, but it is associated with significant morbidity, high rates of mortality and considerable use of mental health services.[62] Elderly people with bipolar disorders fall into two clinically distinct subgroups, namely early and late onset, each with different aetiologies and outcomes.[63] The first group has an initial onset with depressive episode in middle age, which subsequently converts to mania in late life, whereas late-onset cases are sometimes termed secondary mania. Krauthammer and Klerman[64] described secondary mania as a syndrome with multiple causes, including drugs (steroids) and metabolic, infectious and structural cerebro-vascular diseases such as stroke and tumour. Certainly the onset of mania in later life should prompt a search for underlying, often cerebral pathology. The course and presentation of the illness may be less typical, with a picture of pseudodementia, confusion or even depressed mood.[65] Several studies suggest that bipolar disorder may become more persistent and less responsive to treatment in later life, predisposing patients to frequent relapses.[66]

Treatment

As with depressive disorder, establishing and maintaining a therapeutic alliance is vital. Providing education about bipolar disorders, enhancing treatment compliance, identifying new episodes early on and reducing the morbidity and sequelae of bipolar disorder are all important goals.

Pharmacological treatments

Medication for patients with bipolar disorders includes those drugs that decrease symptoms of mania or depression, those that prevent further episodes and those that are helpful at various times during the course of the disorder. These medications may be categorised as *mood stabilisers* (e.g. lithium, carbamazepine, sodium valproate, lamotrigine), *neuroleptics* (typicals and atypicals), *benzodiazepines* and *antidepressants*. Lastly, there are novel and adjunctive treatments such as calcium-channel blockers, clozapine, psychostimulants, thyroxine and ECT.

These, together with benzodiazepines and antidepressants, will not be considered in detail here.

There have been few prospective studies of the treatment of mania in older patients. A number of issues relating to efficacy, side-effects and optimal blood levels of mood stabilisers remain unresolved and await further study. Meanwhile, we have to rely on studies conducted on a younger population. Because the treatment of mania is made difficult by reduced tolerability of drugs such as haloperidol, new treatments such as atypical antipsychotics and the anticonvulsants take on a more important role.[67] The three main mood stabilisers currently available, namely lithium, valproate and carbamazepine, have been studied and used in the treatment of all phases of bipolar disorder.

Lithium

Lithium has been shown to block the metabolism of the intracellular second messenger inositol-1,4,5-triphosphate, which is involved in the increase in ionic intracellular calcium concentration, and which in turn triggers neurotransmitter release and other cellular changes in secretory cells. Its narrow therapeutic window necessitates frequent blood monitoring, and discontinuation may precipitate recurrence, a serious problem in the poorly compliant patient. Lower dosages are required in older people because of the combination of a reduced volume of distribution and decreased renal clearance.[68] There have been no controlled prospective studies of the treatment of manic behaviour in the elderly, but in case studies[69] and retrospective trials[70] lithium has been found to be effective. It has been suggested that lithium may be more efficacious than anticonvulsants (see below) for the treatment of classic mania with minimal or no neurological signs.[71]

It is generally held that older patients manifest toxic effects at lower concentrations.[72] Symptoms include polyuria, gastrointestinal abnormalities, neuromuscular effects, ataxia, cognitive impairment and tremors (see Table 8.4). In the longer term, weight gain, oedema and psoriatic rashes can be troublesome. Bowden[73] concludes that patients who respond best to lithium have mild and uncomplicated illness, pure manic symptomatology and infrequent episodes, whereas those with secondary mania or substance abuse, and adolescent and elderly groups respond less well. The optimum lithium plasma concentration for maintenance therapy for the elderly using prospective studies has not been definitely determined, although a lithium range of 0.4–0.7 mEq/l has been proposed.[54]

Prior to commencing lithium, a typical range of tests (see Table 8.4) should include renal function, electrolytes, electrocardiogram (ECG/EKG), thyroid function and blood glucose.[74] Typical starting doses are 100–200 mg daily.

Valproate

In a randomised, double-blind, placebo-controlled study of 179 younger manic patients, Bowden et al.[75] demonstrated that valproate is effective in the treatment of manic episodes in bipolar patients, although possibly it is not as effective as lithium. Valproate seems to have a broad spectrum of activity, and has significant anti-manic action in mixed affective state, rapid-cycling bipolar disorders and secondary mania, which is particularly relevant to the elderly population.[76] It has therefore been suggested that valproate (either as sodium valproate or as divalproex) is more effective than lithium in the treatment of non-classic mania and secondary mania.[71] In a few open and retrospective case studies, valproate was well tolerated and efficacious.[77] Prior to commencing valproate, liver enzyme tests, a full blood count with platelets and an electrocardiogram should be performed. There is potential for the interaction of valproate with aspirin, phenytoin, fluoxetine and carbamazepine.[74] Starting dosages are typically 125–250 mg daily, with a therapeutic range of 500–1000 mg to achieve blood levels of 65–90 μg/ml.[74] Possible adverse effects include sedation, nausea, tremor and weight gain. Recently, in North America,[78] there has been criticism of the wholesale change away from lithium and towards valproate in older patients, on the grounds that this has little evidence base.

Carbamazepine

There are case reports of the effectiveness of carbemazepine in the treatment of late-life mania.[70] As with valproate, there is some evidence that carbamazepine is more effective than lithium in the treatment of non-classic mania and secondary mania.[71] The data suggest that it may be more efficacious as part of combined drug therapy rather than as monotherapy.[73] However, elderly patients on multiple medications are prone to increased side-effects, as carbamazepine can influence the metabolism of many drugs, such as warfarin, erythromycin, diltiazem, verapamil and valproate.

Prior to commencing carbamazepine, liver enzyme tests, electrolytes, a full blood count with platelets and electrocardiogram should be undertaken. Side-effects include sedation, ataxia, nystagmus, blurred vision, agranulocytosis, anticholinergic effects and hyponatraemia secondary to inappropriate anti-diuretic hormone secretion. Starting dosages are typically 100 mg once or twice daily, with average daily dosages of 400–800 mg to achieve blood levels of 6 to 12 μg/l.[74]

Lamotrigine

Lamotrigine is a phenyltriazine derivative, and is a well-established anticonvulsant agent that has shown efficacy in the prevention of mood episodes in younger patients with bipolar 1 disorder.[79] No drug trial data in elderly populations are available so far. The mechanism of action of the drug may be related to the inhibition of sodium and calcium channels in presynaptic neurons and subsequent stabilisation of the neuronal membrane. Lamotrigine is generally well tolerated, the most common side-effects being headache, nausea, infection and insomnia. It does not cause body-weight gain, and the incidence of diarrhoea and tremors is significantly lower than with lithium, with an incidence of serious rash of about 0.1%. It generally does not require monitoring of serum levels. The dosage should be titrated over a 6-week period to 200 mg/day in order to minimise the incidence of serious rash.

Table 8.4 Mood stabilisers used in bipolar disorder in older people

Drug	Investigations prior to prescribing	Side-effects	Average daily dosages	Target serum levels
Lithium	Renal function Electrolytes ECG/EKG Thyroid function Blood glucose (preferably fasting)	Polyuria, gastrointestinal upset, tremor, neurological disturbance (toxicity), weight gain, oedema, psoriatic rash	400 mg (slow release)	0.4–0.7 mEq/l
Valproate	Liver enzymes Full blood count ECG/EKG	Sedation, nausea, tremor, weight gain	500–1000 mg	65–90 μg/ml
Carbamazepine	Liver enzymes Full blood count ECG/EKG	Sedation, ataxia, nystagmus, blurred vision, agranulocytosis, anticholinergic effects, hyponatraemia	400–800 mg	6–12 μg/l

Other treatments

Other anticonvulsants such as gabapentin and topiramate are used in younger patients with bipolar disorder, but as yet there are no controlled trials concerning older people.

Conventional high-potency antipsychotics such as haloperidol are increasingly being replaced by the newer atypical antipsychotics such as risperidone, olanzapine and quetiapine. However, there is still a place for the use of high-potency typical antipsychotics, with or without a benzodiazepine, in the treatment of the acutely disturbed manic patient.[74] A typical regime is haloperidol, 5 mg intramuscularly, with 1 mg lorazepam repeated in an hour if necessary. Many hospitals have their own rapid tranquillisation drug protocols, which should be consulted.

Olanzapine has a licence for the treatment of acute bipolar mania, and clozapine is used as monotherapy for refractory bipolar disorder in younger adults.[74] However, the latter requires regular monitoring for agranulocytosis, and cardiovascular effects can limit its use. There are reports of the efficacy of all of the atypical antipsychotics in the treatment of older adults with bipolar disorder, but there have been no prospective randomised controlled trials.[74]

Conclusion

Depression in elderly patients often goes unrecognised, and the diagnosis may be complicated by medical comorbidity and cognitive impairment. The consequences of untreated depression include increased disability, morbidity and mortality. Depressive episode in elderly patients responds readily to appropriate treatment, with pharmacotherapy being the mainstay of treatment. Because of the favourable adverse effect profile, SSRIs have in most cases replaced TCAs as first-line therapy. In addition, the advent of other new antidepressants such as venlafaxine and mirtazepine has provided clinicians and patients with more tolerable alternatives to tricyclics and monamine oxidase inhibitors. The prevention of relapse and recurrence in the continuation and maintenance phases of treatment, respectively, are just as important goals as the remission of depressive symptoms in the acute phase of treatment.

Adjunctive treatment with psychotherapy or psychosocial interventions is effective in both acute and continuation therapy. Electroconvulsive therapy is both effective and well tolerated in severe non-responsive depression affecting older people.

Unfortunately, there have been no randomised controlled studies of the treatment of bipolar disorder in old age. However, the limited data that are available support the usefulness of lithium in acute and prophylactic treatment of mania in old age, although with an increased risk of side-effects and toxicity. Increasingly drugs such as sodium valproate, divalproex, carbamazepine and lamotrigine are being used as safe, although not necessarily more effective, alternatives to lithium.

Key points

- The treatment of major depression in older people is complicated by medical comorbidity, yet outcomes in the acute phase of treatment are as good as at other times of life.
- There is no one 'right' antidepressant treatment, but rather treatment should be tailored to the individual patient.
- The goal in acute treatment is full remission of symptoms. Partial recovery is a risk factor for chronic depression and/or increased risk of relapse.
- Keeping the patient well is as important as acute treatment, and evidence exists for prophylaxis with both tricyclics and SSRIs.
- The principles of treatment of mania and bipolar disorder are the same as at other times of life. The main difficulties are with side-effects, especially with lithium salts.

References

1 Macdonald AJD (1986) Do general practitioners 'miss' depression in elderly patients? *BMJ.* **292**: 1365–7.

2 Copeland JRM, Beekman ATF, Dewey ME *et al.* (1999) Depression in Europe: geographical distribution among older people. *Br J Psychiatry.* **174**: 312–21.

3 Hammerlein A, Derendorf H and Lowenthal DT (1998) Pharmacokinetic and pharmacodynamic changes in the elderly: clinical implications. *Clin Pharmacokinet.* **35**: 49–64.

4 Baldwin RC (2001) Depressive disorder. In: R Jacoby and C Oppenheimer (eds) *Psychiatry in the Elderly* (3e). Oxford University Press, Oxford.

5 Lebowitz BD, Oearson JNL, Schneider LS *et al.* (1997) Diagnosis and treatment of depression in late life. *JAMA.* **278**: 1186–90.

6 Baldwin RC, Chiu E, Katona C and Graham N (2002) *Guidelines on Depression in Older People: practising the evidence.* Martin Dunitz, London.

7 Williams JW, Barrett J, Oxman T *et al.* (2000) Treatment of dysthymia and minor depression in primary care: a randomised controlled trial in older adults. *JAMA.* **284**: 1519–26.

8 Folstein MF, Folstein SE and McHugh PR (1975) 'Mini-Mental State': a practical method for grading the cognitive state of patients for the clinician. *J Psychiatr Res.* **12**: 189–98.

9 Yasavage JA, Brink TL, Rose TL *et al.* (1983) Development and validation of a geriatric depression screening scale: a preliminary report. *J Psychiatr Res.* **17**: 37–49.

10 Montgomery SA and Asberg M (1979) A new depression scale intended to be sensitive to change. *Br J Psychiatry.* **134**: 382–9.

11 Hamilton M (1960) A rating scale for depression. *J Neurol Neurosurg Psychiatry.* **23**: 56–62.

12 Mottram P, Wilson K and Copeland J (2000) Validation of the Hamilton Depression Scale and Montgomery and Asberg rating scales in terms of AGECAT depression cases. *Int J Geriatr Psychiatry.* **15**: 1113–19.

13 Chiu E, Ames D, Draper B and Snowdon J (1999) Depressive disorders in the elderly: a review. In: I Maj and N Sartorious (eds) *Depressive Disorders*. John Wiley and Sons, Chichester.

14 Reynolds CF, Frank E, Perel JM *et al.* (1999) Nortriptyline and interpersonal psycho-therapy as maintenance therapies for recurrent major depression: a randomized controlled trial in patients older than 59 years. *JAMA.* **281**: 39–45.

15 Norman TR (1993) Pharmacokinetic aspects of antidepressant treatment in the elderly. *Prog Neuropsychopharmacol Biol Psychiatry.* **17**: 329–44.

16 Georgotas A and McCue R (1989) The additional benefit of extending an anti-depressant trial past seven weeks in the depressed elderly. *Int J Geriatr Psychiatry.* **4**: 191–5.

17 Waugh J and Goa KL (2003) Escitalopram: a review of its use in the management of major depressive and anxiety disorders. *CNS Drugs.* **17**: 343–62.

18 Baumann P (1998) Care of depression in the elderly: comparative pharmacokinetics of SSRIs. *Int Clin Psychopharmacol.* **13 (Suppl. 5)**: S35–43.

19 Stahl S, Lindquist M, Pettersson M *et al.* (1997) Withdrawal reactions with selective serotonin reuptake inhibitors as reported to the WHO system. *Eur J Clin Pharmacol.* **53**: 163–9.

20 Stahl S, Zivkov M, Reimitz PE *et al.* (1997) Meta-analysis of randomised, double-blind, placebo-controlled, efficacy and safety studies of mirtazipine versus amitriptyline in major depression. *Acta Psychiatr Scand.* **96 (Suppl. 39)**: 22–30.

21 Rosenbaum JF, Fava M, Hoog SL *et al.* (1998) Selective serotonin reuptake inhibitor discontinuation syndrome: a randomised clinical trial. *Biol Psychiatry.* **44**: 77–87.

22 Greenblatt DJ, von Moltke LL, Harmatz JS *et al.* (1998) Drug interactions with newer antidepressants: role of human cytochromes P450. *J Clin Psychiatry.* **59 (Suppl. 15)**: 19–27.

23 Von Moltke LL, Greenblatt DJ, Giancarlo GM *et al.* (2001) Escitalopram (S-citalopram) and its metabolites *in vitro*: cytochromes mediating biotransformation, inhibitory effects, and comparison to R-citalopram. *Drug Metab Dispos.* **29**: 1102–9.

24 Spin E and Scardo MG (2002) Clinically significant drug interaction with anti-depressants in the elderly. *Drugs Aging.* **19**: 299–320.

25 Kirby D, Harrigun S and Ames D (2002) Hyponatraemia in elderly psychiatric patients treated with SSRIs and venlafaxine: a retrospective controlled study in an inpatient unit. *Int J Geriatr Psychiatry.* **17**: 231–7.

26 Timmer CL, Paanakker JE and van Hal HJM (1996) Pharmacokinetics of mirtazipine from orally administered tablets: influence of age, gender and treatment regimen. *Hum Psychopharmacol.* **11**: 497–509.

27 Aguglia E (2000) Reboxetine in the maintenance therapy of depressive disorder in the elderly: a long-term open study. *Int J Geriatr Psychiatry.* **15**: 784–93.

28 Mittman N, Herrmann N, Einarson TR *et al.* (1997) The efficacy, safety and tolerability of antidepressants in late-life depression: a meta-analysis. *J Affect Disord.* **46**: 191–217.

29 Wilson K, Mottram P, Sivanranthan A and Nightingale A (2001) Antidepressant versus placebo for depressed elderly (Cochrane Review). In: *The Cochrane Library. Issue 2.* Update Software, Oxford.

30 Edwards JG (1995) Drug choice in depression. Selective serotonin reuptake inhibitors or tricyclic antidepressants? *CNS Drugs.* 4: 141–59.

31 Katona C and Livingston G (2002) How well do antidepressants work in older people? A systematic review of number needed to treat. *J Affect Disord.* 69: 47–52.

32 Perry PJ (1996) Pharmacotherapy for major depression with melancholic features: relative efficacy of tricyclic versus selective serotonin reuptake inhibitor anti-depressants. *J Affect Disord.* 39: 1–6.

33 Gill D and Hatcher S (1999) Antidepressant drugs in depressed patients who also have a physical illness (Cochrane Review). In: *The Cochrane Library. Issue 3.* Update Software, Oxford.

34 Cole MG, Elie LM, McCusker J *et al.* (2000) Feasibility and effectiveness of treatments for depression in elderly medical inpatients: a systematic review. *Int Psychogeriatr.* 12: 453–61.

35 Nyth AL and Gottfries CG (1990) The clinical efficacy of citalopram in treatment of emotional disturbances in dementia disorders. *Br J Psychiatry.* 157: 894–901.

36 Nyth AL, Gottfries CG, Lyby K *et al.* (1992) A controlled multi-centre clinical study of citalopram and placebo in elderly depressed patients with and without concomitant dementia. *Acta Psychiatr Scand.* 86: 138–45.

37 Roth M, Mountjoy CQ and Amrein R (1996) Moclobemide in elderly patients with cognitive decline and depression: an international double-blind placebo-controlled trial. *Br J Psychiatry.* 168: 149–57.

38 Evans M, Hammond M, Wilson K, Lye M and Copeland J (1997) Placebo-controlled treatment trial of depression in elderly physically ill patients. *Int J Geriatr Psychiatry.* 12: 817–24.

39 Zimmer B (1999) Direct and indirect cost of venlafaxine treatment of depression in the elderly with comorbid medical disorders. *Ann Long-Term Care.* 7: 405–9.

40 Gustafson Y, Nilsson I, Mattsson M *et al.* (1995) Epidemiology and treatment of post-stroke depression. *Drugs Aging.* 7: 298–309.

41 Andersen G, Vestergaard K and Lauritzen L (1994) Effective treatment of post-stroke depression with the selective serotonin reuptake inhibitor citalopram. *Stroke.* 25: 1099–104.

42 Anderson IM (1998) SSRIs versus tricyclic antidepressants in depressed inpatients: a meta-analysis of efficiency and tolerability. *Depression Anxiety.* 7 (**Suppl. 1**): 11–17.

43 Wiart L, Petit H, Joseph PA, Mazaux JM and Barat M (2000) Fluoxetine in early post-stroke depression: a double-blind placebo-controlled study. *Stroke.* 31: 1829–32.

44 Trappler B and Cohen CI (1998) Use of SSRIs in 'very old' depressed nursing home residents. *Am J Geriatr Psychiatry.* 6: 83–9.

45 Rosen J, Mulsant BH and Pollock BG (2000) Sertraline in the treatment of minor depression in nursing home residents: a pilot study. *Int J Geriatr Psychiatry.* 15: 177–80.

46 Rosen J, Rogers JC, Marin RS *et al.* (1997) Control-relevant intervention in the treatment of minor and major depression in a long-term care facility. *Am J Geriatr Psychiatry.* 5: 247–57.

47 Mottram P, Wilson KCM, Ashworth L and Abou-Saleh M (2002) The clinical profile of older patients' response to antidepressants – an open trial of sertraline. *Int J Geriatr Psychiatry.* 17: 574–8.

48 Old Age Depression Interest Group (1993) How long should the elderly take anti-depressants? A double-blind placebo-controlled study of continuation/prophylaxis therapy with dothiepin. *Br J Psychiatry.* 162: 175–82.

49 Klysner R, Bent-Hansen J, Hansen HL *et al.* (2002) Efficacy of citalopram in the prevention of recurrent depression in elderly patients: placebo-controlled study of maintenance therapy. *Br J Psychiatry.* **181**: 29–35.

50 Paykel ES (1998) Remission and residual symptomatology in major depression. *Psychopathology.* **31**: 5–14.

51 Flint AJ (1995) Augmentation strategies in geriatric depression. *Int J Geriatr Psychiatry.* **10**: 137–46.

52 Guscott R and Grof P (1991) The clinical meaning of refractory depression: a review for the clinician. *Am J Psychiatry.* **148**: 695–704.

53 Flint AJ and Rifat SL (1996) The effect of sequential antidepressant treatment on geriatric depression. *J Affect Disord.* **36**: 95–105.

54 Baldwin RC (1996) Treatment-resistant depression in the elderly: a review of treatment options. *Rev Clin Gerontol.* **6**: 343–8.

55 Akiskal HS (1985) An approach to chronic and 'resistant' depressions: evaluation and treatment. *J Clin Psychiatry.* **46**: 32–6.

56 Bowskill RJ and Bridges PL (1997) Treatment-resistant affective disorders. *Br J Hosp Med.* **57**: 171–2.

57 Nierenberg AA, Feighner JP, Rudolph R *et al.* (1994) Venlafaxine for treatment-resistant unipolar depression. *J Clin Psychopharmacol.* **14**: 419–23.

58 Austin MPV, Souza FGM and Goodwin GM (1991) Lithium augmentation in anti-depressant-resistant patients: a quantitative analysis. *Br J Psychiatry.* **159**: 510–14.

59 Hoencamp E, Haffmans PMJ, Dijken WA *et al.* (2000) Lithium augmentation of venlafaxine: an open-label trial. *J Clin Psychopharmacol.* **20**: 538–43.

60 National Institute of Health (1992) NIH Consensus panel on diagnosis and treatment of depression in late life *JAMA.* **268**: 1018–24.

61 Weissman MM, Leaf PJ, Tischler GL *et al.* (1988) Affective disorders in five United States communities. *Psychol Med.* **18**: 141–53.

62 Bartels SJ, Forester B, Miles KM *et al.* (2000) Mental health service use by elderly patients with bipolar disorder and unipolar depression. *Am J Geriatr Psychiatry.* **8**: 160–6.

63 Shulman K (1994) Mania in late life: conceptual and clinical issues. In: E Chiu and D Ames (eds) *Functional Psychiatric Disorders of the Elderly*. Cambridge University Press, Cambridge.

64 Krauthammer C and Klerman GL (1978) Secondary mania: manic syndrome associated with antecedent physical illness or drugs. *Arch Gen Psychiatry.* **35**: 1333–9.

65 Fortin L (1990) Manic disorder in the aged: a review of the literature. *Can J Psychiatry.* **35**: 679–83.

66 Ameblas A (1987) Life events and mania. *Br J Psychiatry.* **150**: 235–40.

67 McDonald WM (2000) Epidemiology, etiology, and treatment of geriatric mania. *J Clin Psychiatry.* **61 (Suppl. 13)**: 3–11.

68 Sproule BA, Hardy BG and Shulman KI (2000) Differential pharmacokinetics of lithium in elderly patients. *Drugs Aging.* **16**: 165–77.

69 Charron M, Fortin L and Paquette I (1991) *De novo* mania among elderly people. *Acta Psychiatrica Scand.* **84**: 503–7.

70 Mirchnadani I and Young R (1993) Management of mania in the elderly: an update. *Ann Clin Psychiatry.* **5**: 215–22.

71 Chen ST, Altshuler LL, Melnyk KA *et al.* (1999) Efficacy of lithium vs. valproate in the treatment of mania in the elderly: a retrospective study. *J Clin Psychiatry.* **60**: 181–6.

72 Hirschfield R (1996) *Practice Guidelines for the Treatment of Patients with Bipolar Disorder.* American Psychiatric Association, Washington, DC.

73 Bowden C (1995) Predictors of response to divalproex and lithium. *J Clin Psychiatry.* **56 (Suppl. 3)**: 25–30.

74 Sajatovic M (2002) Treatment of bipolar disorder in older adults. *Int J Geriatr Psychiatry.* **17**: 865–73.

75 Bowden C, Brugger AM, Swann AC *et al.* (1994) Efficacy of divalproex vs. lithium and placebo in the treatment of mania. *JAMA.* **271**: 918–24.

76 Khouzam H, Emery P and Reaves B (1994) Secondary mania in late life. *J Am Geriatr Soc.* **42**: 85–7.

77 Kando JC, Tohen M, Castillo J *et al.* (1996) The use of valproate in an elderly population with affective symptoms. *J Clin Psychiatry.* **57**: 238–40.

78 Shulman KI, Rochon P, Sykora K *et al.* (2003) Changing prescription patterns for lithium and valproic acid in old age: shifting practice without evidence. *BMJ.* **326**: 960–1.

79 Goldsmith DR, Wagstaff AJ, Ibbotson T *et al.* (2003) Lamotrigine: a review of its use in bipolar disorder. *Drugs.* **63**: 2029–50.

Chapter 9

The treatment of psychosis in the elderly

Roger Bullock

Introduction

Age-related deterioration of significant cortical areas with associated neurochemical changes, comorbid physical illnesses, social isolation, sensory deficits and polypharmacy leads to an increased risk of psychosis in the elderly.[1] Thus the prevalence of neuropsychiatric disorders requiring treatment is expected to increase significantly in people above the age of 65 years over the next 20 years, perhaps quadrupling. The Cache County population study found that 5% of all older people had had delusions or hallucinations in the preceding month.[2] Antipsychotic agents are the first-line treatment for psychosis, the symptoms that respond best being hallucinations, delusions, anxiety, verbal and physical agitation and hostility.[3]

Despite this, the elderly population has traditionally been neglected in clinical research, especially where antipsychotics are concerned. Much of the prescribing is technically unlicensed and often unmonitored, especially in primary care. However, the focus of attention has changed, partly due to concern about emerging side-effects, but also because the population is ageing and the increasing presence of psychiatric symptoms in nursing homes has led to widespread use of neuroleptic medication, not always judiciously.[4] Understanding the aetiology of the psychiatric syndromes in which the psychosis occurs in older people, along with the introduction of newer and safer treatments, has helped to improve prescribing.

Psychotic disorders in late life

The conditions most frequently seen in the elderly who present primarily with psychosis or have a psychotic element to their presentation include the following:

- schizophrenia
- delusional disorder
- dementia (every type)
- neurological conditions, especially Parkinson's disease
- delirium
- mood disorder
- substance abuse
- metabolic disturbances

- chronic medical conditions
- drug-induced psychosis.

Antipsychotic medication is always the first-line treatment where psychosis presents in each of these conditions. However, where there are comorbid medical or metabolic conditions contributing to the symptoms (e.g. thyroid disease), these must also be treated to ensure a better recovery.

Schizophrenia

Chronic early-onset schizophrenia

Classical schizophrenia occurring before 45 years of age runs a variable course, with around 50% of patients showing improvement or attenuation of symptoms as they get older.[5] Delusional beliefs and hallucinations become less frequent as the patient ages, and even formal thought disorder may become less bizarre.[6] These patients will have been on antipsychotic medications for many years, as they are the most effective treatment, improving acute symptoms and controlling relapses. Most chronic patients who have been treated for more than 15 years will probably be on typical antipsychotics. These may be at relatively low doses compared with the earlier stages of illness. If these patients are free from unwanted side-effects, they should be left alone, and in particular no attempt should be made to stop what look like ineffective doses. If they do have any unwanted side-effects, especially extrapyramidal effects, then a switch to atypicals may be warranted. This strategy is endorsed by recent guidance from the National Institute for Clinical Excellence.[7]

Schizophrenia in later life

Schizophrenia can occur at any time in life. Most patients are diagnosed early in life, but 15% of patients with schizophrenia or schizophrenia-like illness present after the middle period of life. As these patients age they should be treated in the same way as younger-onset patients.

Late-onset schizophrenia

Around 3% of patients with schizophrenia present after 60 years of age.[8] Late-onset schizophrenia is probably related to cortical degeneration, and so may be a different illness to earlier-presenting schizophrenia. There has been considerable debate about this since the term 'paraphrenia' was dropped. Delusional disorder is a separate diagnosis, but is often used where paraphrenia had been used previously. Another consensus group coined the term 'very-late-onset schizophrenia-like psychosis'. Whatever it is called, the disease follows different demographics to schizophrenia (e.g. a male:female ratio of 8:1), and generally follows a more chronic course.[9] Social isolation and hearing impairment are also associated with the development of late-onset schizophrenia.[10] Complex, well-formed persecutory delusions are especially common, with hallucinations comparatively less frequent.[11] These delusions are often very difficult to treat, partly because the patient usually has little insight and cannot see the need for treatment. In some instances treatment may not be the best option, and this needs to be considered prior to any medication use. The side-effects of typical antipsychotics traditionally alerted suspicious patients, making compliance a problem. This has improved with the use of atypicals, for which it may be expected that lower doses would be needed compared with early-onset patients.[12] However, it is not uncommon for them to require and tolerate equivalent doses.

Psychosis and agitation in elderly patients with dementia

Dementia occurs in approximately 10% of individuals in their seventh decade, and in 20–30% in the eighth and ninth decades.[13] Symptoms of psychosis and agitation such as delusions, hallucinations, aggression and disinhibition occur in about 50% of these patients, and are often challenging to caregivers. Both traditional and atypical antipsychotic agents are effective in treating psychotic symptoms and agitation in elderly patients with dementia. Relatively low dosages of the antipsychotics can be effective,[14] but a meta-analysis of double-blind trials published between 1954 and 1989 found that although traditional antipsychotic agents were significantly more effective than placebo, the effect size was very small ($r = 0.18$) in agitated patients with dementia.[15] No one agent was found to be superior to another.

A more recent meta-analysis of randomised, controlled, double-blind studies in dementia of Alzheimer's type evaluated clinical improvement, side-effects and dropout rates.[16] This included studies published between 1966 and 1995 that were 4 weeks or longer in duration and had a measurable outcome based on a specific rating scale. Again, this study demonstrated a modest effect in the treatment of dementia (61% for treatment compared with 34% for placebo). Dropout rates were the same between groups, with the most frequently reported adverse effects being sedation, movement disorders and orthostasis. A recent review of literature published between 1960 and 2000 again supports the view that conventional antipsychotics are modestly effective.[17] Fewer studies of atypical antipsychotics have been published. Data from clinical trials support the efficacy of risperidone,[18–20] olanzapine,[21] and quetiapine[22,23] in this population. These are discussed in Chapter 14.

Delirium

Delirium is an organic syndrome characterised by acute onset, fluctuating levels of consciousness and global impairment of cognitive functioning. It is more common in the elderly,[24] where 14–56% of those in hospital experience an episode during their stay. It is more prevalent where there is pre-existing cognitive impairment,[25] but other common causes include infections (43%), prescribed medications (20–40%) and endocrine, fluid and electrolyte imbalance. Constipation can also trigger an episode. Non-detection rates are in the range of 33–66%,[25,26] and this increases mortality,[27] hospital length of stay and subsequent risk of residential care.[25]

Treatment of any underlying physical illness and attention to environmental factors are important.[27] If behavioural disturbance such as agitation and hallucinations is prominent, psychotropic medication may be indicated. Antipsychotics are effective where rapid onset of action and little respiratory depression occur. Haloperidol has been widely used in small doses,[25] but there are few data on the use of atypical antipsychotics in delirium. Olanzapine and haloperidol were compared in an uncontrolled case series of 11 patients with delirium due to diverse aetiology.[24] Olanzapine had a similar response, but was better tolerated. This was replicated in a case-report series of post-operative delirium in geriatric patients.[28] There is also limited evidence of clinical benefit with risperidone (1.5–4 mg).[25]

Mood disorders with psychosis

Depression is the commonest psychiatric disorder in the elderly, and psychotic symptoms frequently coexist.[1] Older patients with a psychotic depression have increased rates of relapse, more persistent symptoms, more suicide attempts, and more hospital admissions than those with a non-psychotic depression. Antipsychotic medications are useful in the treatment of psychosis associated with major depression, and also manic episodes in patients with bipolar disorder.[29] In the elderly, often both an antidepressant and an antipsychotic are needed to successfully treat a truly psychotic depression. However, there are few data to support this. In fact, a non-randomised study of 25 patients that compared a tricyclic antidepressant plus antipsychotic with a tricyclic antidepressant and electroconvulsive therapy (ECT) revealed that the former group responded more slowly.[30]

Elderly patients with manic symptoms have a higher prevalence of cognitive dysfunction, with persistence of symptoms and greater mortality.[31] No prospective studies in the elderly have been undertaken, so extrapolations from younger patients' data are all that can be used. Risperidone is reported to reduce psychotic symptoms in elderly patients with mania, although other reports suggest that it may induce mania in some patients.[32] Clozapine appears to be safe and effective in the treatment of mania in the elderly, but does not seem to help the depressed phase in bipolar patients.[33] Olanzapine has been approved for the treatment of mania, so its future use in the elderly should inform practice.

Antipsychotic medication in the elderly

In the elderly, the recommended doses for traditional antipsychotics are much lower than in younger patients. Age-related pharmacokinetic and pharmacodynamic factors, coexisting medical illnesses and concomitant medications increase the risk for both adverse effects and drug interactions in the older patient taking any antipsychotic.[34] Behavioural symptoms tend to respond to lower doses, so the appropriate starting dose of a typical antipsychotic is approximately a quarter of the usual adult dose.[35] To minimise adverse effects (e.g. postural hypotension and sedation), antipsychotics can be given in divided doses and titrated slowly up to the optimum therapeutic effect. For the older patient with schizophrenia, the required dose of antipsychotic correlates inversely with both the patient's current age and the age of onset of illness.[36] In chronically ill patients with schizophrenia, dose requirements often decrease over time.

Patients with schizophrenia have high rates of medical comorbidity and drug–drug interactions because of the high rates of polypharmacy due to coexisting physical illness.[37] Respiratory, cardiovascular, gastrointestinal and neoplastic disorders are more common than in the general population.[38]

Typical antipsychotics

The dopamine hypothesis originated in the 1950s. Delay and Deniker[39] discovered the potential therapeutic effects of chlorpromazine in suppressing hallucinations and delusions in schizophrenic patients. Neurochemical experiments in animal brain demonstrated the dopamine-antagonist properties of neuroleptics.[40–42] Currently, five subtypes of dopamine receptors have been distinguished by gene cloning.[43] They are G-protein-coupled receptors that activate an enzyme or ion channel either to produce an intracellular second messenger or to cause ion fluxes.[44,45] Dopamine receptors have been grouped into two main classes, namely D_1-like (D_1 and D_5) and D_2-like (D_2, D_3 and D_4).[46] D_1 receptors are more abundant in the brain, and seem to be involved in the control of motor, cognitive and cardiovascular functions.[47,48] However, D_1-receptor antagonists do not show any antipsychotic activity. D_2-receptor antagonists are key to the treatment of positive symptoms of schizophrenia. Excessive blockade of these receptors may lead to extrapyramidal symptoms (EPS) and tardive dyskinesia (TD). All of the current antipsychotics have D_2-antagonist activity. Moderate blockade of central D_2 receptors reduces positive symptoms of schizophrenia, but too high a degree of D_2-receptor occupancy gives rise to EPS. Blockade of D_2 receptors in the anterior pituitary causes elevation of blood prolactin levels.[49,50] Interestingly, clozapine has a higher affinity for D_4 than for D_2 receptors. These may play a role in the modulation of gamma-aminobutyric acid (GABA)-ergic neuronal activity by dopamine.[51]

Conventional antipsychotics such as haloperidol, chlorpromazine and promazine are D_2-receptor antagonists that inhibit dopaminergic neurotransmission in a dose-related manner. They virtually decrease the intensity of all psychotic symptoms, although not necessarily to the same extent and with the same time course. Negative symptoms may persist to a much more striking degree than delusions, hallucinations and thought disorders, and there is a dose-related incidence of EPS.

Adverse effects associated with typical antipsychotics

Older patients are particularly vulnerable to the adverse effects associated with conventional antipsychotic agents, such as postural hypotension, sedation and anticholinergic side-effects.[34] In particular they are at risk of developing adverse motor effects and EPS.

Typical antipsychotics are associated with both acute and late-occurring movement disorders, particularly EPS and TD. Dystonia, parkinsonism and akathisia usually occur within a few days or weeks, whereas TD has a delayed onset, occurring months to years after commencing treatment. Movement disorders often impair a patient's quality of life, and TD can lead to speech impairment, falls, feeding problems and depression.[52] Dystonia, dyskinesia, bradykinesia and akathisia can cause gait disturbances, increasing the risk of falls and consequent fractures.

The incidence and prevalence of antipsychotic-induced parkinsonism and TD are significantly increased in older patients (up to 50% in those over 60 years of age).[53,54] After 1 year of treatment with a typical antipsychotic, 26% of elderly patients (mean age 66 years) had TD, compared with 4% of younger patients.[55] This increased risk of movement disorders can be attributed to age-related loss of dopaminergic function. Typically, ascending dopaminergic neurons and post-synaptic dopamine receptors degenerate with age, which means that the dopamine content in the striatum has declined by as much as 50% by the age of 60 years.[56,57] This makes an older individual more susceptible to dopaminergic blockade. In general, this risk is reduced with atypical antipsychotics.[58–60] However, these drugs are not free from side-effects.[61]

Typical antipsychotics are more likely to exhibit a cumulative effect if taken over long periods. Concerns over QT-interval abnormalities, with subsequent ventricular tachycardia and sudden death in patients of all ages, has led to restrictions in the use of thioridazine[62] and withdrawal of droperidol.

Treatment of common movement disorders

Mild cases of antipsychotic-induced movement disorders can be left if the symptoms do not trouble the patient. In more marked cases, reducing the dose to the lowest effective level, choosing a lower-potency antipsychotic or switching to an atypical antipsychotic may reduce or alleviate the symptoms.[53]

Anticholinergic drugs, which have traditionally been used for some EPS, are associated with worse adverse effects in the elderly, including tachycardia, urinary retention, constipation, confusion and memory impairment. They remain the treatment of choice for acute dystonia, which fortunately is rare in the elderly. However, anticholinergic treatment does not usually help acute akathisia, and its traditional use in parkinsonism is now under question. Beta-blockers can help with akathisia, but can cause hypotension and bradycardia.

TD is usually a persistent movement disorder associated with antipsychotic use, but it sometimes occurs spontaneously. Minimising the risk of TD is important, as there is no definitive treatment. Treatment options include using the lowest possible doses, especially in those at high risk of developing TD, and regular review. The incidence of TD appears to be lower in elderly patients who receive atypical antipsychotics rather than typicals.[61]

Atypical antipsychotics

Atypical antipsychotics are drugs with no or minimal EPS and greater efficacy in positive and particularly negative symptoms (and in the original definitions, they should not raise prolactin levels or induce narcolepsy). They have a characteristic mode of action, namely a combination of D_2-receptor antagonism, coupled with $5HT_{2A}$ blockade, which paradoxically reverses the D_2 blockade, especially in the striatum.[63] The enhanced efficacy of atypical antipsychotics is attributed to this high ratio of $5HT_{2A}$ to D_2-receptor blockade, and a greater specificity for the mesolimbic rather than the striatal dopamine system.[64] For example, risperidone shows very potent $5HT_{2A}$ antagonism with weaker D_2 antagonism, and is effective against the positive and negative symptoms of schizophrenia. Its action suggests that negative symptoms may actually derive from overactivity of these excitatory $5HT_{2A}$ receptors, which occur mainly in the telencephalon, and much less in the midbrain and hindbrain.

Atypical antipsychotics also show antagonism at D_3 and D_4 receptors. Although the precise functional significance of these multiple receptors has yet to be clarified, this high D_3 and D_4 selectivity may additionally contribute to the low EPS rates observed with these drugs.[65]

The selectivity of these atypical agents with regard to the limbic system has been demonstrated in electrophysiological studies (percentage of silent dopamine neurons with chronic treatment) and animal tests (low catalepsy in rodents and low EPS in non-human primates).[66]

The biggest issue is the disparity in cost between the older and newer drugs, with sometimes a 30-fold difference in price.[67] This means that cost-effectiveness is a major issue.[68] Because of the improved treatment profile, there seem to be lower relapse rates and fewer admissions to hospital on atypical antipsychotics, coupled with improved quality of life, which make them a more popular choice for patients and clinicians alike.

Adverse events with atypical antipsychotics

The reduced risk of EPS and TD associated with atypical antipsychotics is offset by apparent increases in medical morbidity, including weight gain, abnormal lipid concentrations, hyperglycaemia and consequent type 2 diabetes mellitus.[69] The evidence suggests that some atypical antipsychotic agents, particularly clozapine and olanzapine, may significantly impair glucose metabolism, increasing this diabetic risk. Patients with specific risk factors for diabetes should be closely monitored, particularly if they are on either of these two drugs. Periodic screening for metabolic abnormalities, especially high blood sugar levels, would be best practice regardless of the choice of atypical.[70] As well as weight gain, any atypical antipsychotic agent is capable of causing cardiovascular problems and orthostatic hypotension, while some have anticholinergic effects (e.g. olanzapine) or cause sedation. More recently, risperidone and olanzapine have been shown to be associated with an up to fourfold higher risk of cerebrovascular adverse events in patients with dementia, as a result of which the UK Committee for Safety of Medicines does not recommend their use in this patient group. Thus the profile of some atypical antipsychotics is no better and can often be worse than that of typical antipsychotic drugs.[71] Table 9.1 shows the receptor-binding profiles of the common atypicals compared with haloperidol, and the side-effects that this binding will produce.

Table 9.1 Receptor-binding affinities as predictors of side-effects of antipsychotic drugs

Receptor	Risperidone	Olanzapine	Quetiapine	Haloperidol
Muscarinic M_1	−	+++++	+++	−
Histamine H_1	++	++++	++++	−
α_1-adrenergic	+++	+++	++++	++
Dopamine D_2	++++	+++	++	+++++
Serotonin 5-HT$_2$	+++++	++++	+	+

5-HT = hydroxytryptamine; − = no affinity; + = very low affinity; ++ = low affinity; +++ = moderate affinity; ++++ = high affinity; +++++ = very high affinity.

Drug compliance

Poor uptake of prescribed medication is estimated to occur in up to 50% of any patient population. With antipsychotics this figure can be as high as 70–80%.[72] Breen and Thornhill[73] gave three reasons for this.

1 *Medication-related factors* – e.g. adverse effects, complex schedules of the drug itself or polypharmacy (especially in the elderly), cost and perceived lack of efficacy. Switching medication or treatment of side-effects are both common corrective strategies.
2 *Patient-specific factors* – e.g. psychiatric symptoms, severity of illness and age. These all need to be considered. Older people commonly have visual and auditory impairments, sometimes in combination with cognitive deficit.[74]
3 *Patients' attitudes* – psychosocial rehabilitation, improved patient–clinician relationship (where actively involving patients in treatment decisions can help) and the use of depot antipsychotics may be useful.

A survey by the National Schizophrenia Fellowship in the UK showed that the atypicals are preferred by the people who take them, and this finding was backed up by a survey of European psychiatrists who stated that this is what they would want themselves or their family to receive.

Because of this, together with the lack of superior efficacy and the relative toxicity of the typical antipsychotics, the latter are used infrequently in the elderly. Here the cost of the side-effects outweighs the cost of the drugs, and apart from graduates who remain on treatment, the drugs are rarely initiated as first-line treatment. This has now been endorsed in both the Older Persons' National Service Framework[75] and the National Institute for Clinical Excellence (NICE) guidance on atypical antipsychotics,[7] both of which recommend that new patients start on atypicals. The NICE guidance suggests that those on typicals with no side-effects should be left unchanged, but those with side-effects, especially EPS, should switch to atypicals.

Atypical antipsychotics in the elderly

Further discussion of the use of atypical antipsychotics in the elderly will be restricted to the most commonly prescribed atypical antipsychotics. Each drug will be subdivided as follows:

- schizophrenia and related psychosis
- psychosis in idiopathic Parkinson's disease, where 20–30% of such patients develop psychotic symptoms[76]
- the effect of these drugs on cognitive functioning in the elderly population. Preclinical and clinical studies indicate that an inhibitory effect on dopaminergic, cholinergic and histaminergic neurochemical systems may be responsible for the cognitive effects.[77] This explains the evidence that the use of antipsychotics in the elderly population can cause deleterious cognitive effects in some elderly patients.[78] Atypical antipsychotics may thus possess a more favourable cognitive profile than traditional agents in the elderly population.

The behavioural and psychological symptoms of dementia are discussed in Chapter 14.

Risperidone

Psychosis in the elderly

Risperidone is a benzisoxazole derivative licensed in the UK for the treatment of psychosis, including elderly patients. It followed clozapine on to the market and was rapidly accepted, as it did not carry the risk of agranulocytosis or the need to monitor the leukocyte count frequently. Technically it is not a classical atypical, as it elevates prolactin levels due to inhibition of dopamine in the tubero-infundibular system. The clinical implications of this effect in the elderly are unclear.

Early retrospective reviews and uncontrolled prospective studies indicated the benefits of risperidone treatment for both positive and negative symptoms in late-life schizophrenia.[79] The mean dose varied across the studies, with patients with schizophrenia tending to receive 4–6 mg/day (a very similar dose to the younger adult population). No controlled studies of risperidone in this treatment group have been published.

Jeste et al.[80] and Madhusoodanan et al.[81] reported the inability of elderly patients with schizophrenia to tolerate rapid titration of risperidone (1 mg/day to 3 mg/day twice daily over 3 days) and increased hypotensive episodes, respectively. Risperidone binding potently to α-1 and α-2 adrenergic receptors accounts for these reports of hypotension in some elderly patients. Davidson et al.[82] reported decreased symptoms, continuous improvement and improved EPS in an open-label study of graduate patients switched from typicals to risperidone.

The major metabolite 9-hydroxy-risperidone is active with a similar receptor profile to its parent drug. It remains present in plasma at concentrations 3 to 5 times higher than those of risperidone itself. This means that an elderly patient requires one-third of the risperidone dose needed in younger patients to achieve similar plasma concentrations of active drug. Peak plasma concentrations are reached after oral administration within 1–2 hours, and they are dose proportional.[83,84] Metabolism is via the CYP2D6 hepatic microsomal isoenzyme, which may predict potential drug–drug interactions in clinical use. Risperidone and 9-hydroxy-risperidone have half-lives of about 3 and 24 hours, respectively. A steady state occurs after 1 day for risperidone, and after 4.5 days for 9-hydroxy-risperidone. Excretion is mainly via the kidneys. The half-life of both active compounds is prolonged with age and in patients with hepatic or renal disease.

Consequently, the usual starting dosage in the elderly patient is 0.25–0.5 mg/day given as a single daily dose. This should be titrated to the minimum effective dosage, as anything higher in a susceptible individual may result in loss of atypicality and possible EPS or drug-induced parkinsonism.

Both risperidone and its metabolite 9-hydroxy-risperidone can prolong the QTc interval, so concomitant drugs that are also known to prolong this interval should be either avoided or administered very carefully.

Psychosis associated with idiopathic Parkinson's disease

Psychosis associated with Parkinson's disease poses particular treatment problems. Dopaminergic agents are usually indicated in the treatment of Parkinson's disease, but these agents frequently cause or exacerbate psychotic symptoms. On the other hand, agents that block dopamine can worsen mobility and tremor.

One of the two uncontrolled studies investigating the use of risperidone in Parkinson's disease-related psychosis, by Meco et al.,[85] showed it to be safe and effective without worsening EPS in the dose range 0.25–1.25 mg/day. Case reports by Rich et al.[86] demonstrated that higher doses (in the range 0.5–4 mg/day) exacerbated parkinsonism. However, the authors noted that the lower doses when slowly titrated may have shown better tolerability. A more recent review supports the use of low-dose risperidone in Parkinson's disease.[87] Relatively little information is available to guide physicians in the use of risperidone in dementia with Lewy bodies (DLB). Patients with DLB have been reported to both tolerate and not tolerate risperidone treatment. McKeith et al.[88] have reported rigidity in one patient with DLB.

Cognitive effects in the elderly

Controlled studies

The large double-blind trials by De Deyn et al.[19] and Katz et al.[20] in behavioural and psychological symptoms of dementia (BPSD) examined the cognitive effects of risperidone in patients with dementia. The first flexible dose study reached a mean dose of 1.1 mg/day of risperidone and the second had three fixed doses of risperidone (0.5, 1 or 2 mg/day). None of them found any adverse effect on the cognition of patients with mixed diagnoses of dementia.

Berman et al.[89] conducted a prospective, randomised, double-blind comparison study of risperidone and haloperidol in elderly patients with schizophrenia in order to examine the cognitive effects of these two drugs. They did so because earlier uncontrolled studies of risperidone indicated that the latter improved cognition in elderly patients. Berman et al. concluded that patients who were receiving risperidone improved on the Boston Naming Test (BNT) and Mini-Mental State Examination (MMSE), but not on other cognitive tests. Patients who were receiving haloperidol showed no improvement. This positive cognitive profile of risperidone can be attributed to its lack of significant anticholinergic effects.

Uncontrolled studies

An open-label study by Berman and Merson[90] in elderly patients with schizophrenia treated with risperidone revealed a statistically significant improvement on MMSE scores and also on three of six additional cognitive measures. An open-label study of risperidone by Workman et al.[91] in patients with dementia and idiopathic Parkinson's disease, reaching a mean dose of 1.9 mg/day of risperidone, showed no significant changes in mean MMSE scores. However, reports of the way in which risperidone affects cognition in DLB patients have not shown consistent outcomes.[71]

Conclusion

Risperidone is effective for psychosis in the elderly, but often needs doses equivalent to those used in younger patients. The therapeutic dose/side-effect ratio determines its use here in individual patients, but for most it is an effective treatment. In Parkinson's disease and DLB it has a role, but it must be started at 0.25 mg daily and titrated slowly, with monitoring for side-effects.

Olanzapine

Psychosis in the elderly

Olanzapine is one of the clozapine-derived antipsychotics, and initially looks to be a particularly suitable drug for the elderly, having very few drug–drug interactions and a favourable metabolic profile. It is a thienobenzodiazepine, principally metabolised by hepatic glucuronidation, and there is little evidence of a clinically significant reduction in this metabolic process with age (except in the very old and in patients with Alzheimer's disease). Renal or hepatic impairment does not significantly affect the pharmacokinetics of olanzapine, and dose adjustments are not usually required. Furthermore, with a mean half-life of 30 hours, it can be given once a day, which may be an important factor in aiding compliance. Elderly patients with schizophrenia and bipolar disorders require doses that are usually similar to those of their younger counterparts.

The drug is well absorbed, and peak serum concentrations are reached in approximately 6 hours. There is extensive first-pass metabolism, with about 40% of a dose being metabolised before it reaches the systemic circulation. Steady state occurs after a week. Olanzapine is 93% bound to plasma proteins, with a half-life averaging 30 hours. The commonest side-effects are somnolence (26%), dizziness, agitation, constipation, akathisia, postural hypotension and weight gain. Tardive dyskinesia may occur in about 1% of patients and can be irreversible. Orthostatic hypotension occurs in about 5.5% of patients. Hyperglycaemia, diabetes mellitus and ketoacidosis have been widely reported as drug-induced effects.[92,93]

A potential drawback of olanzapine in the elderly may be its anticholinergic propensity. This is real, although it is unclear how important it is clinically. There are claims that it has agonist activity on the cholinergic receptors as well, but more research is needed to confirm this. In general, drugs with anticholinergic activity are minimised in the elderly, so this may be a factor in some clinicians' judgement.

A prospective, open-label, 8-week trial of olanzapine therapy in elderly schizophrenic patients of mean age 70.6 years showed that olanzapine therapy (at a mean dose of 4.2 mg/day) was effective and well tolerated.[94]

A *post-hoc* analysis of efficacy and safety data from a double-blind, pivotal schizophrenia study comparing olanzapine with haloperidol was conducted on 59 patients aged 65 years or older.[95] This analysis again confirmed the overall efficacy and safety of olanzapine in these geriatric patients. The favourable risk–benefit balance seen at the daily dose of olanzapine used in this geriatric population (12.4 mg/day) was comparable to that seen at the dose used for younger patients with schizophrenia (12.6 mg/day).

Psychosis associated with idiopathic Parkinson's disease

A randomised, double-blind, parallel comparison of olanzapine and clozapine in patients with Parkinson's disease with chronic hallucinations revealed that olanzapine aggravated parkinsonism to such an extent that safety-stopping rules were invoked.[96] The researchers concluded that olanzapine should not be regularly used in the management of hallucinations in patients with Parkinson's disease. Manson et al.[97] conducted a randomised, placebo-controlled, double-blind, cross-over trial to assess the usefulness of low-dose olanzapine (2.5–7.5 mg/day) for levodopa-induced dyskinesias in patients with Parkinson's disease. This study concluded that low-dose olanzapine was effective in reducing dyskinesias in Parkinson's disease, but even at very low doses olanzapine could result in unacceptable increases in parkinsonism and 'off' time.

In an open-label study by Friedman et al.,[98] clozapine was substituted by olanzapine in psychiatrically stable patients with Parkinson's disease. This study revealed that 9 of the 12 patients with Parkinson's disease were unable to make this transition because of worsened parkinsonism with olanzapine. Most of the subjects preferred taking clozapine, despite the onerous monitoring procedure. Another open-label study by Graham et al.[99] concluded that olanzapine was effective in suppressing hallucinosis in patients with Parkinson's disease, but resulted in unacceptable exacerbation of motor disability. Conversely, an open-label, uncontrolled study by Wolters et al.[100] concluded that olanzapine with a mean dosage of 6.5 ± 3.9 mg/day was well tolerated in non-demented patients with psychotic symptoms associated with Parkinson's disease. In this study, patients demonstrated a significant improvement in the psychotic symptoms without worsening of parkinsonism. They were also able to tolerate further increases in the dosages of dopamino-mimetic drugs, with a subsequent improvement in motor functions and no exacerbation of psychosis. Similar results were reported by Aarsland et al.[101] Walker[102] found that 37.5% of patients with DLB who were given olanzapine demonstrated sensitivity reactions, but for the remainder a low dosage (2.5–7.5 mg) was effective.

Cognitive effects in the elderly

A study using olanzapine (5, 10 or 15 mg/day) in elderly patients with dementia looked at the cognitive effects of olanzapine. It reported that MMSE scores were not adversely affected clinically among any of the three groups receiving olanzapine compared with placebo.[21] Similar findings of unchanged MMSE scores compared with baseline were reported in a prospective, open-label study of elderly schizophrenic patients conducted by Sajatovic et al.[94] Other uncontrolled reports suggest that some elderly patients may experience adverse cognitive effects while taking olanzapine.[102,103]

Conclusion

Olanzapine appears to be very effective in elderly psychosis and schizophrenia-like syndromes, using the same treatment regimens as in younger patients. It is also given once daily, which can aid compliance. There are concerns about its anticholinergic profile, and mixed reports on cognition enhance this. In Parkinson's disease it appears to be particularly poorly tolerated, and in DLB it is potentially effective if tolerated. In summary, current evidence makes it one of the first-line choices for primary psychoses in the elderly, but it is perhaps less useful for behavioural problems or psychosis secondary to other organic disease. No controlled studies comparing risperidone with olanzapine in elderly psychotic patients have been published. Madhusoodanan et al.[81] reported data on 151 hospitalised patients treated with risperidone ($n = 114$) and olanzapine ($n = 37$). The response to treatment, interruption of treatment and side-effects were similar in the two groups.

Quetiapine

Psychosis in the elderly

Quetiapine is a dibenzothiazepine that is structurally similar to clozapine, and was introduced into clinical practice in 1997. Its claim was to be an agent efficacious in the treatment of schizophrenia, with exceptionally low potential for EPS even at higher doses and with little anticholinergic or prolactin-elevating action. Therapeutic indications are treatment of psychotic and behavioural disorders.

Quetiapine is administered orally, and is rapidly absorbed, with plasma levels peaking at about 1.5 hours. It is 83% protein bound and metabolised by the liver. Its half-life is about 6 hours, and clearance is reduced in the elderly. The principal adverse effects include drowsiness and postural hypotension.

To date, several abstracts but only limited published literature are available regarding the use of quetiapine in elderly patients. Madhusoodanan et al.[104] demonstrated the efficacy of quetiapine in 4 out of 7 elderly hospitalised patients aged between 61 and 72 years, with schizophrenia-related psychotic symptoms, schizoaffective disorder and bipolar disorder. There are no published controlled studies of quetiapine, but its efficacy in treating both the positive and negative symptoms of schizophrenia has been extrapolated from a number of controlled comparative clinical trials in younger patients.

A 52-week, open-label, multi-centre trial enrolling 184 elderly patients (mean age 76.1 years) was conducted by Tariot et al.[23] to assess the safety and efficacy of long-term quetiapine use in the elderly population. This trial enrolled elderly patients with a variety of neuropsychological disorders. In total, 72% had a psychosis due to general medical conditions such as Alzheimer's disease and 28% had other forms of psychosis, mainly schizophrenia. They were residing in a variety of settings, with a host of comorbid medical conditions and receiving numerous concomitant medications, thus reflecting real-world conditions. With a mean total daily dose of 137.5 mg (range 12.5–800 mg/day), this study concluded that quetiapine was safe and effective for the long-term treatment of psychosis in elderly populations, across all causes. The conclusions from the trial recommended an initial dosage of 25 mg/day, with increases in dose to a target of 100–150 mg, with individualised adjustments as needed. Analysis of the dropouts suggested the use of slow and steady dose escalation in elderly patients, especially when long-term use was anticipated. Quetiapine was associated with negligible EPS, no clinically important changes in laboratory parameters or ECG rates or intervals, and minimal weight gain.

To date, the results extrapolated from the controlled studies in younger patients, in combination with this open-label study in elderly patients, suggest that quetiapine may be beneficial in terms of both efficacy and tolerability in the treatment of elderly patients with psychotic symptoms. On the basis of the clinical literature on quetiapine, Jeste *et al.*[61] recommended that the starting dose of quetiapine in elderly patients should be 12.5 mg to 25 mg daily, with the optimal target dose being 75 mg to 125 mg per day.

Psychosis associated with idiopathic Parkinson's disease

Like other atypical antipsychotics, quetiapine has a clinical advantage in the treatment of psychosis associated with Parkinson's disease. It has a higher affinity for serotonin receptors than for dopamine D_1 and D_2 receptors, and has more affinity for mesolimbic than for nigrostriatal dopamine blockade. The dopamine blockade is only modest. This clinical advantage is reflected in encouraging results from studies using quetiapine in psychosis associated with Parkinson's disease.

An open-label study of the use of quetiapine in 40 patients (mean age 72.6 years) from the Tariot 1-year study who had psychosis associated with Parkinson's disease was reported by Juncos *et al.*[105] These patients were followed up for 1 year with a mean daily dose of 75 mg/day, showing that quetiapine was effective in improving psychotic symptoms in this patient group. This improvement was maintained throughout the 1-year trial period without worsening the motor symptoms of Parkinson's disease. In fact, surprisingly, a significant short-term improvement in motor performance in Parkinson's disease was observed. Similar results have been replicated in other open-label studies where the mean daily dose of quetiapine ranges from 37.5 to 70 mg/day. In DLB, Parsa[106] reported improved psychiatric symptoms with no worsening of confusion or motor symptoms.

Cognitive effects in the elderly

There are no published controlled trials of quetiapine in the elderly. An open-label study of quetiapine in elderly patients by McManus *et al.*[22] did not find any evidence of cognitive impairment in the first 12 weeks of the trial. Similar findings have been reported from case series and case reports.

Conclusion

The benign side-effect profile of quetiapine, along with the ability to use it in very low dosage, has made it an attractive choice in the elderly, but there is relatively little evidence to support it. It has worked well in open-labelled studies, notably the Tariot study, and has earned an anecdotal reputation for being 'motor friendly' – hence it is often favoured in Parkinson's disease and DLB. It seems to do little harm, but more controlled data are needed to show just what its benefits may prove to be.

Clozapine

Psychosis in the elderly

Clozapine is a dibenzodiazepine derivative with greater specificity for the limbic system and a subsequent low incidence of extrapyramidal side-effects. It was the first atypical antipsychotic to be launched, and it changed perceptions about what antipsychotic drugs could do in schizophrenia. Its adverse effects profile prevents it from being prescribed for first-episode patients, but at the time of writing it remains the gold standard for treatment-resistant patients.

Following oral administration, it is rapidly absorbed, but only 27–50% of a dose reaches the systemic circulation, due to an important first-pass metabolism.[107,108] Various individual factors can alter the response, such as smoking, hepatic metabolism, gastric absorption, age and sex. Clozapine is rapidly and extensively distributed, crossing the blood–brain barrier, and 95% is bound to plasma proteins.

Steady state is reached after 7–10 days, with maximum antipsychotic effect occurring several months later. Metabolism occurs primarily via the CYP1A2 and CYP3A4 hepatic microsomal enzymes and leads to two metabolites, namely nor-clozapine and clozapine-N-oxide. The half-life ranges from 6 to 33 hours, and about 50% is excreted in the urine and 30% in the faeces.

Clozapine lowers the seizure threshold and may precipitate grand-mal seizures, particularly in higher doses. It is less likely to cause extrapyramidal side-effects, but can exacerbate prostatic hypertrophy and closed-angle glaucoma due to anticholinergic activity. Tachycardia, orthostatic hypotension and raised glucose levels, with weight gain and diabetes, have all been reported.[109] Excessive sedation and somnolence frequently occur.

Most studies on the use of clozapine in elderly patients are based on retrospective chart reviews, and each seems to agree its place in treating psychosis in the elderly. Clozapine is licensed for this, but side-effects and safety issues limit its use. Elderly patients are not able to tolerate the rapid titration of clozapine dosage (target dose 300 mg/day in 3 weeks). It is recommended that a lower dose should be used to initiate treatment (12.5 mg once on the first day), and to restrict subsequent dose increments cautiously to 25 mg/day. The dosage must be adjusted individually, and for each patient the lowest effective dose should be used. With a mean clozapine dose range of 53–208 mg/day, a marked treatment response was reported in 33–90% of patients receiving the drug by Chengappa et al.,[110] Salzman et al.[111] and Richards et al.[112]

Clozapine is a potent antagonist at α-adrenergic, muscarinic and histaminergic receptors, which explains its ability to cause sedation and delirium in elderly patients. Orthostatic hypotension can occur, and there are reports of tachycardia in elderly patients, which may be sustained. Elderly patients, particularly those with compromised cardiovascular function, may be more susceptible to these effects. In such settings clozapine should be used at the lowest possible dosage, as all of the cardiac effects appear to be dose related.[113] Elderly patients may also be particularly susceptible to the anticholinergic effects of clozapine, such as constipation and urinary retention. Unlike clozapine's action at the other muscarinic receptor subtypes, clozapine is a full agonist at muscarinic M_4 receptors, which may partly explain its ability to cause hypersalivation and salivary gland swelling.

Special attention must be given to the issue of agranulocytosis and the probability of subsequent mortality in elderly patients. Reports indicate that increasing age and female gender are both independently associated with an increased risk of agranulocytosis.[114] As neither clozapine dosage nor plasma drug concentration have been found to be associated with the agranulocytosis risk, it appears that ageing-related changes in clozapine clearance may account for this increased rate of agranulocytosis in the elderly.[115] Thus the elderly appear to be more likely to develop agranulocytosis, and they may be more likely to die if agranulocytosis occurs.

Psychosis associated with idiopathic Parkinson's disease

Case reports, retrospective chart reviews, open-label trials and double-blind, placebo-controlled trials[116] have shown clozapine to be effective overall in the treatment of psychosis associated with Parkinson's disease. The doses required are generally substantially lower than those required for the treatment of patients with a primary psychiatric diagnosis. Several studies have also shown that clozapine can be used to manage psychosis while allowing optimisation of antiparkinsonian treatment and management of motor disability. There is little reported use of the drug in DLB, where caution would be necessary because of clozapine's particular anticholinergic activity. Burke *et al.*[117] have reported increasing confusion in two cases within 48 hours of use.

Cognitive effects in the elderly

Controlled studies

Two large, double-blind, placebo-controlled trials have evaluated the cognitive effects of low-dose clozapine (mean dose 24.7 mg/day and 36 mg/day) given for 4 weeks in patients with Parkinson's disease and drug-induced psychosis, respectively. Neither study found detrimental cognitive effects. Both studies found no differences in MMSE scores between clozapine- and placebo-treated groups.[116,118] A double-blind study of elderly patients with schizophrenia reported half the sedation rate compared with that of a chlorpromazine-treated group.[119]

Uncontrolled studies

In contrast, uncontrolled studies and case reports of clozapine treatment in patients with idiopathic Parkinson's disease and DLB have reported problematic sedation and/or confusion.

Conclusion

In the elderly, clozapine is less frequently utilised, mainly because of its side-effect profile, particularly the anticholinergic activity. It has a place in treatment-resistant psychosis in the elderly, but at much lower doses (< 200 mg) than in younger patients. For Parkinson's disease and BPSD there is evidence that it may help individual cases, but the risk–benefit cost is high, and other treatments should be preferentially tried first. Thus clozapine will usually be used as a last strategy in defined cases.

Amisulpiride

Amisulpiride is a substituted benzamide. No specific data on its use in the elderly have been published, but it is not anticholinergic and it can be initiated in very low doses. It is a pure D_2 antagonist with relative selectivity for the mesolimbic system. This clean profile and the lack of drug–drug interactions are often cited in support of its being a suitable drug for use in older people. It should perform similarly in psychosis in the elderly to that in younger patients,[120] and be safe in the treatment of BPSD. It also has a 15-year record of use in Europe in all age groups. However, the bottom line is that more research needs to be done if specific recommendations are to be made. The same is true of its parent compound, sulpiride.

Aripiprazole

Aripiprazole is an interesting compound that was licensed in the USA in late 2002 and is now available in Europe. It is perhaps the first of a new type of antipsychotic, as it has a different mode of action to anything that has preceded it. It is a partial agonist at the D_2 receptor as well as having the expected $5HT_{2A}$ serotonergic blockade. However, it also has $5HT_{1A}$ agonism, which gives an increased anxiolytic action and may offer some additional cognitive advantages. This profile should have an effect that serves to stabilise dopaminergic function, reducing the effect of dopamine at the receptor through competitive inhibition when dopamine levels are too high, and maintaining adequate dopamine function through its agonist action when levels are low.[121] It has a mild affinity for adrenergic and histaminic receptors, but no muscarinic affinity at all. This profile would make it attractive with regard to all aspects of elderly psychosis.

Aripiprazole is well absorbed, reaching peak plasma concentration at 5 hours. Its oral bioavailability is 87% and it can be taken with or without food. Its major metabolite is dehydro-aripiprazole, which has similar activity to the parent molecule. The half-life of aripiprazole is 75 hours, so it is taken daily. Steady state occurs at 14 days. Elimination is mainly through the hepatic enzymes CYP2D6 and CYP3A4, which means that there are some drug interactions, notably with paroxetine and fluoexetine, which may raise the levels of aripiprazole.

Aripiprazole does not need any dose alteration in renal or hepatic disease. In the elderly, single-dose pharmacokinetic studies showed a 20% lowering in the clearance of aripiprazole, yet multiple-dose studies showed no difference overall. Thus no dose changes are required in older patients. Studies in schizophrenia have shown favourable and consistent results across many studies.[122] Therefore elderly patients with schizophrenia or related psychotic episodes can be treated in the same way as those described. To date, patients treated with aripiprazole have shown a very low incidence of EPS, weight gain, sedation, hyperprolactinaemia, metabolic disorder or QTc changes.

Currently no specific studies have been published concerning aripiprazole use in the elderly. A placebo-controlled study of its use in 208 community-dwelling dementia patients with BPSD over a period of 10 weeks has been conducted. The mean age of patients was 81.5 years, and the mean baseline MMSE was 13.6. A mean dose of 10 mg/day showed that it was significantly more effective than placebo on both the total score and the psychotic subscore (-1.93 vs. -1.27; $P = 0.03$) of the Brief Psychiatric Rating Scale.[123] Discontinuation rates were 8% with aripiprazole and 7% with placebo. Somnolence was mild and not associated with falls or accidental injury. There were no differences in vital signs, laboratory tests, weight gain or ECG. The Neuropsychiatric Inventory was also used as an outcome in the study, but reduction of the total score at 10 weeks was similar in both groups.

The data suggest a favourable effect on psychosis in Alzheimer's disease, as well as schizophrenia. With its daily use, good tolerability profile and lack of any muscarinic activity, this may become an important choice in elderly patients with psychosis.

Ziprasidone

Ziprasidone is a new antipsychotic agent with a high $5HT_2$ to D_2 receptor blockade ratio. It is available orally and in a short-acting injectable form (neither of which is yet available in the UK), and is effective on both positive and negative symptoms. Given orally, it is rapidly absorbed, with steady-state serum levels being reached within 2–3 days,[124] and age does not affect its pharmacokinetics. It does not cause weight gain or orthostatic hypotension, but it has been suggested that it may increase the QTc interval.[125]

There are no published reports of ziprasidone treatment specifically in the elderly. However, as this drug is nearly devoid of anticholinergic activity, it appears that it may have favourable effects in patients with cholinergic dysfunction, including those with Alzheimer's disease. It should be able to be used to treat psychosis in the elderly in a similar fashion to that in younger patients.

Zotepine

Zotepine is a dibenzothiepine licensed for use as an atypical for schizophrenia.[126] It is more difficult to use in the elderly, in whom some severe side-effects have been reported, including tachycardia, hypotension, prolongation of the QTc interval, somnolence and sleep disorders. Parkinsonian side-effects were reported in about 5.3% of the patients treated, and seizures were observed at higher doses.[127] There seems to be little evidence to support its use in the elderly.

Long-acting injectable antipsychotics

To date, low-dose fluphenazine has been the preferred typical depot antipsychotic for elderly patients because it produces less sedation, postural hypotension and anticholinergic effects.[38] Long-acting atypical antipsychotic formulations have long been awaited because of the improved efficacy of the base compounds[128] and the reduced expectancy of EPS and tardive dyskinesia. Risperidone is now the first agent to be approved in a long-acting injectable formulation.

The long delay in formulating this depot has been due to the fact that, because of its lack of a hydroxyl group, risperidone cannot be esterified so it cannot be oil-based. However, the new formulation encapsulates risperidone in 'microspheres' made of a biodegradable polymer that is delivered in a water-based vehicle. This provides a steady release of risperidone, with the polymer dissolving to form water and carbon end-products.

There have been very few studies of the use of depot antipsychotics in elderly patients, but those that exist suggest positive outcomes. A total of 20 patients with chronic schizophrenia (ranging in age from 60 to 73 years) were treated with fluphenazine decanoate, 12.5 mg administered every 21 days for 6 months.[129] This effectively treated emotional withdrawal, blunted affect, suspiciousness and thought disturbances, but not hallucinations. Raskind *et al.*[130] compared 5 mg fluphenazine every 2 weeks with oral haloperidol 2 mg three times daily for 6 weeks in elderly patients with late-onset schizophrenia. In total, 11 out of 13 fluphenazine patients improved, compared with 3 out of 13 in the haloperidol group. This was considered to be due to improved compliance. Low-dose depot zuclopenthixol was effective over a period of 12 weeks in treating persistent psychomotor agitation and psychosis in six patients with Alzheimer's disease.[131] Low doses of fluphenazine enanthate in 10 elderly patients also improved BPSD.[132]

One study involving risperidone in long-acting injectable form has been reported in stable psychotic elderly patients.[133] Patients of mean age of 70.9 years were treated with long-acting risperidone 25 mg ($n = 24$), 50 mg ($n = 17$) or 75 mg ($n = 2$) for up to 50 weeks. Even though patients were clinically stable at entry to the study, 49% showed a 20% reduction in their total positive and negative symptoms in schizophrenia (PANSS) score and 54.5% showed an improvement on the clinical global impression (CGI).[134]

In these elderly patients there were no cases of tardive dyskinesia as assessed by defined research criteria.[135] The most common adverse events were insomnia (10.5%), constipation (10.5%) and bronchitis (12.3%). Weight gain was 0.3 kg on average, and changes in ECG and vital signs were not clinically relevant. This suggests that this new method of delivery is safe and effective over a period of a year in this comparatively frail patient group, even above the current recommendation of 25 mg.

Short-acting injectable antipsychotics

Clopenthixol acetate has been used in the elderly, but no research evidence supports this. It exposes patients to all the risks of typical antipsychotics seen with other formulations. Lorazepam is also used for rapid tranquillisation – again with no controlled data, and there is an increased risk of falls and sedation. A short-acting injectable preparation of olanzapine has been compared with intramuscular lorazepam and placebo in the elderly.[136] Both proved superior to placebo, with olanzapine producing a faster and more sustained response. When available, this may prove a therapeutic choice when rapid tranquillisation is needed, and it may offer a more sensible alternative to the large haloperidol doses that are often prescribed in acute hospitals.

Conclusion

Because the use of typical antipsychotics has fallen out of favour with geriatric psychiatrists, so too has the use of depot medication over the last 10 years, except where there has been an absolute need to trade off potential side-effects against the need for efficacy. The availability of a long-acting injectable atypical antipsychotic will be a welcome addition to the formulary, especially for the late-onset schizophrenia patients who are notoriously resistant to treatment. These patients can tolerate doses similar to those used in younger adults, so are able to tolerate all three doses involved. The lowest dose available delivers a 2 mg/day serum level. However, this may be too high for patients with BPSD, and further research is needed to clarify this.

Key points

The increasing use of atypical antipsychotics in the elderly has highlighted a number of important considerations.

- The use of these drugs needs to be put into individual context. It is not always necessary to treat a patient with late delusional disorder, and cases of BPSD should have non-pharmacological methods tried first. The use of antipsychotics as a panacea has now become much less common.
- The mantra of 'start low, go slow' now has some caveats. Low doses of typicals do not always prove efficacious,[137,138] and low-dose olanzapine has proved no more effective than placebo in one study.[139] Elderly patients with schizophrenia tolerate similar doses to younger ones. Starting too low may not be therapeutic, so rapid escalation to similar doses may be necessary to control symptoms.
- The real issue in using antipsychotics is side-effects. These will determine the outcome of the treatment selected, and the whole rationale of making the choice involves balancing efficacy against side-effects. In an individual patient this means regular review, in the early stages to look for known side-effects in order to minimise them or change the drug, and in the later stages either to look for later-developing side-effects or to review whether continuation is necessary. Clearly, the complexity of titration and subsequent review will also affect clinical preference and choice.
- The cytochrome P450 system can determine drug–drug interactions. How much this affects clinical practice is uncertain, but all attempts to reduce adverse events, especially cardiological ones, should be encouraged. Elongated QTc intervals are a problem with many of the antipsychotics. Care must be taken with patients who have risk factors, especially those who are on polypharmacy.
- Most of these drugs are technically being used off-licence, as apart from risperidone, which is licensed for psychosis, they are all usually licensed for schizophrenia. This increase in indications is being addressed by research. However, as a rule of thumb it is safe to assume that an antipsychotic should treat the common psychotic symptoms, and provided that this remains the rationale for their use, medical opinion will support it.
- Atypical antipsychotic agents have a significant role to play in the treatment of schizophrenia and other psychosis in late life. However, further studies in the elderly population are still required to make certain issues clearer, and until then these agents should be introduced carefully at relevant doses in elderly patients. Conversely, typicals seem to be relatively ineffective in BPSD, problematic with Parkinson's disease and DLB, and for primary psychosis their indefinite use will increase the

risk of TD. Therefore in principle it would seem that their use in the elderly is now severely limited.

- Elderly patients with major comorbidity, such as dementia or other serious physical illnesses, will require doses of atypicals at the lower end of their respective ranges. Conversely, patients with schizophrenia-like illnesses without significant comorbidity will need and tolerate higher doses, similar to the doses used in younger patients.

References

1 Targum SD (2001) Treating psychotic symptoms in elderly patients. *J Clin Psychiatry.* **3:** 156–63.

2 Lyketsos CG, Steinberg M, Tschanz JT *et al.* (2000) Mental and behavioural disturbances in dementia: findings from the Cache County study on memory and aging. *Am J Psychiatry.* **157:** 708–14.

3 Maletta GJ (1990) Pharmacologic treatment and management of the aggressive demented patient. *Psychiatr Ann.* **20:** 446–55.

4 Furniss L, Craig SK and Burns A (1998) Medication use in nursing homes for elderly people. *Int J Geriatr Psychiatry.* **3:** 433–9.

5 Schneider LS (1993) Efficacy of treatment for geropsychiatric patients with severe mental illness. *Psychopharmacol Bull.* **29:** 501–24.

6 Raskind MA and Risse SC (1986) Antipsychotic drugs and the elderly. *J Clin Psychiatry.* **47 (Suppl.):** 17–22.

7 National Institute for Clinical Excellence (2002) *Guidance on the Use of Newer (Atypical) Antipsychotic Drugs for the Treatment of Schizophrenia.* NICE Technology Appraisal No 43. National Institute for Clinical Excellence, London.

8 Harris MJ and Jeste DV (1988) Late-onset schizophrenia: an overview. *Schizophr Bull.* **14:** 39–55.

9 Levy R and Naguib M (1985) Late Paraphrenia. *Br J Psych.* **146:** 451.

10 Ameida OP, Howard RJ, Levy R and David AS (1995) Psychotic states arising in late life (late paraphrenia): the role of risk factors. *Br J Psychiatry.* **166:** 215–28.

11 Tran-Johnson TK, Krull AJ and Jeste DV (1992) Late-life schizophrenia and its treatment: pharmacologic issues in older schizophrenia patients. *Clin Geriatr Med.* **8:** 401–10.

12 Jeste DV, Harris MJ, Peralson GD *et al.* (1988) Late-onset schizophrenia: studying clinical validity. *Psychiatr Clin North Am.* **11:** 1–14.

13 Evans DA, Funkenstein HH, Albert MS *et al.* (1989) Prevalence of Alzheimer's disease in a community population of older persons: higher than previously reported. *JAMA.* **262:** 2551–6.

14 Wragg R and Jeste DV (1989) Overview of depression and psychosis in Alzheimer's disease. *Am J Psychiatry.* **146:** 577–87.

15 Schneider LS, Pollock VE and Lyness SA (1990) A meta-analysis of controlled trials of neuroleptic treatment in dementia. *J Am Geriatr Soc.* **38:** 553–63.

16 Lanctot KL, Best TS, Mittmann N *et al.* (1998) Efficacy and safety of neuroleptics in behavioral disorders associated with dementia. *J Clin Psychiatry.* **59:** 550–61.

17 Kindermann SS, Dolder CR, Bailey A, Katz IR and Jeste DV (2002) Pharmacological treatment of psychosis and agitation in elderly patients with dementia: four decades of experience. *Drugs Aging.* **19:** 257–76.

18 Brodaty H, Ames D, Snowdon J *et al*. (2003) A randomized placebo-controlled trial of risperidone for the treatment of aggression, agitation and psychosis of dementia. *J Clin Psychiatry*. **64**: 134–43.

19 De Deyn PP, Rabheru K, Rasmussen A *et al*. (1999) A randomized trial of risperidone, placebo, and haloperidol for behavioral symptoms of dementia. *Neurology*. **53**: 899–901.

20 Katz IR, Jeste DV, Mintzer JE, Clyde C, Napolitano J and Brecher M (1999) Comparison of risperidone and placebo for psychosis and behavioral disturbances associated with dementia: a randomized, double-blind trial. Risperidone Study Group. *J Clin Psychiatry*. **60**: 107–15.

21 Street JS, Clark WS, Gannon KS *et al*. (2000) Olanzapine treatment of psychotic and behavioral symptoms in patients with Alzheimer disease in nursing care facilities: a double-blind, randomized, placebo-controlled trial. *Arch Gen Psychiatry*. **57**: 968–76.

22 McManus DQ, Arvanitis LA and Kowalcyk BB (1999) Quetiapine, a novel anti-psychotic: experience in elderly patients with psychotic disorders. Seroquel Trial 48 Study Group. *J Clin Psychiatry*. **60**: 292–8.

23 Tariot PN, Salzman C, Yeung PP, Pultz J and Rak IW (2000) Long-term use of quetiapine in elderly patients with psychotic disorders. *Clin Ther*. **22**: 1068–84.

24 Sipahimalani A and Masand PS (1998) Olanzapine in the treatment of delirium. *Psychosomatics*. **39**: 422–30.

25 Meagher DJ (2001) Delirium: optimising management. *BMJ*. **322**: 144–9.

26 Rahkonen T, Makela H, Paanila S *et al*. (2000) Delirium in elderly people without severe predisposing disorders: aetiology and one-year prognosis after discharge. *Int Psychogeriatr*. **12**: 437–81.

27 Cole MG (1999) Delirium: effectiveness of systematic interventions. *Dementia Geriatr Cogn Disord*. **10**: 406–11.

28 Khouzam HR and Gazula K (2001) Clinical experience with olanzapine in the course of post-operative delirium associated with psychosis in geriatric patients: a report of three cases. *Int J Psychiatry Clin Pract*. **5**: 63–6.

29 Glick ID, Murray SR, Vasudevan P, Marder SR and Hu RJ (2001) Treatment with atypical antipsychotics: new indications and new populations. *J Psychiatr Res*. **35**: 187–91.

30 Flint AJ and Rifat SL (1998) The treatment of psychotic depression in later life: a comparison of pharmacotherapy and ECT. *Int J Geriatr Psychiatry*. **13**: 23–8.

31 Shulman KI and Herrmann N (1999) The nature and management of mania in old age. *Psychiatr Clin North Am*. **22**: 649–65.

32 Umapathy C, Mulsant BH and Pollock BG (2000) Bipolar disorder in the elderly. *Psychiatr Ann*. **30**: 473–80.

33 McDonald WM (2000) Epidemiology, etiology and treatment of geriatric mania. *J Clinical Psychiatry*. **61 (Suppl. 13)**: 3–11.

34 Masand PS (2000) Side-effects of antipsychotics in the elderly. *J Clin Psychiatry*. **61 (Suppl. 8)**: 43–9.

35 American Psychiatric Association (1997) Practice guideline for the treatment of patients with schizophrenia. *Am J Psychiatry*. **154 (Suppl. 4)**: 1–63.

36 Jeste DV, Lacro JP, Gilbert PL, Kline J and Kline N (1993) Treatment of late-life schizophrenia with neuroleptics. *Schizophr Bull*. **19**: 17–30.

37 Jeste DV, Gladsjo JA, Lindamer LA and Lacro JP (1996) Medical comorbidity in schizophrenia. *Schizophr Bull*. **22**: 413–30.

38 Sajatovic M, Madhusoodanan S and Buckley P (2000) Schizophrenia in the elderly: guidelines for management. *CNS Drugs*. **13**: 103–15.

39 Delay J, Deniker P and Harl JM (1952) Traitements d'etats confusionnels par le chlorhydrate de diethylaminopropyl-N-chlorophenothiazine (4560 RP). *Ann Med Psychol*. **110**: 398–403.

40 Carlsson A and Lindqvist M (1963) Effect of chlorpromazine or haloperidol on formation of 3-methoxytyramine and normetanephrine in mouse brain. *Acta Pharmacol Toxicol.* **20**: 140–4.

41 van Rossum JM (1966) The significance of dopamine-receptor blockade for the mechanism of action of neuroleptic drugs. *Arch Int Pharmacodyn Ther.* **160**: 492–4.

42 Toru M (1998) Biological research on schizophrenia. *Psychiatr Clin Neurosci.* **52 (Suppl.)**: 170–2.

43 Jackson DM and Westlind-Danielson A (1994) Dopamine receptors: molecular biology, biochemistry and behavioral aspects. *Pharmacol Ther.* **64**: 291–369.

44 Gerfen CR, Engber TM, Mahan LC *et al.* (1990) D_1 and D_2 dopamine receptor-regulated gene expression of nigrostriatal and striatopallidal neurons. *Science.* **250**: 1429–32.

45 Gingrich JA and Caron MG (1993) Recent advances in the molecular biology of dopamine receptors. *Ann Rev Neurosci.* **16**: 299–321.

46 Jaber M, Robinson SW and Missale C *et al.* (1996) Dopamine receptors and brain function. *Neuropharmacol.* **35**: 1503–19.

47 Creese I, Schneider R and Snyder SH (1977) H3 spiroperidol labels dopamine receptors in pituitary and brain. *Eur J Pharmacol.* **46**: 377–81.

48 Demchyshyn LL, Sugamori KS, Lee FJS *et al.* (1995) The dopamine D_1D receptor. Cloning and characterization of three pharmacologically distinct D_1-like receptors from Gallus domesticus. *J Biol Chem.* **270**: 72–6.

49 Hersch SM, Ciliax BJ, Gutekunst CA *et al.* (1995) Electron microscopic analysis of D_1 and D_2 dopamine-receptor proteins in the dorsal striatum and their synaptic relationship with motor corticostriatal afferents. *J Neurosci.* **15**: 5222–37.

50 Nyberg S, Nakashima Y, Nordstrom AL *et al.* (1996) Positron emission tomography of *in vivo* binding characteristic of atypical antipsychotic drugs. Review of D_2 and $5HT_2$ receptor occupancy studies and clinical response. *Br J Psychiatry.* **168**: 40–4.

51 Bristow LJ, Kramer MS, Kulagowski J *et al.* (1997) Schizophrenia and L-745870, a novel dopamine D_4 receptor antagonist. *Trends Pharmacol Sci.* **18**: 186–8.

52 Maixner SM, Mellow AM and Tandon R (1999) The efficacy, safety and tolerability of antipsychotics in the elderly. *J Clin Psychiatry.* **60 (Suppl. 8)**: 29–41.

53 Caligiuri MP, Lacro JP and Jeste DV (1999) Incidence and predictors of drug-induced parkinsonism in older psychiatric patients treated with very low doses of neuroleptics. *J Clin Psychopharmacol.* **19**: 322–8.

54 Hoffman WF, Labs SM and Casey DE (1987) Neuroleptic-induced parkinsonism in older schizophrenics. *Biol Psychiatry.* **22**: 427–39.

55 Jeste DV, Caligiuri MP, Paulsen JS *et al.* (1995) Risk of tardive dyskinesia in older patients: a prospective longitudinal study of 266 outpatients. *Arch Gen Psychiatry.* **52**: 756–65.

56 Volkow ND, Wang GJ, Fowler JS *et al.* (1998) Parallel loss of presynaptic and postsynaptic dopamine markers in normal aging. *Ann Neurol.* **44**: 143–7.

57 Zhang L and Roth GS (1997) The effect of aging on rat striatal D_1 receptor mRNA-containing neurons. *Neurobiol Aging.* **18**: 251–5.

58 Beasley CM, Dellva MA, Tamura RN *et al.* (1999) Randomised double-blind comparison of the incidence of tardive dyskinesia in patients with schizophrenia during long-term treatment with olanzapine or haloperidol. *Br J Psychiatry.* **174**: 23–30.

59 Jeste DV, Okamoto A, Napolitano J, Kane JM and Martinez RA (2000) Low incidence of persistent tardive dyskinesia in elderly patients with dementia treated with risperidone. *Am J Psychiatry.* **157**: 1150–5.

60 Tran PV, Dellva MA, Tollefson GD, Beasley CM Jr, Potvin JH and Kiesler GM (1997) Extrapyramidal symptoms and tolerability of olanzapine versus haloperidol in the acute treatment of schizophrenia. *J Clin Psychiatry.* **58**: 205–11.

61 Jeste DV, Rockwell E, Harris MJ *et al.* (1999) Conventional vs newer antipsychotics in elderly patients. *Am J Geriatr Psychiatry.* **7**: 70–6.

62 Timmell AM (2000) Thioridazine: re-evaluating the risk/benefit equation. *Ann Clin Psychiatry.* **12**: 147–51.

63 Kinon BJ and Lieberman JA (1996) Mechanisms of action of atypical antipsychotic drugs: a critical analysis. *Psychopharmacology.* **124**: 2–34.

64 Bitello B, Martin A, Hill J *et al.* (1997) Cognitive and behavioural effects of cholinergic, dopaminergic and serotonergic blockade in humans. *Neuropsychopharmacology.* **16**: 15–24.

65 Kapur S and Remington G (2001) Atypical antipsychotics: new directions and new challenges in the treatment of schizophrenia. *Annu Rev Med.* **52**: 503–17.

66 Mansour A, Meador-Woodruff JH, Lopez JF and Watson FJ (1998) Biochemical anatomy: insights into the cell biology and pharmacology of the dopamine and serotonergic systems in the brain. In: AF Schatzberg (ed.) *Textbook of Psychopharmacology* (2e). American Psychiatric Press, Washington, DC.

67 Taylor D and Aitchison K (1999) The pharmaco-economics of atypical antipsychotics. *Int J Psychiatr Clin Pract.* **3**: 237–48.

68 Almond S and O'Donnell O (2000) Cost analysis of the treatment of schizophrenia in the UK. A simulation model comparing olanzapine, risperidone and haloperidol. *Pharmacoeconomics.* **17**: 383–9.

69 Masand PS and Gupta S (2000) Long-term adverse effects of novel antipsychotics. *J Psychiatr Pract.* **6**: 299–309.

70 Henderson DC (2002) Atypical antipsychotic-induced diabetes mellitus: how strong is the evidence? *CNS Drugs.* **16**: 77–89.

71 Buckley NA and Sanders P (2000) Cardiovascular adverse effects of antipsychotic drugs. *Drug Safety.* **23**: 215–28.

72 Adams SG and Howe JT (1993) Predicting medication compliance in a psychotic population. *J Nerv Ment Dis.* **181**: 558–60.

73 Breen R and Thornhill JT (1998) Noncompliance with medication for psychiatric disorders. *CNS Drugs.* **9**: 457–71.

74 Wynn Owen PA and Castle DJ (1999) Late-onset schizophrenia: epidemiology, diagnosis, management and outcomes. *Drugs Aging.* **15**: 81–9.

75 Department of Health (2001) *National Service Framework: medicines and older people.* Department of Health, London.

76 Kuzuhara S (2001) Drug-induced psychotic symptoms in Parkinson's disease. Problems, management and dilemma. *J Neurol.* **248 (Suppl. 3)**: 28–31.

77 Byerly MJ, Weber MT, Brooks DL *et al.* (2001) Antipsychotic medications and the elderly: effects on cognition and implication for use. *Drug Aging.* **18**: 45–61.

78 McShane R, Keene J, Gedling K *et al.* (1996) Do neuroleptic drugs hasten cognitive decline in dementia? *BMJ.* **314**: 266–70.

79 Czobor P, Volavka J and Meibach RC (1995) Effect of risperidone on hostility in schizophrenia. *J Clin Psychopharmacol.* **15**: 243–9.

80 Jeste DV, Eastham JH, Lacro JP *et al.* (1996) Management of late-life psychosis. *J Clin Psychiatry.* **57**: 39–45.

81 Madhusoodanan S, Brenner R, Araujo L *et al.* (1995) Efficacy of risperidone treatment for psychosis associated with schizophrenia, schizoaffective disorder, bipolar disorder, or senile dementia in 11 geriatric patients: a case series. *J Clin Psychiatry.* **56**: 514–18.

82 Davidson M, Harvey PD, Vervarcke J *et al.* (2000) A long-term, multicenter, open-label study of risperidone in elderly patients with psychosis. On behalf of the Risperidone Working Group. *Int J Geriatr Psychiatry.* **15**: 506–14.

83 He H and Richardson JS (1995) A pharmacological, pharmacokinetic and clinical overview of risperidone, a new antipsychotic that blocks serotonin $5HT_2$ and dopamine D_2 receptors. *Int Clin Psychopharmacol.* **10**: 19–30.

84 Byerly MJ and De Vane CL (1996) Pharmacokinetics of clozapine and risperidone: a review of recent literature. *J Clin Psychopharmacol.* **16**: 177–87.
85 Meco G, Alessandria A, Bonifati V *et al.* (1994) Risperidone for hallucinations in levodopa-treated Parkinson's disease patients. *Lancet.* **343**: 1370–1.
86 Rich SS, Friedman JH and Ott BR (1995) Risperidone versus clozapine in the treatment of psychosis in six patients with Parkinson's disease and other akinetic-rigid syndromes. *J Clin Psychiatry.* **56**: 556–9.
87 Schweitzer I (2001) Does risperidone have a place in the treatment of nonschizophrenic patients? *Int Clin Psychopharmacol.* **16**: 1–19.
88 McKeith IG, Ballard CG and Harrison RWS (1995) Neuroleptic sensitivity to risperidone in Lewy body dementia. *Lancet.* **346**: 699.
89 Berman I, Merson A, Allan E *et al.* (1995) Effect of risperidone on cognitive performance in elderly schizophrenic patients: a double-blind comparison study with haloperidol. *Psychopharmacol Bull.* **31**: 552–6.
90 Berman I and Merson A (1996) Risperidone in elderly schizophrenic patients. *Am J Geriatr Psychiatry.* **4**: 173–9.
91 Workman R Jr, Orengo CA, Bakey AA *et al.* (1997) The use of risperidone for psychosis and agitation in demented patients with Parkinson's disease. *J Neuropsychol Clin Neurosci.* **9**: 594–7.
92 Bonanno DG, Davydov L and Botts SR (2001) Olanzapine-induced diabetes mellitus. *Ann Pharmacother.* **35**: 563–5.
93 Liebzeit KA, Markowitz JS and Caley CF (2001) New-onset diabetes and atypical antipsychotics. *Eur Neuropsychopharmacol.* **11**: 25–32.
94 Sajatovic M, Perez D, Brescan D *et al.* (1998) Olanzapine therapy in elderly patients with schizophrenia. *Psychopharmacol Bull.* **34**: 819–23.
95 Tollefson GD, Beasley CM and Tran PV (1997) Olanzapine versus haloperidol in the treatment of schizophrenia and schizoaffective and schizophreniform disorders: results of an international collaborative trial. *Am J Psychiatry.* **154**: 457–65.
96 Goetz CG, Blasucci LM, Leurgans S *et al.* (2000) Olanzapine and clozapine: comparative effects on motor function in hallucinating PD patients. *Neurology.* **55**: 789–94.
97 Manson AJ, Schrag A, Lees AJ *et al.* (2000) Low-dose olanzapine for levodopa-induced dyskinesias. *Neurology.* **55**: 795–9.
98 Friedman JH, Goldstein S and Jacques C (1998) Substituting clozapine for olanzapine in psychiatrically stable Parkinson's disease patients: results of an open-label pilot study. *Clin Neuropharmacol.* **21**: 285–8.
99 Graham JM, Sussman JD, Ford KS *et al.* (1998) Olanzapine in the treatment of hallucinosis in idiopathic Parkinson's disease: a cautionary note. *J Neurol Neurosurg Psychiatry.* **65**: 774–7.
100 Wolters EC, Jansen ENH, Tuynman-Qua HG *et al.* (1996) Olanzapine in the treatment of dopaminomimetic psychosis in patients with Parkinson's disease. *Neurology.* **47**: 1082–7.
101 Aarsland D, Larsen JP, Lim NG *et al.* (1999) Olanzapine for psychosis in patients with Parkinson's disease with and without dementia. *J Neuropsychiatry Clin Neurosci.* **11**: 392–4.
102 Walker Z, Grace J, Overshot R *et al.* (1999) Olanzapine in dementia with Lewy bodies: a clinical study. *Int J Geriatr Psychiatry.* **14**: 459–66.
103 Gaile S and Noviasky JA (1998) Speech disturbances and marked decrease in function seen in several older patients on olanzapine. *J Am Geriatr Soc.* **46**: 1330–1.
104 Madhusoodanan S, Brenner R and Alcantra A (2000) Clinical experience with quetiapine in elderly patients with psychotic disorders. *J Geriatr Psychiatry Neurol.* **13**: 28–32.
105 Juncos J, Yeung P, Sweitzer D *et al.* (1999) Quetiapine improves psychotic symptoms associated with Parkinson's disease. *Schizophr Res.* **36**: 283–7.

106 Parsa E (1999) *Quetiapine in Parkinson's disease and dementia with Lewy bodies*. Poster abstract from meeting of World Psychiatric Association, Hamburg. 6–11 August.

107 Taylor D (1997) Pharmacokinetic interactions involving clozapine. *Br J Psychiatry.* **171**: 109–12.

108 Markowitz JS, Brown CS and Moore TR (1999) Atypical antipsychotics. Part I. Pharmacology, pharmacokinetics and efficacy. *Ann Pharmacother.* **33**: 73–85.

109 Mir S and Taylor D (2001) Atypical antipsychotics and hyperglicaemia. *Int Clin Psychopharmacol.* **16**: 63–74.

110 Chengappa KNR, Baker RW, Kreinbrook SB *et al.* (1995) Clozapine use in female geriatric patients with psychosis. *J Geriatr Psychiatry Neurol.* **8**: 12–15.

111 Salzman C, Vaccaro B, Lieff J *et al.* (1995) Clozapine in older patients with psychosis and behavioral disruption. *Am J Geriatr Psychiatry.* **3**: 26–33.

112 Richards SS, Sweet RA and Ganguli R (1996) Clozapine: acute and maintenance treatment in late-life psychosis. *Am J Psychiatry.* **4**: 377–88.

113 Reilly JG, Ayis SA and Ferrier IN (2000) QTc-interval abnormalities and psychotropic drug therapy in psychiatric patients. *Lancet.* **355**: 1048–52.

114 Alvir JJ, Lieberman JA, Safferman AZ *et al.* (1993) Clozapine-induced agranulocytosis: incidence and risk factors in the United States. *NEJM.* **329**: 162–7.

115 Centorrino F, Baldessarini RJ, Flood JG *et al.* (1995) Relation of leukocyte counts during clozapine treatment to serum concentrations of clozapine and metabolites. *Am J Psychiatry.* **152**: 610–12.

116 Parkinson Study Group (1999) Low-dose clozapine for the treatment of drug-induced psychosis in Parkinson's disease. *NEJM.* **340**: 757–63.

117 Burke WJ, Pfeiffer RF and McComb RD (1998) Neuroleptic sensitivity to clozapine in dementia with Lewy bodies. *J Neuropsychiatry Clin Neurosci.* **10**: 227–9.

118 French Clozapine Parkinson Study Group (1999) Clozapine in drug-induced psychosis in Parkinson's disease. *Lancet.* **353**: 2041–2.

119 Howanitz E, Pardo M, Smelson DA *et al.* (1999) The efficacy and safety of clozapine versus chlorpromazine in geriatric schizophrenia. *J Clin Psychiatry.* **60**: 41–4.

120 Waddington J and Casey D (2000) Comparative pharmacology of classical and novel (second-generation) antipsychotics. In: PF Buckley and JL Waddington (eds) *Schizophrenia and Mood Disorders.* Butterworth Heinemann, Oxford.

121 Carlsson A, Waters N, Waters S and Carlsson ML (2000) Network interactions in schizophrenia – therapeutic implications. *Brain Res Rev.* **31**: 342–9.

122 Marder SR, McQuade RD, Stock E *et al.* (2003) Aripiprazole in the treatment of schizophrenia: safety and tolerability in short-term, placebo-controlled trials. *Schizophr Res.* **61**: 121–36.

123 DeDeyn P, Jeste D, Auby P *et al.* (2003) *Aripiprazole in dementia of the Alzheimer's type.* Paper presented at the American Association for Geriatric Psychiatry Sixteenth Annual Meeting, Hawaii, 1–4 March.

124 Wilner KD, Tensfeldt TG, Baris B *et al.* (2000) Single- and multiple-dose pharmacokinetics of ziprasidone in healthy young and elderly volunteers. *Br J Clin Pharmacol.* **49 (Suppl. 1)**: 15–20S.

125 Stimmel GL, Gutierrez MA and Lee V (2002) Ziprasidone: an atypical antipsychotic drug for the treatment of schizophrenia. *Clin Ther.* **24**: 21–37.

126 Cooper SJ, Butler A, Tweed J *et al.* (2000) Zotepine in the prevention of recurrence: a randomised, double-blind, placebo-controlled study for chronic schizophrenia. *Psychopharmacology.* **150**: 237–43.

127 Hori M, Suzuki T, Sasaki M *et al.* (1992) Convulsive seizures in schizophrenic patients induced by zotepine administration. *Jpn J Psychiatry Neurol.* **46**: 161–7.

128 Csernansky JG, Mahmoud R and Brenner R for the Risperidone-USA-79 Study Group (2002) A comparison of risperidone and haloperidol for the prevention of relapse in patients with schizophrenia. *NEJM.* **346**: 16–22.

129 Altamura AC, Mauri MC, Girardi T and Panetta B (1990) Clinical and toxicological profile of fluphenazine in elderly chronic schizophrenia. *Int J Clin Pharmacol Res.* **10**: 223–8.

130 Raskind M, Alvarez C and Herlin S (1979) Fluphenazine enanthate in the treatment of late paraphrenia. *J Am Geriatr Soc.* **27**: 459–63.

131 Robles A, Rodriguez Navarrete FJ, Taboada O, Docasar L, Paramo M and Noya M (1996) A preliminary study of low-dosage zuclopenthixol depot in Alzheimer's disease. *Rev Neurol.* **24**: 273–5.

132 Finkel SI (1998) Antipsychotics: old and new. *Clin Geriatr Med.* **14**: 87–100.

133 Gharabawi G, Erdekens M, Zhu Y and Lasser R (2001) *Long-acting risperidone for the management of elderly patients with psychotic disorders: a favorable benefit/risk ratio.* Paper presented at the First Annual Meeting of the International College of Geriatric Psychoneuropharmacology, Hawaii, 10–12 December.

134 Lasser R, Bossie C, Eerdekens M, Zhu Y and Gharabawi G (2003) *Stable elderly patients with psychotic disorders improve with long-acting risperidone microspheres.* Paper presented at the American Association for Geriatric Psychiatry Sixteenth Annual Meeting, Hawaii, 1–4 March.

135 Lasser R, Bossie C, Zhu Y, Eerdekens M and Gharabawi G (2002) *Long-term assessment of dyskinesia and other movement disorders in elderly patients receiving long-acting injectable risperidone.* Paper presented at the Second Annual Meeting of the International College of Geriatric Psychoneuropharmacology, Barcelona, 22–26 October.

136 Meehan KM, Wang H, David SR *et al.* (2001) Comparison of rapidly acting intramuscular olanzapine, lorazepam, and placebo: a double-blind, randomized study in acutely agitated patients with dementia. *Neuropsychopharmacology.* **26**: 494–504.

137 Devanand DP, Marder K, Michaels KS *et al.* (1998) A randomized, placebo-controlled dose–comparison trial of haloperidol for psychosis and disruptive behaviors in Alzheimer's disease. *Am J Psychiatry.* **155**: 1512–20.

138 Teri L, Logsdon RG, Peskind E *et al.* (2000) Treatment of agitation in AD: a randomised, placebo-controlled trial. *Neurology.* **55**: 1271–8.

139 Satterlee WG, Reams SG, Burns PR *et al.* (1995) A clinical update on olanzapine treatment in schizophrenia and in elderly Alzheimer's disease patients. *Psychopharmacol Bull.* **31**: 534.

Chapter 10

Treatment of anxiety disorders

Srinivas Suribhatla and James Lindesay

Introduction

This chapter gives an overview of the pharmacological management of anxiety symptoms and disorders in old age. Epidemiological studies show that anxiety disorders are common in the elderly population, with prevalence rates of up to 13.7–15.0% if comorbid cases are included.[1,2] At all ages, individuals with anxiety and depression are significant consumers of health and social services.[3] One UK study has estimated the annual health and care cost of anxiety in old age to be £750 million,[4] although this figure is not adjusted for medical and psychiatric comorbidity. Much of this cost is associated with general medical and social care. This might be reduced if anxiety disorders in old age were more effectively identified and treated.

Drugs are still the most common form of treatment for anxiety in elderly patients, despite the growing body of evidence that psychological interventions (e.g. cognitive behavioural therapy, anxiety management) are effective in this age group, and probably safer than long-term medication. This may reflect the current limited availability of health professionals skilled in the delivery of these therapies. This chapter focuses on pharmacological management, but it should be emphasised at the outset that drugs should only be prescribed as part of a comprehensive plan that includes psychological and social interventions.

General principles

- Thorough assessment in order to reach an accurate diagnosis is the essential first task in determining the most appropriate management strategy. As discussed below, anxiety is often comorbid with depression and physical illness. Elderly people are more likely to have concurrent medical illnesses and to be on a number of medications that may exacerbate or cause apprehension and agitation.
- Consider the available non-pharmacological alternatives, in particular cognitive behavioural and environmental interventions. Patient education, lifestyle advice (cutting down on alcohol and caffeine, encouraging exercise, etc.) and supportive counselling also play an important role, and in some cases are sufficient for the effective management of anxiety disorders.
- It is important to be mindful of physiological differences between elderly and younger populations. Medications are metabolised less effectively and eliminated more slowly in some elderly individuals (*see* Chapter 5). 'Start low and go slow' whenever possible is the rule.

- Set clear goals for the treatment – for example, symptom relief with minimum sedation, improvement in sleep, freedom from autonomic and cognitive toxicities, freedom from physical dependence and drug interactions.[5]
- Ensure that there is an adequate trial of treatment. Some drugs (e.g. anti-depressants) can take several weeks to produce their full effect.
- When starting an anxiolytic drug, decide how long the course of treatment will be. Too many patients end up on long-term prescriptions simply because no consideration is given as to whether the drug is still required.
- Be aware of the possible adverse effects of the drug treatment, including side-effects, interactions with other drugs, potential for dependency and abuse, and toxicity in overdose.

Comorbidity

The widespread occurrence of psychiatric and physical comorbidity among patients with anxiety disorders has been well documented. It is often difficult to differentiate anxiety from coexisting depression and cognitive disorders.

Depression

Among elderly patients with major depression, 30–80% may have significant anxiety symptoms, although in many cases these do not meet the criteria for an anxiety disorder. Similarly, 33–70% of elderly patients with anxiety disorders are depressed.[1] As in many younger patients, the commonest presentation of anxiety in elderly patients is in the context of depression.[6] Depressed elderly patients with comorbid anxiety symptoms present with more severe pathology and have a more difficult course of illness, including decreased or delayed treatment compliance and response.[7,8]

Dementia

Anxiety occurs at all stages of dementia, although it is not clear to what extent its frequency differs from that in the non-demented elderly population. Estimates of its prevalence in demented individuals range from 3.3% to 38%.[9,10] Mildly affected individuals are understandably concerned about the future, and their social functioning may be impaired by anxiety and loss of confidence. Later in the course of the dementia, anxiety may be associated with depression or psychosis.[11] Agitation may be the expression of anxiety in severely demented patients.[12] Individuals with vascular dementia may be more liable to develop anxiety symptoms than those with Alzheimer's disease.[13]

Physical illness

In elderly community populations, anxiety disorders are associated with increased physical morbidity and mortality.[14,15] This association is even more marked in psychiatric and medical patients,[16,17] which highlights the importance of careful history taking and physical examination, particularly in late-onset cases. This issue is reviewed in detail elsewhere.[18]

Drugs

Classification of anxiolytics

Several classes of compounds are used as anxiolytics in elderly patients:

- benzodiazepines
- azapirones
- antidepressants:
  - tricyclic antidepressants (TCAs)
  - monoamine oxidase inhibitors (MAOIs)
  - selective serotonin reuptake inhibitors (SSRIs)
  - serotonin and noradrenaline reuptake inhibitors (SNRIs)
  - 5 hydroxytryptamine ($5HT_2$) antagonists
- antipsychotics
- beta-blockers
- anticonvulsants
- antihistamines
- chloral hydrate
- barbiturates.

There are surprisingly few formal controlled trials of any drug treatment for anxiety in elderly patients, and those that have been published are difficult to interpret because of the diverse nature of the subjects included and the methods used to investigate them.[19] Prescribing practice in this age group is still based primarily on clinical experience, case reports, extrapolation from studies of younger adults, and studies of pharmacokinetics in elderly patients.

Benzodiazepines

Benzodiazepines are the most frequently used drugs for the acute and long-term management of anxiety disorders in elderly patients. They act as allosteric modulators at the benzodiazepine receptor linked to gamma-aminobutyric acid (GABA)-A, causing hyperpolarisation through chloride ion influx, and they have anxiolytic, hypnotic, muscle relaxant and anticonvulsant actions. Long-acting benzodiazepines undergo both oxidative and conjugative metabolic phases. The oxidative phase tends to be prolonged in elderly patients, and it produces active metabolites that stay in the system even longer. Short-acting benzodiazepines only undergo a conjugative metabolic phase, which is not affected by age, and they produce no active metabolites. They should therefore be used preferentially in elderly patients.

Benzodiazepines are undoubtedly effective anxiolytics. They have a rapid onset of action, and with some important exceptions (e.g. patients with respiratory depression) they are safe both at therapeutic doses and in overdose. However, there are problems associated with their prolonged use, including dependence, memory impairment, poor motor co-ordination, depression of respiratory drive and paradoxical excitement.[20–22] Elderly people are particularly sensitive to these adverse effects, and the accumulation of drugs with long elimination half-lives also leads to drowsiness, delirium, incontinence, falls and fractures. Benzodiazepines with long half-lives (e.g. diazepam, flurazepam, chlordiazepoxide) are on the Beers list of medications deemed inappropriate for elderly patients.[23]

Patients will experience the maximum benefit from benzodiazepines within 6 weeks, so their use should be restricted to the management of short-term anxiety symptoms, and drugs with short half-lives and no active metabolites, such as oxazepam and lorazepam, are recommended (*see* Table 10.1). Maintenance treatment may be appropriate in a few elderly cases, but long-term use of benzodiazepines should be avoided and established users weaned off their medication whenever possible.[24]

Table 10.1 Half-lives of benzodiazepines

Name	Half-life (hours)	Dose (mg)
Long acting		
Diazepam	20–100	2–15
Chlordiazepoxide (Librium)	5–30	5–50
Clorazepate (Tranxene)	30–200	7.5–15
Alprazolam (Xanax)	12–15	0.25–3
Clonazepam* (Rivotril)	18–56	0.5–4
Short acting		
Lorazepam	8–24	1–2
Oxazepam	5–15	10–20

* Not as an anxiolytic in the UK.

Azapirones

Buspirone, an azapirone anxiolytic, is a $5HT_{1A}$ partial agonist that differs both chemically and pharmacologically from the benzodiazepines. Its pharmacokinetics, safety and efficacy in elderly patients are similar to those in younger adults,[25–28] and it appears to be well tolerated by those with chronic medical conditions,[29] although it should be used with care in patients with renal and hepatic disease. Its short-term use is not associated with rebound, dependence or abuse.[30] There is no cross-tolerance with benzodiazepines, so buspirone should not be used to cover benzodiazepine withdrawal. For the same reason, initiation of buspirone therapy in patients with generalised anxiety who have only recently terminated benzodiazepine treatment should be undertaken cautiously and combined with appropriate patient education. Unlike other anxiolytics, it takes about 2 to 4 weeks to become effective, which limits its role in the management of acute anxiety states.

Antidepressants

There is now good evidence, at least in younger adults, that generalised anxiety disorder, obsessive-compulsive disorder (OCD) and panic disorder respond to antidepressant drugs. If depression is a prominent feature of an anxiety disorder, then treatment with antidepressant medication should be considered. Both tricyclics and the SSRIs are effective, but the latter are preferable because they can be used safely in severely physically ill and suicidal patients.[31] It has been suggested that SSRIs may be better suited for treating panic disorder and OCD, whereas nefazodone may be the treatment of choice for generalised anxiety disorder comorbid with depression.[5] MAOIs are relatively well tolerated by elderly patients, although their use has declined in recent years. Moclobemide is a specific MAO-B inhibitor with much less peripheral activity than the older MAOIs, and there is consequently less need for dietary restrictions. Whether or not it has any particular role in the treatment of anxiety in old age is not known. Although some neurotic symptoms may remit along with the depression follow-ing antidepressant medication, others such as established phobic avoidance will usually require a separate psychological intervention.[32] The use of antidepressant drugs in elderly patients is discussed in more detail in Chapter 8.

Antipsychotics

The risk of disabling extrapyramidal side-effects means that typical antipsychotic drugs such as haloperidol are not indicated for the management of anxiety symptoms in most elderly patients. The newer atypical antipsychotics may have a limited, short-term role in the management of anxiety disorders in some elderly patients, as they possess a more favourable cognitive[33] and extrapyramidal side-effect profile than that of traditional agents in this age group. However, as yet there is no evidence for their effectiveness in the management of anxiety disorders, and they should only be used as adjunctive therapy for non- or partial responders. Short courses of these drugs are also of benefit when fear and agitation are secondary to psychotic experiences, as in delirium. The use of neuroleptic drugs in the management of agitation in dementia is discussed in Chapter 9.

Beta-blockers

In some patients, the sympathetic somatic symptoms of anxiety, such as tachy-cardia, sweating and tremor, are particularly troublesome, and low doses of a beta-blocking drug (e.g. propranolol) may be useful in controlling these. However, there is no published evidence of their effectiveness in elderly patients. They should not be used in patients with asthma, chronic obstructive airways disease, cardiac conduction defects or heart failure. These restrictions, together with side-effects such as nightmares and insomnia, limit their usefulness in elderly patients.

Anticonvulsants

There are some case reports and uncontrolled studies which suggest that anticonvulsant drugs such as sodium valproate and gabapentin may be effective in the treatment of anxiety disorders.[34] As yet there is no evidence to support their use in elderly patients.

Antihistamines

Antihistamine drugs such as hydroxyzine have a long history of use as anxiolytic agents in elderly patients. Their effect is probably due to their sedative action. They are relatively safe, although hypotension and drowsiness can be problem-atic, and they have significant anticholinergic activity. They can be useful in patients in whom respiratory depressant drugs are contraindicated.

Chloral hydrate

This is another time-honoured sedative drug that is sometimes used in sub-hypnotic doses as an anxiolytic in patients who cannot tolerate the alternatives.

However, there is no evidence to support this, and the drug is not licensed for this indication in the UK. It has a rapid onset of action and a short elimination half-life, and is relatively safe to use in frail elderly patients, although gastric irritation can sometimes be a problem. It induces liver enzymes, which may increase the rate of metabolism of other drugs that the patient is taking.

Barbiturates

The only reason for mentioning barbiturates in this context is to reiterate that they no longer have any place in the management of anxiety disorders at any age. They are highly addictive, have a poor side-effect profile and are dangerous in overdose. Clinicians occasionally encounter elderly long-term users of these drugs. In such cases, careful withdrawal as an inpatient is advisable.

Generalised anxiety disorder (GAD)

GAD is characterised by persistent anxious mood accompanied by motor tension, autonomic symptoms, apprehensiveness and hypervigilance. Estimates of the prevalence of GAD in elderly people range from 0.7% to 4.7%.[35] Benzodiazepines are the most frequently prescribed drug in the management of GAD. In the younger adult population they have been proved to be effective for short-term treatment of generalised anxiety, with no significant difference in effectiveness between different members of the class, or drugs from other classes (e.g. buspirone, SSRIs). In the elderly population the limited available evidence also indicates that they are more effective than placebo.[36,37]

Antidepressant drugs, including paroxetine and venlafaxine, are also effective anxiolytics and resolve the symptoms of depression in younger patients with GAD.[38] The benefit of venlafaxine can be sustained long term, enabling increased numbers of patients to achieve remission from symptoms and experience restoration of normal functioning. In a pooled analysis of five randomised placebo-controlled clinical trials, venlafaxine ER was found to be safe and well tolerated, and showed similar efficacy in younger and older patients in the treatment of GAD.[39] Early uncontrolled studies involving younger adults suggest that citalopram may also be an effective treatment for GAD, particularly for patients who have failed previous treatment with other SSRIs.[40]

In younger adults with GAD, the response rate with buspirone has been found to be greater than that with placebo, and equivalent to that with venlafaxine[41] and benzodiazepines.[42] Acute-phase treatment lasts for up to a few weeks, where the aim is resolution of symptoms, and the chronic phase aims to optimise the use of medication with minimal side-effects. It is recommended that short-acting benzodiazepines (e.g. oxazepam, lorazepam) are used to avoid drug accumulation and troublesome side-effects such as daytime drowsiness, cognitive impairment, ataxia, fatigue, paradoxical reactions and respiratory depression. In chronic cases of GAD, benzodiazepines should be avoided and the use of an anxiolytic antidepressant or buspirone is recommended. However, because of the delayed onset of action of the antidepressants and buspirone, short-term treatment with a benzodiazepine is sometimes needed as an adjunct in order to alleviate marked symptoms of anxiety. Benzodiazepines work quickly but may cause rebound anxiety on tapering or withdrawal.

Panic disorder

Panic disorder is characterised by recurrent attacks of intense fear, accompanied by severe somatic anxiety symptoms. Little is known about panic disorder in the elderly population, as it is relatively rare in this age group, with a 1-month prevalence rate of 0.1–0.2%. The limited evidence from case reports, volunteer samples and non-psychiatric populations suggests that panic in old age is less common than in adulthood, is commoner in women and widows, and late-onset cases are symptomatically less severe than those whose disorder started earlier in life.[43]

The paucity of published research on the treatment of panic disorder in old age is probably a consequence of its relative rarity in this population. One short-term randomised controlled study has shown comparable efficacy of alprazolam and imipramine in older adults with panic disorder.[44] However, SSRIs are fast emerging as the drugs of first choice for panic disorder at all ages. Paroxetine, citalopram and escitalopram are currently licensed for use in panic disorder in the UK. A number of controlled trials have demonstrated that SSRIs have short-term efficacy in treating panic attacks in young adults. Some patients with panic disorder experience an initial feeling of increased anxiety and jitteriness when beginning treatment with an SSRI. For that reason, the initial dose should be lower than that usually prescribed to patients with depression.[45] It is generally accepted that a response with SSRIs does not occur for at least 4 weeks, and some patients will not show a full response before 8 to 12 weeks.

Many controlled studies in young adults have shown that tricyclic antidepressants, benzodiazepines and the MAOI phenalzine are also effective in panic disorder. However, an increase in QT variability[46] and other side-effects, especially anticholinergic ones, limits the usefulness of tricyclic agents in this group. Short-acting benzodiazepines tend to act more rapidly in patients with panic attacks, but sedation is the most frequent side-effect. Although a substantial proportion of anxiety-disordered patients use benzodiazepines, little is known about the influence of long-term benzodiazepine use on treatment outcome. There is evidence that venlafaxine, nefazadone and valproate may also be effective treatments for panic disorder in young adults.

Obsessive-compulsive disorder (OCD)

OCD is characterised by obsessive thoughts and/or compulsive acts which are a significant source of distress, or which interfere with social functioning. The mean age of onset for OCD is 20–25 years, and it is unusual for first onset to occur after the age of 50 years. However, OCD is a chronic disorder, and a significant proportion of cases persist into old age, when they may present to services for the first time.[47]

In practice, drug treatment and behavioural therapy are often given in combination. Studies of OCD in younger adults show that 30–60% of patients respond to appropriate medication, with a better response for obsessional thoughts than for compulsive behaviours.[47] Clomipramine is the most extensively studied treatment for OCD, and has been shown to be superior to placebo in younger adults. However, lack of receptor specificity and significant anticholinergic and antihistaminic side-effects limit its usefulness in elderly patients. In this age group, one of the SSRIs is the drug treatment of first choice. Fluoxetine, sertraline, fluvoxamine and paroxetine have all been found to be equal in efficacy to clomipramine in controlled trials involving younger adults. None of the clinical trials supporting this indication specifically involved elderly patients. The effective dose for the treatment of OCD with SSRIs tends to be higher than that required for depression, and the time taken to respond is typically much longer (18–20 weeks). Studies suggest that long-term therapy is required, as discontinuation of medication leads to relapse of symptoms. Buspirone, fenfluramine, pimozide, clonazepam and behaviour therapy may augment the effects of SSRIs in partial responders. There are case reports which suggest that MAOIs may also be useful in OCD patients with concomitant panic and anxiety. However, side-effects and dietary restrictions make their use more problematic in elderly patients.

Phobic disorders

Phobias are defined as the persistent and irrational fear of an object, activity or situation, resulting in a compelling desire to avoid the phobic stimulus. Phobic disorders are the commonest anxiety disorders in the elderly population, with 1-month prevalence rates of 5–10%.[43] However, it is rare for elderly people to seek help for these problems. This may explain the relative lack of controlled trials investigating the usefulness of different therapeutic interventions.

As in younger patients, cognitive behavioural therapy is the mainstay of management of phobic disorders in old age. There is evidence of the effectiveness of pharmacological interventions in younger populations, in whom the treatment of combined panic disorder and agoraphobia has received particular attention. However, no controlled studies to date have demonstrated the efficacy of any pharmacological interventions in specific phobias. Anecdotal evidence suggests that low-dose benzodiazepines may be useful.

SSRIs, MAOIs, benzodiazepines (e.g. alprazolam) and buspirone have been shown to be effective in younger patients with social phobias. Beta-blockers (e.g. propranolol) and benzodiazepines may be useful in controlling autonomic symptoms associated with this condition in young adults. However, it is not clear how far these findings can be applied to elderly people.

Post-traumatic stress disorder (PTSD)

PTSD occurs following exposure to an extreme stressor, and the syndrome includes re-experiencing of the trauma, avoidance, numbing and increased arousal. Little is known about the prevalence and characteristics of PTSD in the elderly population, but it can persist for many years, sometimes manifesting itself for the first time in old age.[48,49] SSRIs such as paroxetine and sertraline have been shown to be of benefit in the treatment of PTSD in younger adults.

Measurement of response and progress

There are very few instruments that have been specifically developed for the identification and measurement of anxiety in old age, and most studies to date have used scales validated in younger populations. However, in recent years, some scales have been developed for use with elderly patients, such as the 10-item Short Anxiety Screening Test (SAST),[50] the 4-item FEAR, an instrument developed as a screen for generalised anxiety in elderly primary care attenders,[51] and the Rating Anxiety in Dementia (RAID) scale for assessing anxiety in the context of dementia.[52]

Key points

- The effective management of anxiety disorders in the elderly population is limited by three different and important issues.
- First, although anxiety disorders are common, some hard-pressed health professionals regard their treatment as a relatively low priority.
- Second, pharmacotherapy for anxiety disorders is often an easy and convenient means of avoiding a more detailed and painstaking assessment of patients' symptoms and circumstances. Drugs are still the mainstay of management, despite the availability of effective psychosocial treatment strategies.
- Third, we still lack an adequate evidence base for the effectiveness of pharmacological treatments.
- Not surprisingly, anxiety disorders in old age are absent from various databases of systematic reviews, such as the Cochrane Library. Current treatment strategies are therefore mainly based on knowledge gleaned from the adult literature and from clinical experience.
- We need clinical trials that demonstrate the effectiveness (or otherwise) of the various pharmacological agents in the elderly population, and we need to establish their safety and tolerance profiles, and any significant additive effects or interactions that they may have in this age group.

References

1 Lindesay J, Briggs K and Murphy E (1989) The Guy's/Age Concern Survey: prevalence rates of cognitive impairment, depression and anxiety in an urban elderly community. *Br J Psychiatry.* **155**: 317–29.

2 Manela M, Katona C and Livingston G (1996) How common are the anxiety disorders in old age? *Int J Geriatr Psychiatry.* **11**: 65–70.

3 Kennedy BL and Schwab JJ (1997) Utilization of medical specialists by anxiety disorder patients. *Psychosomatics.* **38**: 12.

4 Livingston G, Manela M and Katona C (1997) Cost of care for older people. *Br J Psychiatry.* **171**: 56–9.

5 Weiss KJ (1996) Optimal management of anxiety in older patients. *Drugs Aging.* **9**: 191–201.

6 Doraiswamy PM (2001) Contemporary management of comorbid anxiety and depression in geriatric patients. *J Clin Psychiatry.* **62 (Suppl. 12)**: 30–5.

7 Flint AJ and Rifat SL (1997) Two-year outcome of elderly patients with anxious depression. *Psychiatr Res.* **66**: 23–31.

8 Lenze EJ, Mulsant BH, Shear MK *et al.* (2001) Comorbidity of depression and anxiety disorders in later life. *Depression Anxiety.* **14**: 86–93.

9 Forsell Y and Winblad B (1997) Anxiety disorders in non-demented and demented elderly patients: prevalence and correlates. *J Neurol Neurosurg Psychiatry*. **62**: 294–5.

10 Wands K, Merskey H, Hachinski V *et al*. (1990) A questionnaire investigation of anxiety and depression in early dementia. *J Am Geriatr Soc*. **36**: 535–8.

11 Ballard CG, Patel A, Solis M *et al*. (1996) One-year follow-up study of depression in dementia sufferers. *Br J Psychiatry*. **168**: 287–91.

12 Mintzer JE and Brawman-Mintzer O (1996) Agitation as a possible expression of generalized anxiety disorder in demented elderly patients: toward a treatment approach. *J Clin Psychiatry*. **57 (Suppl. 7)**: 55–63.

13 Sultzer DL, Levin HS, Mahler ME *et al*. (1993) A comparison of psychiatric symptoms in vascular dementia and Alzheimer's disease. *Am J Psychiatry*. **150**: 1806–12.

14 Kay DWK and Bergmann K (1966) Physical disability and mental health in old age. *J Psychosom Res*. **10**: 3–12.

15 Lindesay J (1990) The Guy's/Age Concern Survey: physical health and psychiatric disorder in an urban elderly community. *Int J Geriatr Psychiatry*. **5**: 171–8.

16 Bergmann K (1971) The neuroses of old age. In: DWK Kay and A Walk (eds) *Recent Developments in Psychogeriatrics*. Headley Bros, Ashford.

17 Burn WK, Davies KN, McKenzie FR *et al*. (1993) The prevalence of psychiatric illness in acute geriatric admissions. *Int J Geriatr Psychiatry*. **8**: 175–80.

18 Hocking LB and Koenig HG (1995) Anxiety in medically ill older patients: a review and update. *Int J Psychiatry Med*. **25**: 221–38.

19 Salzman C (1991) Pharmacologic treatment of the anxious elderly patient. In: C Salzman and BD Lebowitz (eds) *Anxiety in the Elderly*. Springer, New York.

20 Tyrer P (1980) Dependence on benzodiazepines. *Br J Psychiatry*. **137**: 576–7.

21 Curran HV (1986) Tranquillising memories: a review of the effects of benzodiazepines on human memory. *Biol Psychiatry*. **23**: 179–213.

22 Fancourt G and Castleden M (1986) The use of benzodiazepines with particular reference to the elderly. *Br J Hosp Med*. **5**: 321–5.

23 Beers MH (1997) Explicit criteria for determining potentially inappropriate medication use in nursing home residents. *Arch Intern Med*. **157**: 1531–6.

24 Higgitt A (1992) Indications for benzodiazepine prescriptions in the elderly. *Int J Geriatr Psychiatry*. **3**: 239–49.

25 Robinson D, Napoliello MJ and Shenck L (1988) The safety and usefulness of buspirone as an anxiolytic drug in elderly versus young patients. *Clin Ther*. **10**: 740–6.

26 Steinberg JR (1994) Anxiety in elderly patients. A comparison of azapirones and benzodiazepines. *Drugs Aging*. **5**: 335–45.

27 Pecknold JC (1997) A risk–benefit assessment of buspirone in the treatment of anxiety disorders. *Drug Safety*. **16**: 118–32.

28 Mahmood I and Sahajwalla C (1999) Clinical pharmacokinetics and pharmaco-dynamics of buspirone, an anxiolytic drug. *Clin Pharmacokinet*. **36**: 277–87.

29 Bohm C, Robinson DS, Gammans RE *et al*. (1990) Buspirone therapy in anxious elderly patients: a controlled clinical trial. *J Clin Psychopharmacol*. **10**: 47–51S.

30 Lader M (1991) Can buspirone induce rebound, dependence or abuse? *Br J Psychiatry*. **159 (Suppl. 12)**: 45–51.

31 Evans ME and Lye M (1992) Depression in the physically ill: an open study of treatment with the 5-HT reuptake inhibitor fluoxetine. *J Clin Exp Gerontol*. **14**: 297–307.

32 Blazer DG, Hughes DC and Fowler N (1989) Anxiety as an outcome symptom of depression in elderly and middle-aged adults. *Int J Geriatr Psychiatry*. **4**: 273–8.

33 Byerly MJ, Weber MT, Brooks DL *et al*. (2001) Antipsychotic medications and the elderly: effects on cognition and implications for use. *Drugs Aging*. **18**: 45–61.

34 Ghaemi SN, Katzow JJ, Desai SP *et al*. (1998) Gabapentin treatment of mood disorders: a preliminary study. *J Clin Psychiatry*. **59**: 426–9.

35 Krasucki C, Howard R and Mann A (1999) Anxiety and its treatment in the elderly. *Int Psychogeriatr.* **11**: 25–45.

36 Bresolin N, Monza G, Scarpini E *et al.* (1988) Treatment of anxiety with ketazolam in elderly patients. *Clin Ther.* **10**: 536–42.

37 Koepke H, Gold RL, Linden ME *et al.* (1982) Multicenter controlled study of oxazepam in anxious elderly outpatients. *Psychosomatics.* **23**: 641–5.

38 Gorman JM (2002) Treatment of generalized anxiety disorder. *J Clin Psychiatry.* **63 (Suppl. 8)**: 17–23.

39 Katz IR, Reynolds CF, Alexopoulos GS *et al.* (2002) Venlafaxine ER as a treatment for generalized anxiety disorder in older adults: pooled analysis of five randomized placebo-controlled clinical trials. *J Am Geriatr Soc.* **50**: 18–25.

40 Varia I and Rauscher F (2002) Treatment of generalized anxiety disorder with citalopram. *Int Clin Psychopharmacol.* **17**: 103–7.

41 Gale C and, Oakley-Browne M (2000) Anxiety disorder. *BMJ.* **321**: 1204.

42 Gould RA, Otto MW, Pollack MH *et al.* (1997) Cognitive behavioural and pharmacological treatment of generalised anxiety disorder: a preliminary meta-analysis. *Behav Ther.* **28**: 285–305.

43 Lindesay J and Marudkar M (2001) Neurotic disorders. *Rev Clin Gerontol.* **11**: 51–70.

44 Sheikh JI and Swales PJ (1999) Treatment of panic disorder in older adults: a pilot study comparison of alprazolam, imipramine, and placebo. *Int J Psychiatry Med.* **29**: 107–17.

45 American Psychiatric Association (1998) *Practice Guideline for the Treatment of Patients with Panic Disorder.* American Psychiatric Association, Washington, DC.

46 Yeragani VK, Pohl R, Jampala VC *et al.* (2000) Effects of nortriptyline and paroxetine on QT variability in patients with panic disorder. *Depression Anxiety.* **11**: 126–30.

47 Lindesay J (2002) Obsessive-compulsive disorder. In: JRM Copeland, MT Abou-Saleh and DG Blazer (eds) *Principles and Practice of Geriatric Psychiatry* (2e). John Wiley and Sons, Chichester.

48 Kluznik JC, Speed N, van Valkerberger C *et al.* (1996) Forty-year follow-up of United States prisoners of war. *Am J Psychiatry.* **143**: 1443–5.

49 Kaup BA, Ruskin PE and Nyman G (1994) Significant life events and PTSD in elderly World War II veterans. *Am J Geriatr Psychiatry.* **2**: 239–43.

50 Sinoff G, Ore L, Zlotogorsky D *et al.* (1999) Short Anxiety Screening Test – a brief instrument for detecting anxiety in the elderly. *Int J Geriatr Psychiatry.* **14**: 1062–71.

51 Krasucki C, Ryan P, Ertan T *et al.* (1999) The FEAR: a rapid screening instrument for generalized anxiety in elderly primary care attenders. *Int J Geriatr Psychiatry.* **14**: 60–8.

52 Shankar KK, Walker M, Frost D *et al.* (1999) The development of a valid and reliable scale for rating anxiety in dementia. *Aging Ment Health.* **3**: 39–49.

Chapter 11

Sleep disturbance and its management in older patients

Alison Diaper and Ian Hindmarch

Introduction

Insomnia is one of the most democratic of disorders, and while there is no particular physical constitution or psychological trait which confers immunity, it is well established that advancing age increases the frequency of reports of insomnia. Indeed, the population with the highest prevalence and severity of insomnia is the elderly.[1–7] In a classic survey of sleep disturbance, Karacan *et al.*[8] found that while only 9% of those aged 20–29 years reported sleep problems, around 21% of those aged 60–69 years complained of 'often having trouble sleeping'. It is important to manage and treat insomnia in the older adult, especially as the proportion of the elderly population continues to expand.[9]

Poor sleep in the elderly is associated with excessive daytime sleepiness, irritability and increased nocturnal activity, which increases the risk of accidents and falls.[10–12] Martikainen *et al.*[13] surveyed 1600 middle-aged people and found that daytime sleepiness was associated with disturbed nocturnal sleep, and also those suffering from tiredness complained more of poor health than other respondents. Traffic accidents and other mishaps attributable to tiredness had occurred in 1.3% of cases, and almost 5% of male respondents had dozed off while driving at least five times in their lives. Pollak *et al.*[14] suggest that these daytime sequelae of nocturnal sleep disturbance may even result in the institutionalisation of the elderly individual. It is particularly the daytime consequences of disturbed sleep which achieve importance in the elderly, and the amelioration and reduction of such activity are the main objectives behind the management of sleep-related disorders. Young *et al.*[15] found that accidents in the elderly had an increased risk of mortality and cost to society when compared with accidents involving younger individuals. Cwikel[16] found that among individuals aged over 65 years, 24% reported a fall in the last year, 37% of which involved hospitalisation. Advancing age was associated with repeated falls, an increase in cycle and pedestrian accidents, bone fractures and errors of judgement while driving.[17,18]

Insomnia and other sleep-related disturbances impact on both subjective well-being and physical health.[19,20] Foley *et al.*[6] found that between 7% and 15% of those aged over 65 years rarely or never felt rested in the morning, and that sleep complaints were associated with an increased number of respiratory symptoms, physical disabilities and depressive symptoms. Sleep problems were also related to breathing problems and self-perceived health,[21] and have been linked to an increased risk of mortality.[6,14,22] Indeed, sleep problems have been linked to poorer health in various surveys.[4,5,23–31] In general, functional physical limitations were linked to earlier bedtime, increased sleep duration, increased likelihood of a prolonged sleep latency (over 30 minutes), and a decreased likelihood of feeling rested in the morning. A history of heart attack and stroke in women was associated with not feeling rested in the morning, and in men it was associated with a prolonged sleep latency.[3]

Poor sleep is also associated with arthritis,[3,32] angina and hypertension,[33] psychiatric disorders[32,34,35] and physical pain.[36]

In any discussion of the relationship between sleep and health it is difficult to establish causality and to know whether poor health leads to poor sleep, or whether poor sleep leads to poor health. However, the close relationship between overall physical and psychological health is of major importance in considering sleep disturbance in the elderly.

The origin of sleep problems in older people

Studies in Sweden,[7] the USA,[8] England[27] and Japan[37] show that sleep problems in older age appear to be global and pancultural. However, a major problem in the elderly is what an individual patient might perceive insomnia to be. For example, Weinstein et al.[38] found that 4–5% of those surveyed in San Francisco would report 'insomnia', but 13–16% would then admit to difficulty in initiating or maintaining sleep, and other aspects of 'insomnia' itself. This may be indicative of a possible stigma associated with 'insomnia'.[39] Alternatively, older adults may experience events such as nocturnal awakenings or extended sleep onset latency, but may not consider this to be 'insomnia' per se. Indeed, some may enjoy a period of wakefulness at the beginning of the night as an opportunity to read and relax.[40] It has been suggested[41,42] that insomnia will only be reported if daytime activities are affected by sleep problems. A change in sleep pattern may only be a problem if subsequent daytime sleepiness interferes with daytime activities. The prevalence of insomnia in the older population has been variously reported in many countries. In the USA, the figures range from 10.4% of those over 60 years old[21] to just over 20% for those aged over 50 years.[8,43] In Italy, 45% of those aged over 65 years reported suffering insomnia,[44] while in Sweden only 18.6% of a similar population complained of insomnia.[7] In England, Morgan et al.[45] found that 12.8% of those over 65 years of age reported insomnia, and Beaman[46] found the prevalence of 'insomnia during the last week' to be 76% of those aged over 60 years. The most striking difference in the reported prevalence of insomnia is between old and young patients. For example, in Iceland, Gíslason et al.[47] found that 68% of the population aged over 65 years complained of insomnia, whereas Janson et al.[20] found in a younger age group (20–45 years) from the same country that only 9% complained of sleep problems.

Females tend to complain of increased frequency and severity of sleep disturbance,[3,36,37,45] with typically almost twice as many females aged over 64 years (24%) complaining of sleep problems, compared with 13% of males of the same age.[7] The reason for the sex difference in reporting sleep problems is unclear, but females do seem to be subjectively more affected by changes in sleep patterns. Hoch et al.[48] demonstrated that although both males and females showed a higher concordance between subjective estimates and polysomnographic recordings for sleep-onset latency and sleep duration, only females showed significant correlations between EEG measures and subjective 'restlessness', and 'soundness' of sleep.

It has also been suggested that females are more able to talk about unpleasant experiences and have a more accurate perception of those experiences,[48,49] and Briscoe[50] suggested that females are more likely to talk about their feelings and emotional problems. Urponen et al.[51] found that females tended to be more bothered at night by thoughts about human relationships, arguments and social worries, whereas males were more preoccupied by work-related worries (when in employment) and generalised stress. Males were also more likely to be under the influence of alcohol (which disrupts sleep in the later part of the night and suppresses rapid eye movement [REM] sleep).[52]

Depression in the elderly can lead to poor sleep,[3,6,44,53] and given that females report more depressive symptoms than males,[3,54] the over-reporting of sleep problems in females could simply be a reflection of the higher incidence of psychological distress. However, there are more attempted suicides by older males than females,[55] indicating that in the elderly the prevalence of depressive symptoms might be more similar between the sexes. The higher prevalence of sleep complaints in females compared with males may thus be due to older females being more willing to talk about sleep problems[56] as well as other more frequently reported physical ailments.[3]

Physical and psychological health in normal ageing

Although sleep disturbance is a presenting symptom in many of the physical disorders of old age, complaints about sleep problems are just as likely[57] to be related to whether or not 'successful ageing' has occurred. Successful ageing can be regarded as the maintenance of appropriate levels of 'mental and physical health', 'vitality' (active engagement in life) and 'resilience' (being able to 'bounce back' from stressors). Successful adaptation to ageing is best demonstrated by normal sleep efficiency.[32,48]

Physical aspects of ageing that influence sleep

A high number of health problems are associated both with increasing age and with increasing reports of sleep problems.[30,33,46,47,56,58]

Pain is cited in many surveys as a major cause of poor sleep.[46,52,54,59–62] Poor sleep worsens the subjective experience of pain,[63] and nocturnal pain as a cause of sleep problems has been found to be experienced by 23–29% of elderly sleep-disturbed patients.[7,60]

Gastro-oesophageal reflux and general indigestion have also been highlighted in surveys as a cause of disturbance to sleep.[34,64,65] Maggi et al.[44] also noted that indigestion occurs in 4.9% of the elderly who are unable to get to sleep, in 1.1% of those who wake in the night, and in 0.9% of those who wake too early in the morning.

It is perhaps too simplistic to propose that physical ailments must necessarily result in poor sleep, and indeed it has been proposed[6] that sleep deprivation due to disturbed or poor sleep can itself lead to ill health (e.g. angina).[33] The available evidence[26] suggests that patients who present with a sleep problem may have an underlying physical problem, and the complaint of poor sleep may distract physicians from the correct diagnosis and precipitate the prescribing of hypnotics without necessarily considering what might really be causing the sleep problems.[52,63] The lack of a reasoned diagnosis might well result in unnecessary hypnotics being used, which may in turn exacerbate undiagnosed but underlying physical and respiratory problems[12] and cause adverse effects.[66]

One of the major contributors to sleep disturbance (by disrupting sleep continuity and maintenance) in the elderly is the frequent need to use the toilet at night.[6,30,47,59,65,67–69] Too few physicians recognise this as a problem,[39] even though 91% of elderly males and 90% of elderly females need to use the toilet at night.[30] The nocturnal need to urinate increases with age[56] due to an age-related decrease in night-time levels of the antidiuretic hormone (ADH), especially in males. It is possible that managing the ADH levels in patients may result in less nocturnal waking and increased sleep continuity, without the need for hypnotic medication,[70] which would certainly not improve the need to urinate and might cause inco-ordination and clumsy movement in patients walking to the bathroom.

Environmental influences on sleep are well known and remain important causative agents in many individual cases. Noise, an uncomfortable bed/bedroom, heat, cold, alcohol, nicotine and caffeine have all been shown to have a demonstrable effect on sleep induction and/or maintenance.[6,44,46,51,52,58,60,71]

It is clear that health problems may affect sleep, and may increase or result in sleep problems. Pain, indigestion and the need to urinate have all been shown to influence the sleep of the elderly patient. This demonstrates the importance of considering the whole sleep situation of a particular patient when assessing and diagnosing sleep-related problems and deciding on an appropriate management strategy.

Psychological aspects of ageing which influence sleep

Good 'psychological adjustment' to ageing is important for good sleep. Problems occur when the elderly fail to accept that the changes in their sleep patterns are normal and natural for their age. Some elderly patients have unrealistic expectations of how they should be sleeping,[28,46,53,54,58,61,67,72–74] and poor sleepers have a larger discrepancy between current sleep patterns and their expected sleep requirements. An individual who is not fulfilling their expected sleep requirement or who believes that their sleep is poorer than that of their peers[32] may experience psychological distress or anxiety over sleep,[75] which leads to increased arousal and, in turn, to more sleep problems. 'Worries',[3,47,51,61,76] 'grief'[6,77] and 'tension'[7,61,62,72] are all found to be significant causes of sleeping problems in elderly populations. Worrying late at night has been found to affect sleep initiation to a greater extent than either sleep maintenance or early-morning waking.[7,44,51,59] The subjective nature of the perception of poor sleep in the elderly has led some[61] to diagnose the *complaint* of insomnia, rather than actual insomnia. Poor sleepers will only complain of sleeping badly if they suffer concomitant psychological distress from it,[78] and those individuals with poor sleep who do not suffer any psychological distress do not complain of insomnia. This may explain why those in good health might still report sleeping badly, and why many who, to a casual observer, have a bizarre sleep pattern might not complain of a sleep problem. Evidence of psychological distress seems to be the most reliable indicator for distinguishing between good and poor sleepers.[75]

'Vitality' is another aspect that is thought to be necessary for 'successful ageing'. Habte-Gabr et al.[3] found that the more 'engaged with life' elderly had better sleep and less illness. Inactivity has been thought to be a problem of retirement, as the elderly become less active and more lethargic,[30] although Kronholm and Hyyppä[54] suggested that sleep is worse just before retirement, due to an increased effort to cope at work. However, Fichten et al.[61] found no difference in the amount of physical activity between good and poor elderly sleepers, nor were there differences in the diversity of activities, or in how busy the patients perceived themselves to be. Yet, differences in sleep occurred between insomniacs and non-insomniacs when they rated how 'pleasant' they found their day. Sleep problems appear to arise when subjectively more unlikeable activities are carried out during the day than subjectively perceived pleasant ones. Whether individuals are active or not, Fichten et al.[61] suggest that better sleep will occur if the self-perception of the patient's own lifestyle is favourable.

Qualitative measurements of sleep

Insomnia is usually categorised into one of three types, namely a difficulty initiating sleep (DIS), a difficulty maintaining sleep (DMS) or early-morning awakening (EMA).[6,7]

DIS includes a long sleep latency, and is consistently found to increase with age.[79] The prevalence of DIS in the elderly has been variously estimated to be 49%,[80] 51%,[46] 53%[8] and 40%,[81] and to involve almost half of the elderly population. Elderly women complain more frequently than men about DIS,[7,21,33,36,37,44,54,56,72,82,83] which again demonstrates the increase in reported sleep problems in females.

DMS is also thought to increase with age,[2,8,32,46,47,60] with a prevalence in the elderly variously reported to be 30%,[61] 21%,[8] 33%,[47] 34%[7] and 49%.[46] The relationship between DMS and general psychological health in the elderly was demonstrated by Newman et al.[33] in a study of the cardiovascular health of 5201 ageing adults. The survey gathered information on cardiopulmonary symptoms and disease, ECG, depression, social support, activities of daily living, physical activity, cognitive function, current medications and sleep disturbance. The authors found that approximately 67% of the participants experienced disturbed sleep at night, and proposed that increased DMS in older adults is mainly due to the association between DMS and concurrent illness. Although the severity and extent of sleep problems are closely associated with health states,[6,36,45,47] several authors[59,84,85] have emphasised the role of the psychological effects of poor health rather than the physical illness itself, in that depressed mood due to ill health may be more influential in poor sleep. Some authors[56] suggest that DMS increases with age more in males than in females, primarily because of waking due to habitual snoring, as males tend to snore more than females, and Gislason et al.[47] found that DMS was habitually reported by 37% of elderly men but only 19% of elderly women. However, other studies suggest that more females than males suffer from DMS.[46,83]

EMA has also been shown to be related to increasing age,[20,46,47,58,60,61] although some authors have failed to find a relationship.[54] The prevalence of habitual EMA has been found to be 14–33% of the elderly.[33,44,47,67]

Quantitative measurements of sleep

Time in bed (TIB)

TIB generally increases with age,[3,45,56,59,86] with elderly women in general tending to remain in bed for longer (7 hours) than men (6.7 hours).[7] Seppälä et al.[59] suggest that this may be due to an attempt to compensate for degradation in sleep quality due to ageing,[87] because staying in bed for a longer time may provide more opportunity for restful or restorative sleep. Alternatively, it may simply be a method of staying warm.[20] Several researchers[4,28,45,61,70,79,88] have demonstrated similar age-related decreases in total sleep time (TST), with males and females being similarly affected.[3]

Sleep efficiency (SE)

Sleep efficiency (SE) is the result of dividing the total sleep time (TST) (from lights out to rising in the morning) by the time in bed (TIB). Thus a patient who was asleep for 6 hours (TST), but who was in bed for 8 hours (TIB), would have a sleep efficiency of 6/8 or 75%. Sleep efficiency scores range from 72% to 83% in various populations of older adults,[5,61,75,89] with no significant difference in objective sleep efficiency between the sexes, although there is evidence of an age-related deterioration in SE.

It is perhaps important to remember that although there may be a decrease in nocturnal SE, TST and TIB related to advancing age, there is no obvious age-related change when a 24-hour period is considered. Sleep requirement seems to be relatively constant with regard to age. It is simply that the sleep of the elderly becomes more dispersed around the 24-hour period and more fragmented.[32,52,86,90] One explanation for sleep fragmentation in the elderly is that there is a reduction in the effectiveness of nocturnal sleep control mechanisms,[32,52,91] and the natural circadian rhythms which regulate sleep become 'out of phase', leading to irregular and polyphasic sleep patterns. Stampi[92] has suggested that 'normal' monophasic adult sleep/wake cycles only apply when there are social or occupational constraints, and that when these are removed, as in retirement, sleep reverts to the polyphasic patterns seen in infants.

Napping

With advancing age, sleep fragmentation seen in reduced SE and increased nocturnal wake time seems to become more pronounced, and the occurrence of daytime napping increases.[32,46,48,54] Good and poor sleepers seem to nap equally often,[32,61] indicating that napping does not interfere with sleep in the elderly as much as it does in younger adults. Beh[93] has suggested that daytime napping reduces the number of complaints of poor sleep, because the naps help to alleviate daytime sleepiness and the associated decline in cognitive function. Also, when naps are habitual, nocturnal sleeplessness and its alleviation become less important to the sufferer.[86] The prevalence of napping in the elderly ranges from 22–25%[6,7] to 42–56%.[54,59] It seems that elderly males tend to nap more than elderly females,[26,30,86] which may be due in part to snoring and sleep apnoea[30] being more prevalent in older males.[30,33]

Daytime sleepiness

Daytime sleepiness (DS) is the inevitable consequence of sleep disturbance from whatever cause, or indeed as a consequence of the side-effects of pharmacological intervention used to manage insomnia or other medical conditions. The prevalence of DS in the elderly ranges from 15%[58] to 80%,[33] and while there is some evidence of an age-related increase,[56] this is regarded as an epiphenomenon of nocturnal pain and physical illness[2,30] and not due to sleep-related variables *per se.*

Diagnosis and management of insomnia in the elderly

From the foregoing review of insomnia in the elderly, it is evident that much of the sleep disturbance that is manifested in elderly patients is a consequence of physical and/or psychological disturbance. Primary or 'idiopathic' insomnia, where there is no obvious or readily discernible cause or reason for the sleep disturbance, can only be regarded as a definitive diagnosis following polysomnographic analysis in a sleep laboratory.

Insomnia usually involves difficulty in maintaining sleep or a difficulty in initiating sleep, although many patients complain of both prolonged sleep onset and sleep fragmentation.

Although the *International Classification of Sleep Disorders*[94] lists some 88 identifiable and diagnosable sleep disorders, it is true to say that outside the sleep disorder centres, such a finesse of diagnosis is impractical. Diagnosis then depends on a clinical interview with the patient to exclude primary causes of the reported insomnia.

Nocturnal pain due to physical illness and trauma, and skin irritation and discomfort brought about by dermatological disorders, will usually benefit from analgesia and appropriate use of antihistamines. Hypnotics should not be used as primary treatments in such circumstances. Antihistamines need not necessarily be sedatives, for removal of the itching and irritation is the primary promoter of sleep.

Similarly, respiratory problems and sleep apnoea should be treated without recourse to hypnotics, especially benzodiazepines with their intrinsic myorelaxant action. Sleep apnoea responds well to the use of constant positive airway pressure (CPAP) machines, and those patients with suspected sleep apnoea (evidence from bed-partner including complaints of loud snoring, fighting for breath, excessive daytime sleepiness, etc.) should be referred to an appropriate sleep or respiratory clinical centre.

Patients with evidence of a psychological disorder should be treated appropriately with antidepressants and/or anti-anxiety agents and observed for a few weeks to see whether the accompanying insomnia is ameliorated as the clinical effects of the drugs take effect. Some patients might find a week's treatment with an effective hypnotic useful to counteract the sleep disruption produced by many SSRIs at the start of drug treatment regimens. The SSRIs are now widely indicated for a range of psychiatric disorders, including generalised anxiety disorder, post-traumatic stress disorder, social phobia, panic disorder and obsessive-compulsive disorder, many if not all of which psychological states are characterised by sleep problems. However, the continued use of hypnotics after the first week of SSRI treatment is not necessarily automatic, and this restricted treatment regimen must only be extended if the individual patient's need demands it.

There are no general rules for the use of hypnotics within neurological disorders (e.g. Parkinson's disease), and much will depend on the symptoms and progress of the disorder on an individual patient basis. However, restless legs syndrome (RLS), an increasingly recognised cause of sleep disturbance in patients of all ages, but especially in the elderly, in whom the frequency of RLS increases, does respond to low doses of dopaminergic agents (e.g. pramipexol, ropinerol).

Primary insomnia needs careful diagnosis, but this does not necessarily mean that a large amount of clinic time needs to be expended on the initial interview of an acute presentation.

Patients who present with an acute and identifiable transient problem (e.g. bereavement, home relocation, acute stress or even a 'flare-up' of a physical condition, such as arthritis, for no apparent reason) may be safely prescribed up to 7 nights' treatment with a standard hypnotic at the appropriate clinical dose for the elderly (e.g. zolpidem 5 mg, zopiclone 3.75 mg, nitrazepam 2.5 mg, temazepam 10 mg). Such a practice is usually without any significant adverse effects, but care must be exercised if benzodiazepines are to be given to patients with respiratory/apnoeic conditions.

Patients without such transient problems must first be screened to enable the physician to ensure that the reported insomnia is not simply an aspect or symptom of a pre-existing or newly diagnosed psychiatric or physical disorder. The majority of chronic physical and psychological disorders progress in a cyclical manner where symptoms of insomnia may occur from time to time. Although it is permissible for these acute problems to be treated as described above, the use of hypnotics for a longer period must never be permitted without a full clinical evaluation of the case.

If a patient passes the psychiatric and physical screen, the next step is to eliminate lifestyle changes as a source of the reported disorder. Insomnia due to major changes in lifestyle is not uncommon. Its management is probably non-pharmacotherapeutic and involves a simple restoration of the patterns of sleep hygiene, which most probably have been severely disrupted. Proper sleep hygiene is essential for good sleep induction and sound sleep continuity. The consumption of drinks containing caffeine, smoking tobacco, vigorous exercise, mental excitement (from violent/horror films), a noisy or intemperate (too hot or too cold) bedroom environment, an incompatible bed-partner (snoring or periodic limb movements, leading to frequent nocturnal arousals) and existential anxieties and worries will all individually and in combination contribute to a non-optimal sleep environment. However, even if a patient has bad sleep hygiene habits, this does not necessarily indicate that they have a 'clinical problem'. The patient's perceived insomnia might well be due to an unrealistic perception of sleep needs and requirements in the older patient. The 'problem' could also be simply an aspect of peer-group comparison and reaction to advertising of over-the-counter sleep products.

The acid test of whether a subjective report of insomnia is a realistically valid symptom is that the report of sleep disturbance is coincidental to reports of daytime sleepiness and impaired behaviour. Whereas in younger patients the sequelae of a poor night's sleep are manifested as daytime impairment of cognitive and psychomotor function, in the elderly patient it is difficult to distinguish the daytime impairment produced by poor nocturnal sleep from that produced by either the adverse effects of medicines currently in use for physiological or psychological disorder, or the fragmentation of sleep–wake patterns caused by advancing age.

Excessive daytime sleepiness leading to impairment of cognitive and psychological function is important for a younger population of car-driving, computer-operating and otherwise active individuals in domestic, work and road-using scenarios. Daytime sleepiness can be reduced by daytime napping, an option that is not readily available to the younger patient in employment. However, elderly unemployed or retired patients are usually able to structure their day to take advantage of napping. Indeed, many elderly people with insomnia manage the daytime consequences of the complaint by taking late-morning or mid-afternoon naps without recourse to any other treatment stratagem. Daytime naps as part of the management of the elderly patient constitute an effective *modus operandi*, but only if the full consequences of such a practice are made clear to the patient. Daytime naps will necessarily cause a reduction in the total nocturnal sleep time, or a fragmentation of nocturnal sleep. This is a problem if the patient cannot adjust their circadian behaviours to account for a short night's sleep with one or two further sleep/rest periods during the day. Patients who live in cities may find the increasing '24/7' society helpful in permitting a range of activities (e.g. supermarket shopping, food outlets, theatres) which will aid a 'siesta-style' approach to coping with insomnia.

In the case of patients who are unable or unwilling to adopt such a behavioural solution, every effort must be made to reduce daytime napping in order to concentrate the need and drive for sleep at night-time. This is best achieved by adherence to the principles of sleep hygiene.

Sleep hygiene will not in itself manage insomnia, other than those sleep problems which are a direct result of inadequate attention being paid to it. However, it can be used as an aid to establishing a clear division between daytime activity and nocturnal sleep, and allowing the natural sleep tendency to accumulate during the day. To achieve this, patients should refrain from caffeine-containing drinks from mid-afternoon, avoid excess alcohol consumption in the evening, reduce pre-bed stimulation (including watching television, especially if the material is provoking or exciting) and also refrain from physiological arousal caused by exercise. Attention should be given to the bedroom and sleeping facilities to make them as compatible as possible with the requirements of the individual. Although there is little scientific evidence that ear plugs, eye shades, herbal pillows, etc. have a robust effect in aiding sleep, their psychological impact may be useful in certain cases.

Sleep restriction schedules, whereby patients with sleep induction problems remain awake for an extra hour and, most importantly, rise the next morning half an hour or an hour earlier, are quite useful techniques for consolidating night-time sleep. However, it is important to emphasise that sleep-restriction scheduling will only help within the context of a nap-free day.

These behavioural techniques and patient manipulation of awake–sleep cycles to enhance the discrimination between waking and sleep can also be adopted to help to regulate the 'siesta-style' management of insomnia.

When considering pharmacotherapeutic management of insomnia in the elderly, the first principle is to cause no harm, or in treating the disorder use drug treatment regimens which might decrease the patient's overall quality of life by increasing side-effects due either directly to the particular medication used or to its interaction with other medication(s) which may need to be co-administered.

It is, of course, evident that insomnia as a secondary symptom of another disorder or disease must not be treated in isolation until the patient's response to prescribed treatment for the primary presenting symptoms has been evaluated.

This is particularly important in the case of sleep apnoea and other respiratory conditions, where the myorelaxant properties of some (particularly benzodiazepine) hypnotics will exacerbate rather than improve the underlying condition.

In depressed patients with insomnia, the slight improvement noted with regard to some aspects of cognitive arousal[95,96] following SSRIs can be utilised with a breakfast-dosing regimen to augment normal daytime arousal and add contrast to day/night rhythmicity. Periodicity in depression is well known,[97] but it is not yet possible to unequivocally link depression to a disturbance of a circadian or biological clock.[98] However, some antidepressants may disrupt sleep, and then hypnotics may be employed briefly at the beginning of therapy as described previously. Regular concurrent use of hypnotics with any other concomitant therapy must be regarded as the exception rather than the rule.

There are three main classes of drugs with the potential to be used as hypnotics.

Gamma-aminobutyric acid (GABA)–chloride-ion receptor agonists

The GABA–chloride-ion receptor agonists are the classic sedative agents and range from chloral hydrate through barbiturates, chlormethiazole, benzodiazepines (temazepam and nitrazepam) and non-benzodiazepine ligands of the GABA–chloride-ion receptor complex (zopiclone, zolpidem and zaleplon) to newer substances (indiplon and gaboxadol) which have a specific effect on GABA but not benzodiazepine receptors.

Anticholinergic antihistamines

Low doses (c. 25 mg) of anticholinergic antidepressants (e.g. amitriptyline) have been used extensively within general practice for the management of insomnia, but there have been few formal studies of the effectiveness of such therapy, and given the anticholinergic as well as antihistaminic activity of these drugs, long-term usage must give rise to concerns over accelerated cognitive decline and xerostoma (resulting from prolonged dry mouth).

Conventional first-generation antihistamines (e.g. promethazine, triprolidine, chlorpheniramine) are well-established sedative agents, due directly to the inverse agonism of central H_1 receptors. Although many of them are effective as sleep inducers, they do generally cause significant residual sequelae.[99]

Herbals and miscellaneous products

There is a great deal of anecdotal evidence and a strong historical lineage to suggest the utility and efficacy of herbal products (e.g. valerian, passiflora, hops), but controlled clinical investigations do not provide unequivocal evidence of efficacy.[100,101]

Some substances (e.g. trazodone) have become popular for 'off-label' use as hypnotics in the elderly, without the benefit of a supportive database of appropriate trials. The use of sedative antidepressants, tricyclics, trazodone, mianserin and mirtazepine on nocturnal administration schedules to aid sleep while producing the desired antidepressant effect is, as far as hypnotic activity is concerned, based on an erroneous understanding of the effects of such drugs on sleep. Sedation *per se* is not necessarily what is required for an effective hypnotic, and although the administration of sedative antidepressants at night might help to allay the untoward side-effects of daytime sedation, they cannot be recommended of themselves as first-line hypnotics.

Within the next few months, new hypnotics will appear on the market which have been specially developed with elderly patients' needs in mind. Some (e.g. eszopiclone and modified-release zolpidem) are variants of existing efficacious molecules. Others (e.g. pregabalin) are thought to exert their effects on sleep by acting on calcium channels (i.e. outside the sedative hypnotic tradition of GABA-ergic agonists). Intriguingly, $5HT_2$-receptor antagonists have also been shown to have effects in increasing the amount of slow-wave sleep, which may prove beneficial in promoting sleep without the consequences of nocturnal sedation and its daytime sequelae.

Although there are major differences between hypnotics with regard to their intrinsic toxicity and levels of residual sedation, there would seem to be little difference between them with regard to sleep induction properties. Choosing an appropriate hypnotic for an elderly patient initially entails a relatively straightforward elimination of those compounds which are pharmacologically toxic (i.e. barbiturates, chloral derivatives, chlormethiazole and tricyclic antidepressants). Lack of proven efficacy precludes herbal remedies and aromatherapy from serious consideration as first-line medications.

In practice, the choice of effective hypnotics means a selection from benzodiazepine and non-benzodiazepine ligands of the GABA–chloride-ion receptor complex, as the antihistamines as currently formulated lack consistency in clinical efficacy, and those that are effective seem to possess residual activity as a matter of course.

There are many misconceptions regarding the use of benzodiazepine hypnotics, and the risks of abuse and dependency have clearly been overplayed,[102] as has the contribution of benzodiazepine hypnotics to car-driving accident statistics.[103] Broadly speaking, the benzodiazepines remain safe and well-tolerated drugs for the treatment of insomnia in elderly patients unless it is anticipated that the therapy will be other than acute or short term (1 or 2 months at most). Although much is made of the long elimination half-life of some derivatives (e.g. nitrazepam and flurazepam), the clinical evidence only suggests a longer duration of action than other drugs, and does not mean that these drugs necessarily produce a hangover of sedation. However, the use of benzodiazepines with elimination half-lives of well under 24 hours (e.g. temazepam, loprazolam, lormetazepam) does ensure that there is little or no parent drug or active metabolite present during the day following nocturnal use, and the issues of accumulation of the drug are obviated, which is important when patients are receiving polypharmaceutical intervention for a variety of clinical conditions. The largest single factor determining residual effects with benzodiazepines is the dose of drug administered, and as the elimination half-life and duration of action are not always in concordance, residual effects can be found following high doses of drugs with a short elimination half-life.

To minimise the risk of daytime accumulation and residual effects, all drugs should be used at half their adult dose level (e.g. nitrazepam 2.5 mg, lormetazepam 0.5 mg, temazepam 10 mg, loprazolam 0.5 mg, flurazepam 15 mg).

The non-benzodiazepine ligands of the GABA–chloride-ion receptor complex should also be used at reduced dose regimens (i.e. zopiclone 3.75 mg, zolpidem 5 mg), although in the case of zaleplon, 10 mg seems to be the appropriate dose for both young and elderly patients. The major advantages of the 'Z-drugs' are their proven lack of residual effects and their lack of influence on EEG-sleep architecture.

The choice of which agent to use from those mentioned above is determined as much by the patient's response as by any other pharmacological or side-effect variable. There is also, once primary illness and disorder are managed, no clear clinical advantage of one hypnotic over another, and no particular insomnia or sleep disturbance which responds to one particular drug and not another.

Insomnia, as has been shown, is prevalent in the elderly, and strikingly more so than in younger patients. The effective management of such reported problems is relatively straightforward.

Key points

- Manage the primary illness first (this is especially true for depression and anxiety states) without using hypnotics (unless they are used as short-term co-medication with SSRIs at the start of antidepressant therapy).
- If the insomnia is due to sleep apnoea or respiratory disease, do not use hypnotics, but refer the patient for appropriate assessment/treatment.
- If the insomnia is primary or idiopathic without an evident cause, then initially attempt to manage the complaints by means of behavioural/ lifestyle changes.
- If there is an identifiable cause of an acute insomnia (e.g. bereavement), up to 7 nights of medication may be prescribed.
- In cases where the reported insomnia is sufficiently severe to cause daytime impairment of cognitive or behavioural integrity, low doses of effective hypnotics should be given on a regimen that encourages the patient to use the drug sporadically and only when absolutely needed. Regular and especially regular prolonged use of hypnotics is not a good therapeutic option in the long term, and patients whose insomnia persists for periods in excess of 2 months should be referred for evaluation in a clinical sleep disorders unit, as it is only via an appropriate polysomnographic assessment that an appropriate diagnosis of the aetiology of a particular sleep disturbance can be made.

References

1 Webb WB (1982) The measurement and characteristics of sleep in older persons. *Neurobiol Aging*. **3**: 311.

2 Braz S, Hirshowitz M, Tufik S, Neumann BG and Karacan I (1990) Survey of sleep complaints among 1000 residents of Sao Paulo. *Sleep Res*. **19**: 198.

3 Habte-Gabr E, Wallace RB, Colsher PL *et al.* (1991) Sleep patterns in rural elders: demographic, health and psychobehavioral correlates. *J Clin Epidemiol*. **44**: 5–13.

4 Bliwise DL, King AC, Harris RB and Haskell WL (1992) Prevalence of self-reported poor sleep in a healthy population aged 50–65. *Soc Sci Med*. **34**: 49–55.

5 Hoch CC, Dew MA, Reynolds CF *et al.* (1994) A longitudinal study of laboratory- and diary-based sleep measures in healthy 'old old' and 'young old' volunteers. *Sleep*. **17**: 489–96.

6 Foley DJ, Monjan AA, Brown SL *et al.* (1995) Sleep complaints among elderly persons: an epidemiologic study of three communities. *Sleep*. **18**: 425–32.

7 Mallon L and Hetta J (1997) A survey of sleep habits and sleeping difficulties in an elderly Swedish population. *Ups J Med Sci*. **102**: 185–98.

8 Karacan I, Thornby JI, Anch M *et al.* (1976) Prevalence of sleep disturbance in a primarily urban Florida county. *Soc Sci Med*. **10**: 239–44.

9 Office for National Statistics (1999) *Population Trends (Quarterly). Summer 1999 issue.* The Stationery Office, London.

10 Ray WA, Griffin MR, Schaffner W, Baugh DK and Melton LJ (1987) Psychotropic drug use and the risk of hip fracture. *NEJM*. **316**: 363–9.

11 Pollak CP and Perlick D (1991) Sleep problems and institutionalization of the elderly. *J Geriatr Psychiatry Neurol*. **4**: 204–10.

12 Swift CG and Shapiro CM (1993) ABC of sleep disorders: sleep and sleep problems in elderly people. *BMJ*. **306**: 1468–71.

13 Martikainen K, Hasan J, Urponen H, Vuori I and Partinen M (1992) Daytime sleepiness: a risk factor in community life. *Acta Neurol Scand*. **86**: 337–41.

14 Pollak CP, Perlick D, Linsner JP, Wenston J and Hsieh F (1990) Sleep problems in the community elderly as predictors of death and nursing home placement. *J Commun Health*. **15**: 123–35.

15 Young JS, Cephas GA and Blow O (1998) Outcome and cost of trauma among the elderly: a real-life model of a single-payer reimbursement system. *J Trauma-Injury Infect Crit Care*. **45**: 800–4.

16 Cwikel J (1992) Falls among elderly people living at home: medical and social factors in a national sample. *Is J Med Sci*. **28**: 446–53.

17 Kazar G, Bauer O, Kosa J and Pestessy J (1996) Accidents of the elderly. *Orvosi Hetilap*. **137**: 1245–9.

18 Daigneault G, Joly P and Frigon JY (2002) Previous convictions or accidents and the risk of subsequent accidents of older drivers. *Accid Anal Prev*. **34**: 257–61.

19 Kripke DF, Ancoli-Israel S, Fell RL. *et al.* (1991) Health risk of insomnia. In: JH Peter, T Penzel, T Podzus *et al.* (eds) *Sleep and Health Risk*. Springer Verlag, New York.

20 Janson C, Gíslason T, De Backer W *et al.* (1995) Prevalence of sleep disturbances among young adults in three European countries. *Sleep*. **18**: 589–97.

21 Schmitt FA, Phillips BA, Cook YR, Berry DTR and Wekstein DR (1996) Self-report of sleep symptoms in older adults: correlates of daytime sleepiness and health. *Sleep*. **19**: 59–64.

22 Wingard DL and Berkman LF (1983) Mortality risk associated with sleeping patterns among adults. *Sleep*. **6**: 102–7.

23 Ford DE and Kamerow DB (1989) Epidemiological study of sleep disturbances and psychiatric disorders. *JAMA*. **262**: 1479–84.

24 McGhie A and Russell SM (1962) The subjective assessment of normal sleep patterns. *J Ment Sci*. **108**: 642–54.

25 Cirignotta F, Mondini S, Zucconi M, Lenzi PL and Lugaresi E (1985) Insomnia: an epidemiological survey. *Clin Neuropharmacol*. **8**: S49–54.

26 Gíslason T and Almqvist M (1987) Somatic diseases and sleep complaints. *Acta Med Scand*. **221**: 457–81.

27 Morgan K, Dallosso H, Ebrahim S, Arie T and Fentem PH (1988) Prevalence, frequency and duration of hypnotic drug use among the elderly living at home. *BMJ*. **296**: 601–2.

28 Monk TH, Reynolds CF, Buysse DJ *et al.* (1991) Circadian characteristics of healthy 80-year-olds and their relationship to objectively recorded sleep. *J Gerontol Med Sci*. **46**: M171–5.

29 Regestein QR (1980) Insomnia and sleep disturbances in the aged: sleep and insomnia in the elderly. *J Geriatr Psychiatry*. **13**: 153–71.

30 Asplund R (1996) Daytime sleepiness and napping amongst the elderly in relation to somatic health and medical treatment. *J Intern Med*. **239**: 261–7.

31 DeGraaf W, Poelstra PAM and Visser P (1983) The relations between the sleep quality and the patient's morbidity history. *Sleep Res*. **12**: 306.

32 Morin CM and Gramling SE (1989) Sleep patterns and aging: comparison of older adults with and without insomnia complaints. *Psychol Aging*. **4**: 290–4.

33 Newman AB, Enright PL, Manolio TA, Haponik EF and Wahl PW (1997) Sleep disturbance, psychosocial correlates, and cardiovascular disease in 5201 older adults: the Cardiovascular Health Study. *J Am Geriatr Soc*. **45**: 1–7.

34 Reynolds CF, Kupfer DJ, Taska LS *et al.* (1985) EEG sleep in elderly depressed, demented, and healthy subjects. *Biol Psychiatry*. **20**: 431–42.

35 Kales JD, Kales A, Bixler EO *et al.* (1984) Biopsychobehavioral correlates of insomnia. V. Clinical characteristcs and behavioral correlates. *Am J Psychiatry*. **141**: 1371–6.

36 Schechtman KB, Kutner NG, Wallace RB, Buchner DM, Ory MG and the FICSIT Group (1997) Gender, self-reported depressive symptoms, and sleep disturbance among older community-dwelling persons. *J Psychosom Res*. **43**: 513–27.

37 Yamaguchi N, Matsurbara S, Momonoi F, Morikawa K, Takeyama M and Maeda Y (1999) Comparative studies on sleep disturbance in the elderly based on question-naire assessments in 1983 and 1996. *Psychiatry Clin Neurosci*. **53**: 261–2.

38 Weinstein L, Dement W, Redington D, Guilleminault C and Mitler M (1983) Insomnia in the San Francisco Bay area: a telephone survey. In: C Guilleminault and E Lugaresi (eds) *Sleep/Wake Disorders: natural history, epidemiology and long-term evaluation*. Raven Press, New York.

39 Friedman LF, Bliwise DL, Tanke ED, Salom SR and Yesavage JA (1991/1992) A survey of self-reported poor sleep and associated factors in older individuals. *Behav Health Aging*. **2**: 13–20.

40 Hindmarch I (1984) Subjective aspects of the effects of benzodiazepines on sleep and early morning behaviour. *Ir J Med Sci*. **153**: 272–8.

41 Von Faber M, Bootsma-van der Wiel A, van Exel E *et al.* (2001) Successful aging in the oldest old. *Arch Int Med*. **161**: 2694–700.

42 Chambers MJ and Keller B (1993) Alert insomniacs: are they really sleep deprived? *Clin Psychol Rev*. **13**: 649–66.

43 Mellinger GD, Balter MB and Uhlenhuth EH (1985) Insomnia and its treatment. *Arch Gen Psychiatry*. **42**: 225–32.

44 Maggi S, Langlois JA, Minicuci N *et al.* (1998) Sleep complaints in community-dwelling older persons: prevalence, associated factors, and reported causes. *J Am Geriatr Soc*. **46**: 161–8.

45 Morgan K, Dallosso H, Ebrahim S, Arie T and Fentem PH (1988) Characteristics of subjective insomnia in the elderly living at home. *Age Ageing*. **17**: 1–7.

46 Beaman P (1989) Factors affecting sleep in the non-institutionalised elderly: a questionnaire approach. *Commun Psychiatry.* **August:** 19–20.

47 Gíslason T, Reynisdóttir H, Kristbjarnarson H and Benediktsdóttir B (1993) Sleep habits and sleep disturbances among the elderly – an epidemiological survey. *J Intern Med.* **234:** 31–9.

48 Hoch CC, Reynolds CF, Kupfer DJ, Berman SR, Houck PR and Stack JA (1987) Empirical note: self-report versus recorded sleep in healthy seniors. *Psychophysiology.* **24:** 293–9.

49 Blay SL and Mari JJ (1990) Subjective sleep reports of sleep disorders in the community elderly. *Behav Health Aging.* **1:** 143–9.

50 Briscoe ME (1978) Sex differences in perceptions of illness and expressed life satisfaction. *Psychol Med.* **8:** 339–45.

51 Urponen H, Vuori I, Hasan J and Partinen M (1988) Self-evaluations of factors promoting and disturbing sleep: an epidemiological survey in Finland. *Soc Sci Med.* **26:** 443–50.

52 Moran MG, Thompson TL and Nies AS (1988) Sleep disorders in the elderly. *Am J Psychiatry.* **145:** 1369–78.

53 Ohayon MM and Caulet M (1996) Psychotropic medication and insomnia complaints in two epidemiological studies. *Can J Psychiatry.* **41:** 457–64.

54 Kronholm E and Hyyppä MT (1985) Age-related sleep habits and retirement. *Ann Clin Res.* **17:** 257–64.

55 Pearson JL (2002) Recent research on suicide in the elderly. *Curr Psychiatry Rep.* **4:** 59–63.

56 Middelkoop HAM, Smilde-van den Doel DA, Neven AK, Kamphuisen HAC and Springer CP (1996) Subjective sleep characteristics of 1485 males and females aged 50–93: effects of sex and age, and factors related to self-evaluated quality of sleep. *J Gerontol Med Sci.* **51A:** M108–15.

57 Rowe JW and Kahn RL (1987) Human aging: usual and successful. *Science.* **237:** 143–9.

58 Lack L, Miller W and Turner D (1988) A survey of sleeping difficulties in an Australian population. *Commun Health Stud.* **11:** 200–7.

59 Seppälä M, Hyyppä MT, Impivaara O, Knuts L-R and Sourander L (1997) Subjective quality of sleep and use of hypnotics in an elderly urban population. *Aging.* **9:** 327–34.

60 Henderson S, Jorm AF, Scott LR, Mackinnon AJ, Christensen H and Korten AE (1995) Insomnia in the elderly: its prevalence and correlates in the general population. *Med J Aust.* **162:** 22–4.

61 Fichten CS, Creti L, Amsel R, Brender W, Weinstein N and Libman E (1995) Poor sleepers who do not complain of insomnia: myths and realities about psychological and lifestyle characteristics of older good and poor sleepers. *J Behav Med.* **18:** 189–223.

62 Waters WF, Adams SG, Binks P and Varnado P (1993) Attention, stress and negative emotion in persistent sleep onset and sleep maintenance insomnia. *Sleep.* **16:** 128–36.

63 Moffitt PF, Kalucy EC, Kalucy RS, Baum FE and Cook RD (1991) Sleep difficulties, pain and other correlates. *J Intern Med.* **230:** 245–9.

64 Gerard P, Collins KJ, Doré C and Exton-Smith AN (1978) Subjective characteristics of sleep in the elderly. *Age Ageing.* **7 (Suppl.):** 55–9.

65 Mant A and Eyland EA (1988) Sleep patterns and problems in elderly general practice attenders: an Australian survey. *Commun Health Stud.* **12:** 192–9.

66 Clark BG, Jue SG, Dawson GW and Ward A (1986) Loprazolam: a preliminary review of its pharmacodynamic and pharmacokinetic properties and therapeutic efficacy in insomnia. *Drugs.* **31:** 500–16.

67 Englert S and Linden M (1998) Differences in self-reported sleep complaints in elderly persons living in the community who do or do not take sleep medication. *J Clin Psychiatry.* **59:** 137–44.

68 Zepelin H and Morgan LE (1981) Correlates of sleep disturbance in retirees. *Sleep Res.* **10**: 120.

69 Barker J and Mitteness L (1988) Nocturia in the elderly. *Gerontologist.* **28**: 99–104.

70 Prinz PN, Vitiello MV, Raskind MA and Thorpy MJ (1990) Geriatrics: sleep disorders and aging. *NEJM.* **323**: 520–6.

71 Smith A (2002) Effects of caffeine on human behaviour. *Food Chem Toxicol.* **40**: 1243–55.

72 Liljenberg B, Almqvist M, Hetta J, Roos BE and Ågren H (1988) The prevalence of insomnia: the importance of operationally defined criteria. *Ann Clin Res.* **20**: 393–8.

73 Fichten CS, Creti L, Amsel R, *et al.* (1995) Poor sleepers who do not complain of insomnia: myths and realities about psychological and lifestyle characteristics of older good and poor sleepers. *J Behav Med.* **18**(2): 189–223.

74 Hohagen F, Kappler C, Schramm E *et al.* (1994) Prevalence of insomnia in elderly general practice attenders and the current treatment modalities. *Acta Psychiatr Scand.* **90**: 102–8.

75 Libman E, Creti L, Amsel R, Brender W and Fichten CS (1997) What do older good and poor sleepers do during periods of nocturnal wakefulness? The Sleep Behaviors Scale: 60+. *Psychol Aging.* **12**: 170–82.

76 Mayers AG, van Hooff JC and Baldwin DS (1999) *Are inefficient sleepers more depressed than efficient sleepers?* Paper presented at the 1999 Conference of the British Sleep Society, Sleep and its Disorders from Childhood to Old Age, Oxford. 16–17 September.

77 Breckenridge JN, Gallagher D, Thompson LW and Peterson J (1986) Characteristic depressive symptoms of bereaved elders. *J Gerontol.* **41**: 163–8.

78 Stepanski E, Koshorek G, Zorick F, Glinn M, Roehrs T and Roth T (1989) Characteristics of individuals who do or do not seek treatment of chronic insomnia. *Psychosomatics.* **30**: 421–7.

79 Weyerer S and Dilling H (1991) Prevalence and treatment of imsomnia in the community: results from the Upper Bavarian Field Study. *Sleep.* **14**: 392–8.

80 Kim K, Uchiyama M, Okawa M, Liu X and Ogihara R (2000) An epidemiological study of insomnia among the Japanese general population. *Sleep.* **23**: 41–7.

81 Bixler EO, Kales A, Soldatos CR, Kales JD and Healey S (1979) Prevalence of sleep disorders in the Los Angeles Metropolitan Area. *Am J Psychiatry.* **136**: 1257–62.

82 Dodge R, Cline MG and Quan SF (1995) The natural history of insomnia and its relationship to respiratory symptoms. *Arch Intern Med.* **155**: 1797–800.

83 Domino G (1986) Sleep habits in the elderly: a study of three Hispanic cultures. *J Cross-Cult Psychol.* **17**: 109–20.

84 Rodin J, McAvay G and Timko C (1988) A longitudinal study of depressed mood and sleep disturbances in elderly adults. *J Gerontol: Psychol Sci.* **43**: 45–53.

85 Kennedy GJ, Kelman HR, Thomas C *et al.* (1989) Hierarchy of characteristics associated with depressive symptoms in an urban elderly sample. *Am J Psychiatry.* **146**: 220–5.

86 Seppälä M (1993) Sleep and hypnotics in the elderly: epidemiological and pharmacological studies in an urban community and in nursing homes. *Psychiatr Fenn.* **24**: 177–92.

87 Brabbins CJ, Dewey ME, Copeland JRM *et al.* (1993) Insomnia in the elderly: prevalence, gender differences and relationship with morbidity and mortality. *Int J Geriatr Psychiatry.* **8**: 473–80.

88 Hayter J (1983) Sleep behaviours of older persons. *Nurs Res.* **32**: 242–6.

89 Riedel BW and Lichstein KL (1998) Objective sleep measures and subjective sleep satisfaction: how do older adults with insomnia define a good night's sleep? *Psychol Aging.* **13**: 159–63.

90 Dement WC, Miles LE and Carscadon MA (1982) 'White Paper' on sleep and aging. *J Am Geriatr Soc.* **30**: 25–50.

91 Shock N (1977) Biological theories of aging. In: J Birren and K Schaie (eds) *Handbook of the Psychology of Aging.* Van Nostrand Reinhold, New York.

92 Stampi C (1992) Evolution, chronobiology, and functions of polyphasic and ultrashort sleep: main issues. In: C Stampi (ed.) *Why We Nap: evolution, chronobiology and functions of polyphasic and ultrashort sleep.* Birkhauser, Boston, MA.

93 Beh H (1994) A survey of daytime napping in an elderly Australian population. *Aust J Psychol.* **46**: 100–6.

94 American Sleep Disorders Association (1990) *The International Classification of Sleep Disorders Diagnostic and Coding Manual.* American Sleep Disorders Association, Rochester.

95 Hindmarch I and Bhatti JZ (1988) Psychopharmacological effects of sertraline in normal, healthy volunteers. *Eur J Clin Pharmacol.* **35**: 221–3.

96 Kerr JS, Sherwood N and Hindmarch I (1991) The comparative psychopharmacology of 5HT reuptake inhibitors. *Hum Psychopharmacol: Clin Exp.* **6**: 313–17.

97 Wirz-Justice A and Van den Hoofdekker RH (1999) Sleep deprivation in depression. What do we know, where do we go? *Biol Psychiatry.* **46**: 445–53.

98 Bolvin DB (2000) Influence of sleep–wake and circadian rhythm disturbances in psychiatric disorders. *J Psychiatry Neurosci.* **25**: 446–58.

99 Soldatos CR and Diekos DG (1995) Neuroleptics, antihistamines and antiparkinsonian drugs: effects on sleep. In: A Kales (ed.) *Pharmacology of Sleep.* Springer-Verlag, Berlin.

100 Donath F, Quispe S, Diefenbach K, Maurer A, Fietze I and Roots I (2000) Critical evaluation of the effect of valerian extract on sleep structure and sleep quality. *Pharmacopsychiatry.* **33**: 47–53.

101 Kuhlmann J, Berger W, Podzuweit H and Schmidt U (1999) The influence of valerian treatment on 'reaction time, alertness and concentration' in volunteers. *Pharmacopsychiatry.* **32**: 235–41.

102 Allgulander C (2000) The benzodiazepine addiction story. In: Trimble M and Hindmarch I (eds) *Benzodiazepines.* Wrightson Biomedical Publishing, Petersfield.

103 Barbone F, McMahon AD, Davey PG and Morris AD (1998) Association of road traffic accidents with benzodiazepine use. *Lancet.* **352**: 1331–6.

Chapter 12

Drug treatment in dementia

Roger Bullock

Introduction

Pharmacological intervention is now playing an increasing role in the management of dementia, especially in Alzheimer's disease (AD). After the cautious
introduction of the cholinesterase inhibitors, the prospect of future more effective
treatments is now eagerly anticipated as the understanding of relevant neurobiological processes unfolds.

This chapter will focus on the neurodegenerative dementias, primarily AD,
vascular dementia (VaD) and dementia with Lewy bodies (DLB), rather than
dementia due to reversible causes. In the latter case, treatment of the underlying
condition wherever possible is the most important intervention. In most cases
there is little evidence to demonstrate any impact on cognition through any
primary intervention, and there are no adequate data in the literature to support
treatment of the secondary cognitive impairment with any specific therapy.

Three types of drug intervention are possible:

- *symptomatic* – where the effect of the treatment continues for as long as the
  drug continues to be taken, but is rapidly lost when the drug is discontinued
- *disease modifying* – where the treatment alters the course of the illness while
  being taken, and continues to show the alteration in the course of the illness
  after it is stopped
- *cure* – where the disease is eradicated as a result of the treatment.

Finding a cure for dementia is the obvious aim, but in the absence of achieving
that goal, current treatments are predominantly symptomatic, with a suggestion
in some instances of possible disease modification. Something as simple as
vitamin E has been shown to delay institutionalisation in patients with AD,[1]
while the more complex and experimental strategy of the amyloid vaccine[2]
showed early promise, but is currently suspended following complications that
arose in the phase II study.

In the absence of cure, drug therapy remains just part of the total service
provision for people with dementia. The price of these new drugs can create a
tension between what they cost and what is spent on other service provision. On
average, in the UK only 2–3% of mental health revenue is spent on drugs. This
must be increased over the ensuing years to facilitate the introduction of more
new drugs and combinations of therapy. At present only 20% of patients who are
eligible for cholinesterase inhibitors are treated across the Western world, due to a
mixture of low detection rates, early stopping of treatment due to disappointment
with the results, and contained prescribing. As treatments improve in efficacy,

screening and demand will radically alter this picture, so services must be in a position to respond to this.

Primary treatments

Cholinesterase inhibitors

The cholinergic hypothesis of AD[3] led to a number of strategies to enhance failing cholinergic neurons and the consequent reduction of the neurotransmitter acetylcholine (ACh). The most consistent therapeutic effect to date has been via the use of inhibitors of the enzyme acetylcholinesterase (AChEIs), which cleaves the transmitter through hydrolysis in the cholinergic synapse to form choline and acetate, which are recycled. This enzyme inhibition in part compensates for the hypofunctioning cholinergic system. Four such compounds have now been licensed for the treatment of AD, namely tacrine (now largely discontinued because of its four times daily regimen and associated liver toxicity), donepezil, rivastigmine and galantamine. These drugs have increased awareness of AD, with increasing numbers of referrals (to the point now that in some areas 50% of expected cases have been detected). As a result, UK centres are now reporting consistent results with these treatments [4-6] and their efficacy is looking more robust.[7] AChEIs were initially regarded as an interim measure before better disease-modifying compounds became available.[8] However, despite many compounds being in development, only memantine, an N-methyl-D-aspartate (NMDA) inhibitor, represents a new and different pharmacological class to enter the market. Protocols were rapidly established to enable treatment with cholinesterase inhibitors.[9] However, these have now been superseded in the UK by the National Institute for Clinical Excellence (NICE) guidance[10] on the use of these three drugs.

Donepezil

Donepezil is a long-acting piperidine-based selective acetylcholinesterase (AChE) inhibitor. AChE has an active site that contains two subsites – an ionic one and an esteratic one. The ionic site binds the quaternary amine group of ACh, bringing its ester group into apposition with the catalytic esteratic site, which then cleaves ACh by acylation. Inhibition can occur at either of these subsites. Tacrine and donepezil act at the ionic subsite. This gives selective AChE inhibition, with no effect on the butyrylcholinesterase (BuChE) enzyme. Rivastigmine and galantamine act at the esteratic subsite.

Absorption after an oral dose is almost 100%, with maximal plasma concentration reached at 4 hours. The half-life is 70 hours, so steady state should occur at 16 days. Metabolism is via the liver, through P450 enzymes, where the active metabolite is 6-O-desmethyl donepezil. Excretion also occurs via the kidneys, although renal disease is not a contraindication. Not all of the drug is excreted, suggesting that there is some accumulation. The pharmacokinetics are linear to 10 mg, so doses of 5 mg and 10 mg are recommended, although clinical studies of 20 mg are ongoing.

Controlled studies

In the initial studies, donepezil was found to have a significant effect on cognition at 5 mg (but not at 1 mg or 3 mg), which was then replicated equally at both 5 mg and 10 mg in the second study.[11,12] The first phase III study was of placebo vs. 7 days of 5 mg, followed by 24 weeks of 5 or 10 mg donepezil, finishing with a 6-week placebo washout.[13] Again donepezil was more effective than placebo on the Alzheimer's Disease Assessment Scale (cognitive section) (ADAS-cog) (3.1 points on 10 mg), Mini-Mental State Examination (MMSE) (1.36 points on 10 mg) and Clinical Global Impression Scale (0.44 units on 10 mg). Much of the effect size was due to placebo deterioration rather than pure improvement, and as before there was no difference between 5 mg and 10 mg doses. During the placebo washout, the treatment group scores fell to the same values as those for subjects who had always been on placebo. This is the basis on which donepezil is considered to be a symptomatic therapy.

The European, South African and Australasian study was identical to the US study and reported very similar results, namely ADAS 2.9 points on 10 mg and 0.4 units on the Global Impression Scale.[14] This time 10 mg did appear to be superior to 5 mg in terms of cognition. There was also an improvement in function as measured by the Interview for Deterioration in Daily Living Activities in Dementia at 10 mg but not 5 mg. As before, the washout led to the loss of effect.

Tariot *et al.*[15] reported a study in nursing homes of patients with AD and AD with cerebrovascular disease. This did not show any cognitive or behavioural effect. In the Nordic countries a 52-week placebo-controlled study was performed.[16] This used the Gottfries, Brane and Steen scale (GBS) rather than the standard regulatory instruments. The study showed a benefit for donepezil in terms of cognition, and using the global deterioration scale, a difference in terms of decline. Function improved with donepezil on the Progressive Deterioration Scale (PDS) but not the activities of daily living (ADL) subscale of the GBS. Once more there was no evidence to support a behavioural effect. Although this was a positive study, there were significant dropouts in both groups, making interpretation of the results more difficult.

Another 1-year randomised study looked at the effect of donepezil on MMSE and ADL in patients with moderate AD.[17] Patients were followed up until a predetermined worsening in ADL occurred, and a survival analysis was performed. This meant that 57% of the combined patient numbers did not complete the study. At 48 weeks, 51% of the donepezil-treated patients remained in the study, compared with 35% of the placebo-treated patients. This was a statistically significant result, but if the actual scale scores were used, there was no difference between the groups.

An outpatient group with moderate to severe AD showed improvement in terms of cognition (on the MMSE and Severe Impairment Battery, SIB) and global impression.[18] This study did show significant improvements in behaviour, as measured by the Neuropsychiatric Inventory, an effect driven by the apathy, anxiety and depression subscales.

Recent evidence suggests that exposure to donepezil does have an effect in delaying admission to a nursing home,[19] although the study has methodological problems that weaken its conclusions. However, these are the first real-time data to be published that attempt to support the economic models that have been used before to demonstrate the cost utility of this class of drugs.

Summary

Eight published studies covering mild, moderate and severe AD have been published (*see* Table 12.1). In each one donepezil was associated with significant cognitive improvement over placebo. The Cochrane Review finds donepezil modestly effective, at 5 mg and 10 mg, in improving both cognition and global impression, with a minimal reduction in the rate of functional decline only at the higher dose.[20] No clear benefits in the treatment of behaviour have yet been established. Using the numbers needed to treat (NNT) paradigm, across all of the studies and both doses, donepezil shows the following NNTs:

- cognition   8–14
- clinical global impression   5–16
- function/behaviour   no interpretable data.

Table 12.1 Placebo-controlled studies with donepezil in AD

Author	Duration (weeks)	Number of patients	Mean age (years)	Phase	Dose (mg/day)
Rogers and Friedhoff[11]	12	161	71.8	II	1, 3, 5
Rogers et al.[12]	12	468	73.7	III	5, 10
Rogers et al.[13]	24	473	73.4	III	5, 10
Burns et al.[14]	24	818	72.0	III	5, 10
Tariot et al.[15]	24	208	85.6	IV	5, 10
Winblad et al.[16]	52	286	72.5	IV	5, 10
Mohs et al.[17]	52	431	75.4	IV	5, 10
Feldman et al.[18]	26	207	74.3	IV	5, 10

Rivastigmine

Rivastigmine is a pseudo-irreversible, selective AChE subtype inhibitor that is particularly selective for the G1 monomeric form of AChE. This form is particularly concentrated in the cortex and hippocampus, and is also found on postsynaptic membranes, degrading ACh independently from its presynaptic release. This differs from the more common G4 tetramer, which is found on presynaptic membranes and cleaves the enzyme while inhibiting further ACh release. G4 decreases with age (and more so in AD). G1 does not alter with time or disease, which suggests that this is a more selective site of action, and offers a differentiating factor for rivastigmine.

Rivastigmine also inhibits butyrylcholinesterase (BuChE), which is found in increasing amounts in the brain as AD progresses. Studies have demonstrated that specific inhibition of BuChE can produce similar cognitive improvements to AChE inhibition.[21] This dual enzyme inhibition may prove to have some clinical relevance, with rivastigmine continuing to produce a positive effect until late into the illness.

Absorption of rivastigmine is rapid, but after a first-pass effect only 35% of the dose is available. Peak plasma levels occur at 1 hour, with peak activity at 6 hours and duration of action of 12 hours. Rivastigmine is not plasma protein bound, nor is it metabolised in the liver, but it is broken down by AChE itself. The carbamate portion of rivastigmine is slowly hydrolysed after binding to the enzyme, and is then cleaved, conjugated to a sulphate and excreted via the kidneys. The principal metabolite is essentially inert. This metabolism makes it unlikely to interact with other medications.

Controlled studies

Early studies showed a significant improvement in cognition in patients with dementia.[22] Four similarly designed phase III studies with differing dose regimens were conducted in patients with mild to moderate AD. These were all 26-week randomised studies as shown in Table 12.2. The two published studies[23,24] were flexible dose-range studies, with rapid titration to a low-dose group (1–4 mg) or a high-dose group (6–12 mg) vs. placebo over 7 weeks, followed by a 19-week flexible dosing regimen. A fixed-dose study of 3, 6 or 9 mg and a broad 2–12 mg dose-range study have never been published, although some results from the former have been included in secondary reports.[25,26] Patients entering all of these studies were allowed to have a wide range of comorbid illnesses (77–96%) and subsequent concomitant medication (77–98%).

In both of the published studies, rivastigmine was superior to placebo on cognitive (ADAS-cog), functional (PDS) and global scales. The effect sizes in the Corey-Bloom study were 3.78 on the ADAS, 0.19 on the PDS and 0.29 on the Clinicians' Interview-Based Impression of Change (CIBIC). Similar findings were obtained in the Rosler study (2.28, ADAS; 2.73, PDS; 0.44, CIBIC. In the fixed-dose study, the 6 and 9 mg groups were more effective than placebo on the ADAS and global rating. Behaviour was not measured in these studies.

Table 12.2 Controlled studies with rivastigmine in AD

Author	Duration (weeks)	Number of patients	Phase	Dose
B103 (unpublished)	13	405	II	3 or 2 mg
Forette et al.[22]	18	114	II	Maximum tolerated
Corey-Bloom et al.[23]	26	699	III	1–4 mg (3.5), 6–12 mg (9.7)
Rosler et al.[24]	26	725	III	1–4 mg (3.7), 6–12 mg (10.4)
B351 (unpublished)	26	702	III	3, 6 or 9 mg
B304 (unpublished)	26		III	

The clinical trial data have been amalgamated in several reports. The Cochrane Review is the most systematic pooled evidence. Using this method, the ADAS-cog scores ranged between a 1.7 and 4.2 point improvement and the PDS having a 2.4 point gain. For both, only the higher dose range was significant vs. placebo. This was also the case with global measures. Another pooled analysis by Schneider *et al.*[25] had previously reported similar findings. Farlow *et al.*[27] have reported an increased effect of rivastigmine in those who are declining more rapidly, suggesting that rivastigmine may be particularly effective when a person is experiencing a noticeable change in their condition.

Summary

The mixture of published and unpublished studies initially makes the overall interpretation appear difficult. However, it seems clear that 1–4 mg is not usually a therapeutic dose, but at 6–12 mg there is a modest improvement in cognition, function and global measures. As yet no clear behavioural benefit has been demonstrated in controlled studies. Using the NNT methodology, then, for rivastigmine:

- cognition: 8–20
- function: 6–15
- global: 8–17
- behaviour: no interpretable data.

Galantamine

Galantamine is an alkaloid extract from *Galanthus woronowi* (Caucasian snow-drop). It is a reversible, competitive inhibitor of AChE with partial (50-fold less) BuChE activity. It competes with ACh at the binding site on AChE, so will be most effective in areas of low transmitter concentration, producing a selective effect on the areas most affected by AD. Galantamine is also an allosteric modulator at nicotinic cholinergic receptor sites, which further enhances cholinergic trans-mission [28] and may have positive effects on other neurotransmitter systems.

Allosteric modulation is the method of action of benzodiazepines, and is thus a powerful and recognised pharmacological action. Galantamine is a relatively weak cholinesterase inhibitor compared with donepezil and especially rivastig-mine. To achieve results similar to the inhibitors, it is proposed that the allosterically potentiating ligand (APL) effect makes a significant contribution to the observed efficacy of the drug.

Galantamine is rapidly absorbed with linear pharmacokinetics, slowed by ingesting with food. Bioavailability is 80–100%, protein binding is 15% and the half-life is 8 hours. Metabolism is via the liver P450 system to inactive metabolites, which are excreted with unchanged drug in the urine.

Controlled studies

Several early studies to determine sample sizes have been reported.[29–31] Seven randomised studies have also been reported, and one unpublished study (*see* Table 12.3). A 3-month dose-finding study showed that statistically signific-ant improvements in cognition and side-effects were both dose related.[32] Another study allowed doses of up to 50 mg/day, and patients were then randomised to placebo or continuation.[33] The treatment group faired 3.06 points better on the ADAS. A 3-month study again showed that 24 mg and 32 mg galantamine were effective for cognition, ADL and global measures.[34] A titration study of 29 weeks' duration with a fixed titration to 32 mg remains unpublished.

Three pivotal phase III studies have been published. Two of them used a fixed-dose treatment regimen of 24 or 32 mg/day in divided doses.[35,36] The other study used 8, 16 and 24 mg doses and was only 20 weeks in duration.[37] In all of these studies, galantamine was significantly better than placebo in terms of cognitive function at doses above 16 mg/day (ADAS 3.5 points at 24 mg and 4.1 points at 32 mg). With function, the Tariot study showed benefit for galantamine on the ADCS-ADL at 16 mg (3.5 points) and 24 mg (2.4 points). This benefit was due to placebo deterioration and stabilisation of the treatment group. The other studies used different scales and only showed significance at 32 mg. Global measures in all of the studies were significant at all doses except 8 mg/day. Uniquely, to date, behavioural data were captured in the galantamine studies. The Rockwood study failed to show significance, but the Tariot trial showed benefit on the NPI at 16 mg (2.4 points) and 24 mg (2.4 points).

Table 12.3 Controlled studies of galantamine in AD

Author	Duration (weeks)	Number of patients	Age (years)	Phase	Dose
Kewitz and Berzewski[31]	13	94	60–87	II	15–20 mg
Rainer[33]	13	167	Not applicable	II	Up to 50 mg
Wilkinson et al.[32]	12	285	73.7	II	18, 24 or 36 mg
Rockwood et al.[34]	12	386	75	III	24 or 32 mg
Gal-95–05	29	554	72.9	II	32 mg
Wilcock et al.[36]	26	653	72.2	III	24 or 32 mg
Raskind et al.[35]	26	636	72.2	III	24 or 32 mg
Tariot et al.[37]	20	978	77.7	III	16, 24 or 32 mg

Summary
Galantamine has shown modest benefits in all of the domains of AD at doses of 16, 24 and 32 mg. The latter dose is associated with a higher incidence of side-effects and so is not recommended within the license. The Cochrane Review[38] agrees with these findings, reporting an overall improvement on the ADAS of 3.5 points at 24 mg. NNTs were calculated from the review as follows:

- cognition: 5–10
- global: 5–12
- function/behaviour: not enough data to calculate reliably.

Adverse events with cholinesterase inhibitors

The commonest adverse events are due to the cholinomimetic effects, namely nausea, diarrhoea, vomiting, muscle cramps, insomnia, fatigue and anorexia. These effects are mostly mild and transient and do not significantly interrupt treatment. The most likely times when these side-effects may occur are during initiation and dose escalation. Slower titration and taking these drugs with food are both reported to reduce the likelihood and intensity of side-effects. If necessary, anti-emetic drugs can be used in conjunction with cholinesterase inhibitors to assist in achieving relevant treatment levels.

It is suggested that inhibition of the G4 tetramer AChE is more likely to produce insomnia, muscle cramps and cardiac effects than inhibition of G1. This would imply some advantages for rivastigmine, but in turn it does appear to have a worse profile for anorexia, so it would seem that the common adverse events for these three drugs are broadly similar (*see* Table 12.4). This is borne out by initial Food and Drug Administration (FDA) monitoring, which reports similar numbers of notifications of adverse events for both donepezil and rivastigmine.[39]

Table 12.4 Number needed to harm (NNH) of common adverse events with donepezil, rivastigmine and galantamine

Adverse event	Donepezil	Rivastigmine	Galantamine
Nausea	7	5	5
Diarrhoea	10	9	10
Vomiting	12	9	10
Anorexia	17	10	30
Withdrawals from studies	17	8	13

Patient selection

Clinical studies have mainly been performed on patients with mild to moderate AD, and apart from the rivastigmine studies, without significant comorbidity or concomitant medication. This means, in general, that the patients are younger and fitter than the population that is usually seen in the standard memory clinic. They are also selected on the basis that they have less behavioural symptoms. It is therefore often claimed that the studies are not representative. However, a crossover, placebo-controlled, clinical practice study of donepezil in the USA[40] usefully demonstrated similar findings to those in the pivotal studies.

What has not been demonstrated yet is how these drugs fare in mild cognitive impairment (MCI) and severe AD. MCI remains a research-based concept, and in a patient without dementia, no treatment is yet proven, and so currently none should be offered. However, MCI is not a clearly established concept and is very memory biased. Many of the patients who are seen also have executive problems and mild functional change – factors that would fulfil the criteria for dementia, making treatment possible. MCI is a political as well as a clinical entity. In the USA, a diagnosis of AD means a significant loss of rights. Starting treatment within a non-dementia framework is an appealing option there.

Severe AD is difficult to study because of issues relating to informed consent and sensitivity of instruments. The cholinergic deficit may be worse at this stage,[41] suggesting that the drugs may prove particularly beneficial. Studies in both MCI and severe dementia are ongoing. Although there continues to be a lack of evidence, the National Institute for Clinical Excellence (NICE) in the UK has placed certain restrictions on treating more advanced sufferers, suggesting that their use would normally be discontinued below an MMSE score of 12. Usual practice is to continue while clear benefit remains, but severe AD must be studied properly in order to clarify best practice and allay concerns that the drugs could also extend the period of decline, which would make some cost-effectiveness predictions less robust.

Patients with pre-existing gastrointestinal disease (especially peptic ulceration), asthma, obstructive airways disease and conduction defects may theoretically have these conditions exacerbated by the vagotonic effects of the AChEIs, so caution is required if these drugs are considered to offer benefit. Donepezil and galantamine are metabolised by the liver, so care should be taken in patients with hepatic impairment. Also, any patient with potential anorexia or weight loss should be monitored while on these compounds. Less frequent problems may include urinary retention, seizures and prolongation of muscle relaxant recovery after anaesthesia. Clearly, patients with hypersensitivity to any of these drugs or their derivatives should not take them.

Practical dilemmas with regard to the use of anticholinesterase inhibitors in AD

Response

In all cholinesterase inhibitor trials, a 'response', as measured by the scales used, was found in approximately 40% of the patients studied. This sounds low, but compares favourably with most drugs used in chronic illness. The problem is that it is offset by a high placebo response. This placebo effect is common in mental health studies, where it encompasses numerous non-drug as well as drug factors, including the treatment effect of multiple lengthy assessment visits for both patient and carer, that do not occur routinely in the clinical setting. Although this responder and non-responder division is reported in the literature, current criteria may be too harsh. Over-extensive seeking for indicators of who will respond in clinical practice may be premature, as true response rates may be higher. Anecdotal and published memory clinic data sets suggest 60–80% response rates when all domains are considered.

While valid biological markers for AD are still sought, relevant proxy measures will continue to be used, so they must have acceptable reliability and validity. Defining such outcome measures for clinical practice continues to need more research and definition, as currently no hard predictors of response or non-response have yet been identified that meet the need.[42] Patients should receive a chosen treatment for a reasonable length of time – at least 3 months after titration to maximal doses. During this time, care must be taken to ensure that the drugs are actually taken properly, or symptomatic effects will not be detected. Decisions can then be made on the best available data collected. Some patients may take longer to demonstrate a drug effect. However, pragmatism dictates that a decision about continuation of therapy should be made by the 6-month mark.

Switching

If one cholinesterase inhibitor produces intolerable side-effects or fails to produce efficacy, another should be tried, as although they are classed together they have clearly different modes of action. There are few published data on switching these drugs, but what there is suggests that it is safe to do so, and that the presence of side-effects or lack of efficacy in one drug does not predict that either will occur in

Table 12.5 Comparison of the three licensed cholinesterase inhibitors

	Donepezil	Rivastigmine	Galantamine	Clinical relevance
Efficacy in primary outcome measures – cognition and global impression	Proven in pivotal clinical trials	Proven in pivotal clinical trials	Proven in pivotal clinical trials	All work in a similar way
Safety	No serious issues reported in first 6 years. Caution with active peptic ulceration, severe asthma and bradycardia below 50 years	No serious issues reported in first 5 years. Caution with active peptic ulceration, severe asthma and bradycardia below 50 years	No serious issues reported in first 3 years. Caution with active peptic ulceration, severe asthma and bradycardia below 50 years	None have safety limitations – good practice may suggest that patients should have ECGs
Tolerability	No serious issues. Insomnia, agitation and leg cramps have been reported	No serious issues. Agitation reported	No serious issues. No clinical reports as yet	No difference in dropout rates in clinical studies, adverse event monitoring or clinical surveys. No evidence that one drug is any better than another
Side-effects	Gastrointestinal. No difference from placebo otherwise	Gastrointestinal. No difference from placebo otherwise	Gastrointestinal. No difference from placebo otherwise	Gastrointestinal effects can be limited by slow titration and taking the drug with food. No evidence in studies suggesting any difference in tolerability across the three drugs
Dosing	Daily	Twice a day	Twice a day (daily due shortly)	Compliance issues – especially where patients live alone

Titration	Two doses: go from lower to higher at 4 weeks	Multiple dose: slow titration to maximum tolerated dose	Three doses: slow titration to maximum tolerated dose	Complex titration may influence decisions by the patient, carer and service
Pricing	Two level	Flat rate	Three level	Cost implications, titration practice and reimbursement strategies
Inhibition	Reversible	Pseudo-irreversible	Reversible/competitive	Competitive inhibitor may act in more AD-specific areas
Half-life	72 hours	8 hours	7 hours	Easier to switch from shorter half-life compounds
Metabolism	Liver	By anticholinesterase itself	Liver	Liver metabolism involves P450 system – potential drug interactions
Butyrylcholinsterase inhibition	No	Yes	Mild	Possible longer duration of effect in AD and effect on plaque maturation
Nicotinic modulation	No	No	Yes	Improved attention, prevention of cell death and possible neuroprotection
Specific AChE subtype inhibition	G4 subtype	G1 subtype	G4 subtype	Possible reduction in insomnia, muscle cramps and cardiac effects if G1 specific
Data in behavioural symptom response	Some data to support a benefit with apathy, anxiety and depression	Open-label data in nursing homes. Some data from *post-hoc* analyses	Proven benefit as part of pivotal trials	Will be used in BPSD as well as primary dementia treatment

another.[43,44] The convention when switching drugs is to leave five times the half-life between drugs (making it 60 hours after stopping rivastigmine or galantamine and 15 days for donepezil). The data suggest that this is unnecessary except where the switch is due to tolerability.[45] Consensus suggests that the change can be overnight, with early titration to therapeutic doses of the new choice, so as not to lose the symptomatic effect. No controlled data support this as yet.

What is more controversial is what to do when a person who has responded successfully then starts to fail. In the absence of evidence to the contrary it could be argued that continuation on current therapy is the best option, but there are other options (e.g. increasing the dose, switching cholinesterase inhibitor, or using memantine, among others). Most of the published evidence is on switching from donepezil to rivastigmine. In the Auriocombe study, this open-label design showed new benefits in 55% of patients. It is intuitive to switch therapies, as happens elsewhere in medicine, but this requires careful consideration in terms of risk and cost. Further research will clarify best practice.

Choice

The cholinesterase inhibitors appear similar yet have quite different individual characteristics (*see* Table 12.5). Donepezil is very selective for acetylcholinesterase (AChE), which is claimed to reduce its side-effect profile. However, no clinical data have been published to show increased tolerability. It is given once daily, which may favour its use in patients who live alone, and where external supervision is required. However, there is evidence to suggest tolerance with donepezil and up-regulation of acetylcholinesterase,[46] meaning that the initial effect would wear off. Paradoxically, it is known that in AD the level of AChE falls as the disease progresses,[47] matched by a rise in butyrylcholinesterase (BuChE), which appears to contribute to plaque formation after being released from the activated glial cells. What BuChE inhibition means clinically is unclear, but those with an inert genetic variant appear to run a more benign course in AD,[48] which does suggest a certain cause and effect. Rivastigmine inhibits BuChE, donepezil does not, and galantamine does so non-significantly, so perhaps rivastigmine does work differently in later disease, although no published evidence supports this. A 2-year blinded comparison between rivastigmine and donepezil in patients with moderate AD is currently ongoing and will be reported by the end of 2005.

Galantamine is both a cholinesterase inhibitor and an allosteric potentiating ligand (APL). It may be that this modulation at a different site on the nicotinic receptor rather than a direct agonist effect at the acetylcholine site protects against tolerance, allowing the drug to work for much longer. Further studies are needed to confirm this. Allosteric nicotinic modulation should also preferentially improve aspects of attention. This has been demonstrated in a comparison study where galantamine showed superiority over donepezil in terms of computerised attentional tasks.[49] Nicotine is putatively neuroprotective, and the fact that galantamine behaves like nicotine *in vitro*, and now in a clinical study, may give an indication that these *in-vitro* effects (e.g. reducing apoptosis and up-regulation of bcl) may be expected to apply *in vivo* as well.

In practice, there seems to be little difference in the cholinesterase inhibitors for the treatment of mild to moderate AD, which is not surprising given the similar studies performed and the already advanced nature of the condition being treated. Comparison between different studies is difficult, as the conditions are always different. An example is claiming that donepezil has better tolerability than galantamine on the basis of clinical trial dropout, when in fact during the donepezil studies no other treatment existed, but when galantamine entered trials, licensed drugs for AD offered an alternative, changing the nature of the patients included and increasing the likelihood of withdrawal of consent from the study.

Comparative studies

Three comparative studies have been completed. Two of these were 12-week studies comparing donepezil with rivastigmine and galantamine, respectively.[50,51] The rivastigmine study demonstrated no difference in efficacy outcomes, but showed that twice daily administration and complex titration were less acceptable to clinicians and carers. Side-effects were also seen more with rivastigmine, partly due to the 2-weekly forced titration regimen. The galantamine study again showed no difference in primary outcomes, but while galantamine performed as expected compared with previous clinical trial data, donepezil outperformed it with regard to both cognition and function. The significance of this is unclear, as donepezil also outperformed anything it had done itself in previous randomised controlled trials.[49] The third study was a 1-year pilot comparison of galantamine and donepezil with function as a primary endpoint. Again this showed no difference in primary endpoint, but galantamine proved to have superiority on most cognitive tests, especially those with known nicotinic activity.

All of these studies are difficult to interpret, as they involved small samples, insensitive tests and, in two of the three studies, a relatively short time period. It would seem that once again these data suggest that there is little to choose between the three licensed drugs in mild to moderate AD. Belief in the modes of action, tolerability data and past experience will influence which of these drugs will be the first choice for the individual clinician.

Other cholinergic therapies

Muscarinic agonists were thought to be a logical option, as they would preclude the need for an intact presynaptic neuron, and muscarinic receptors are not lost in AD. They have been tried in clinical trials, but these drugs have a narrow therapeutic window before side-effects become intolerable, and to date no clinical trial has shown significant effects on cognition at the doses used. Nicotine analogues show marked tolerance, and none of the small studies in the literature suggest that anything to date will prove of use. New nicotinic agonists are currently in development.

Cholinesterase inhibitors in other dementias

Cholinesterase inhibitors arose from the cholinergic hypothesis for AD. However, cholinergic deficits exist in vascular dementia (VaD),[52,53] dementia with Lewy bodies (DLB) and Parkinson's disease dementia (PDD), and recent studies are now showing that cholinergic therapies improve cholinergic function whatever the aetiology of the deficit, and so have a role beyond AD alone. The relationship between AD and VaD is not distinct, and often both pathologies coexist. The Nun study suggests that it is the number of strokes that actually predicts the intensity of the AD syndrome,[54] making it even more likely that cholinesterase inhibitors will work in the presence of even quite marked cerebrovascular disease.

Cholinesterase inhibitors in VaD

Galantamine

The first published study in a mixed population of patients with both AD plus cerebrovascular disease (CVD) and pure VaD was designed to evaluate the use of 24 mg galantamine vs. placebo over 6 months in patients excluded from AD studies because of the presence of CVD.[55] Overall, the galantamine group improved by 1.7 points on the ADAS-cog while the placebo group deteriorated by 1.0 point (a statistically significant improvement). The global, functional and behavioural measures also achieved superiority over placebo, and anxiety and apathy were noticeably improved.

The study design was for a mixed population with patients recruited as they presented. It was expected that the numbers of VaD cases would be relatively low, but the group was divided almost equally between AD plus CVD and VaD. Thus even though the study was not powered for subgroup analysis, such an analysis was performed. This showed that the AD plus CVD group behaved in a similar way to the overall study (and to studies in pure AD), and achieved a statistically significant effect on the cognitive and global scales. However, while the VaD group showed a 2.4-point improvement on the ADAS from baseline, the placebo group remained unchanged, so statistical significance was not reached.

Rivastigmine

In a large randomised controlled trial of patients with mild to moderately severe AD, participants were subsequently stratified according to the presence of vascular risk factors using the Hachinski scale. Treatment with rivastigmine resulted in significantly greater reductions in ADAS-cog scores in patients with AD plus cerebrovascular risk factors compared with those with pure AD. Rivastigmine has also demonstrated efficacy in 8 patients with subcortical ischaemic vascular dementia over 52 weeks, where it maintained or improved cognitive ability. In contrast, 8 patients receiving cardioaspirin for 52 weeks showed cognitive deterioration.[56] These VaD patients receiving rivastigmine also showed improvements in behavioural symptoms without needing additional treatment for behavioural and social problems. The control group showed worsening behaviour and caregiver stress, with increased use of sedatives or neuroleptics.

No large-scale, randomised, placebo-controlled trials have yet been completed with rivastigmine, but they are ongoing.

Donepezil

Two identical, 600-patient, placebo-controlled, double-blind trials of donepezil in patients with probable or possible VaD have been conducted.[57,58] Both studies demonstrated efficacy at 5 and 10 mg over placebo in terms of cognition (on ADAS and MMSE) and function, but one did not reach significance on the global score, which may explain the lack of licensed indication to date. Around 90% of these VaD patients had very high levels of concomitant cardiovascular or cerebrovascular disease, with 65% having suffered stroke disease. This is the first evidence for one of the cholinesterase inhibitors in a pure VaD sample.

For all three compounds, safety and tolerability were very similar to that reported in the AD studies, with (reassuringly) no increase in cardiovascular or cerebrovascular morbidity even where pre-existing levels of both were significant.

One concern is the use of the CIBIC in VaD. This is a fairly blunt instrument, showing little change even in AD studies, where the placebo group is deteriorating. This effect will be even smaller where the placebo group remains stable, and so may account for why two out of three VaD studies have missed the global endpoint. With three more VaD studies ongoing with the same outcome measure, it may be that the use of AChEIs in this condition may be held up in clinical practice, for want of a better instrument.

Dementia with Lewy bodies (DLB) and Parkinson's disease dementia (PDD)

DLB is a dementia with a profoundly cholinergic deficit (74% reduction in cholinergic markers, compared with 60% in AD).[59] This would support the use of AChEIs for this condition. An open-label tacrine study reported cognitive but not global improvement.[60] Donepezil has been shown to reduce hallucinations,[61] but the only controlled study published to date was with rivastigmine.[62] This study of 120 patients showed a significant cognitive and behavioural response, with the total NPI and NPI-4 (delusions, hallucinations, depression, apathy) both showing a 30% reduction in symptoms. Neuroleptic sensitivity in DLB is widely reported, and many of the case series described are discussed in Chapter 14. It is therefore felt that first-line therapy for the psychiatric phenomena in DLB should be rivastigmine, although titration should be as slow as usual, as the number of rivastigmine dropouts in the McKeith study was relatively high compared with the placebo group.

Concomitant use of anti-parkinsonian agents in DLB is controversial, and there are no conclusive data either way. These drugs can make psychiatric phenomena worse, but in the absence of evidence, a pragmatic balance between control of physical and psychological symptoms needs to be pursued.

GABA interneurons are important in motor control and receive inputs from the cholinergic basal forebrain nuclei. Carbamazepine has been shown to improve hallucinations and fluctuations,[63] while chlormethiazole and benzodiazepines have been proposed as helpful, but with little data to support this view. Rapid eye movement (REM) sleep disorder is common in DLB. Low-dose clonazepam (0.5 mg) is a recognised treatment for this.[64] Baclofen has been reported to relieve rigidity in DLB.[65]

Parkinson's disease involves a loss of nicotinic receptors equal to that in AD, and Parkinson's disease dementia (PDD) is increasingly recognised. A case series has suggested the benefits of rivastigmine,[66] and AChEIs do not seem to make the motor symptoms worse. Good practice seems to be to establish relatively high doses of cholinesterase inhibitor and reduce all PD medication down to the lowest dose of dopamine possible. Formal studies with donepezil and rivastigmine in PDD are currently ongoing. A recent large controlled study of the latter reported encouraging early results with regard to cognition, function and behaviour, which may lead to the licensing of rivastigmine for this disorder.

Frontotemporal dementia (FTD)

There is no evidence to support the use of cholinesterase inhibitors in FTD, which is not surprising, as this condition does not have a cholinergic deficit. No other treatment is currently licensed in FTD, which is usually managed symptomatically with antidepressants and antipsychotics, although there are no controlled data to support any particular one.

These findings are summarised in Table 12.6.

Table 12.6 Primary treatments for the common dementias

Dementia	Recommended treatment	Reference
Alzheimer's disease (ICD-10 F00):		
Mild/moderate (F00.0, F00.1)	Donepezil	Rogers (1998),[12] Burns (1999)[14]
	Rivastigmine	Corey-Bloom (1998)[23], Rosler (1998)[24]
	Galantamine	Raskind (2000),[24] Tariot (2000),[39] Wilcock (2002)[70]
Moderate/severe (F00.0, F00.1)	Memantine	Winblad (1999),[67] Reisberg (2003)[68]
AD plus cerebrovascular disease (F00.2)	Donepezil Galantamine	Feldman (2001)[18] Erkinjuntti (2002)[55]
Vascular dementia (ICD-10 F01)	Donepezil Galantamine	Black,[57] Wilkinson (2003)[58] Erkinjuntti (2002)[55]
Dementia with Lewy bodies	Rivastigmine	McKeith (2000)[62]
Parkinson's disease dementia (F02.3)	Rivastigmine	Bullock (2002) case series[43]
Frontotemporal dementia	Nil recommended	None

Glutamatergic therapies

Glutamatergic neurons are the predominant type found in the human brain, and glutamate over-stimulation may lead to neuronal damage. It is not surprising that glutamate is increasingly implicated in dementia pathogenesis, with N-methyl-D-aspartate (NMDA) blockade being a putative therapy. Memantine, an NMDA-receptor blocker, has been shown to protect against amyloid neurotoxicity and improve learning in rats.

Memantine

Two studies and over 20 years of use as a licensed medication in Germany have led to the licensing of memantine as a treatment for moderate to severe AD.[67,68] The former study was a 3-month trial in 166 patients with a diagnosis of dementia in nursing homes in Latvia. The scores on both functional and overall scales were superior in the treatment group. These data were sufficient to initiate a full programme to evaluate the use of memantine in AD.

The Reisberg study was a placebo-controlled study in 252 patients with moderate to severe AD. It showed a significant reduction in the rate of decline compared with placebo in all domains, with effect sizes comparable to those seen in the Feldman study of donepezil (e.g. 5.7 points difference on the severe impairment battery(SIB)). The results were diminished by a 28% dropout rate, but show that another neurochemical strategy can now be used in AD. Studies in patients with mild to moderate AD are expected to be reported in late 2005.

Memantine is now in use for moderate to severe AD. It is difficult to calculate NNTs and NNHs from the data available to date, but both look broadly similar to the cholinesterase inhibitors, confirming that memantine is a good alternative, especially where cholinesterase inhibitors are either contraindicated or not indicated.

Two studies have also been conducted in VaD.[69,70] In both, memantine was superior to placebo on the ADAS-cog (2 and 1.75 points; $P = 0.01$), with the largest benefit being seen in patients with an MMSE of <15. Unfortunately, the global end points were not statistically different to placebo, although this may be a reflection of the instrument rather than of memantine itself.

Vitamin E

Injury to cell structures caused by highly reactive oxygen agents generated in normal cell metabolism has been thought to play a role in many age-related diseases,[71] and this oxidative stress is implicated in amyloid generation in AD.[72] Antioxidants such as vitamins E and C may prevent amyloid deposition[73] and reduce its neurotoxicity.[74] This protection may extend to stroke[75] and so impact on vascular dementia as well. Sano et al.[1] showed a delay in institutionalisation in AD, but no cognitive effect. Despite the relatively small effect size in this study, the fact that vitamin E is relatively inexpensive and free from side-effects has led to its widespread use. The American Academy of Neurology includes its use in their practice guidelines for treating AD.[76] It is less frequently used in Europe, where it is felt that better evidence is needed before adopting what could be little more than a placebo response. A longitudinal study of Japanese–American men in Hawaii, using a combination of vitamins E and C, showed an 88% reduction in expected vascular dementia over a period of 5 years.[77] The reason is postulated to be protection of neuronal damage after ischaemic events, rather than a reduction in the number of events. Together with the study by Sano et al., it does seem that a primary prevention study of these two vitamins in dementia is now needed.

Oestrogen

Although observational studies suggested a protective role for oestrogen,[78] three controlled studies of diagnosed AD have now proved negative. The first was a 16-week, placebo-controlled study using equine oestrogen in 42 women,[79] which showed no difference between drug and placebo on the cognitive or global primary outcome measure. The second study was a 1-year, placebo-controlled study of two doses of oestrogen by the AD Cooperative Study in 120 hyster-ectomised women.[80] This again failed to demonstrate a difference between drug and placebo, even suggesting a worsening with oestrogen on the Clinical Dementia Rating scale. The third study involved 50 women in a 12-week, randomised study using premarin.[81] Again no difference was found between drug and placebo.

These findings are disappointing, as the oestrogen model has some appeal.[82] Laboratory evidence suggests that oestrogen may improve cholinergic transmission, have neurotrophic effects[83] and possess anti-amyloidogenic properties.[84] It may be that using classic regulatory AD trial methods is inappropriate, with a long-term prevention study being more valid. However, a large prospective Women's Health study was discontinued in 2003 because of increased adverse events in the treatment group, including no clear cognitive advantage and perhaps even inferior performance compared with placebo.

One small positive study using transdermal patch oestrogen over a period of 8 weeks[85] may suggest that the method of delivery of oestrogen is important – where avoiding the first-pass effect significantly increases bioavailability. Some observational data suggest that oestrogen may enhance the effects of cholinesterase inhibitors, and this may be clarified in current studies. However, a recent study shows that after 1 year premarin does improve oestradiol and oestrone levels, but this increase does not correlate with cognitive functioning at either 2 or 12 months.[86,87] The current evidence therefore does not support routine usage of oestrogens in dementia treatment. Ongoing, better-designed studies may provide evidence that alters this position. However, oestrogens remain useful for other conditions and, where this use is applicable, there is no contraindication to using them in AD.

Anti-inflammatory drugs

A significant inflammatory reaction occurs in AD, and arthritic patients who are taking long-term anti-inflammatory medication appear to have some protection.[87,88] This observation was reconfirmed with the publication of the Cache County Population Study,[89] which confirmed the inverse relationship between AD and the use of both non-steroidal anti-inflammatory drugs (NSAIDs) and H_2-receptor antagonists. This was replicated more recently by Landi et al.,[90] who suggest that this association is only for non-aspirin NSAIDs. A smaller population sample from Sydney demonstrated a reduced frequency of AD, but not other dementias, at both high and low doses of anti-inflammatory drugs.[91]

Inflammation does seem to be implicated in the neurodegenerative process, correlating with free-radical formation, oxidative stress and disruption of both mitochondrial and calcium homeostasis. This effect may be due to inhibition of cyclo-oxygenase (COX), which converts arachidonic acid into prostaglandins, prostacyclins and thromboxane-A_2, all of which are involved in inflammatory mechanisms. Two types of COX exist. COX-1 inhibitors are the constitutive form and cause the gastrointestinal problems that are so commonly observed. COX-2 is a mitogen-inducible form which some believe is the main factor in inflammation. It is up-regulated in the brains of people with dementia compared with non-cognitively-impaired controls, and it may be involved in subsequent neurodegeneration. These COX-2 inhibitors seem to have fewer side-effects, so longer-term studies are now under way. However, a prospective follow-up study of neuropathology and inflammatory reaction in AD patients who either had or had not taken anti-inflammatory drugs showed an enhanced cognitive effect, but no change in the progression of pathological changes.[92] Thus the proposed mode of action may not be as simple as was first thought, with platelet and endothelium dysfunction perhaps being important contributors to the AD process as well.

One randomised study of 138 AD patients using 10 mg prednisone showed no improvement over placebo[93] in slowing cognitive decline. This may be due to too low a dosage, but anything higher in the elderly is associated with serious toxicity, and a high serum cortisol level may itself be associated with memory deficits. NSAIDs do seem to be a better option than steroids, as they inhibit microglial activation[94] and two small randomised studies have shown a trend towards cognitive protection.[95]

The current evidence does not provide conclusive proof that NSAIDs should be used to treat any dementia, although some clinicians have treated mild AD with COX-2 inhibitors as a secondary preventative measure, especially in the USA. It appears that the observed neuroprotective effect is not a class effect (at least *in vitro*), and that certain NSAIDs have better cognitive effects than others.[96] An enantiomer of flurbiprofen appears to act as a putative gamma-secretase inhibitor with little NSAID activity, again supporting the notion that these drugs may act in more ways than is currently considered to be the case. However, although these drugs seem to be relatively safe, there are not enough long-term data on them to support their use in primary prevention. If conclusive evidence that they do not work in AD is ever published, then all treatment given for that sole purpose to date should be discontinued.

Statins

A study comparing 284 patients treated with lipid-lowering agents with 1080 untreated controls showed an estimated 70% lower risk of dementia than in patients who did not receive drug or need it.[97] This has led to a particular interest in the role of statins in dementia treatment, and combination studies with cholinesterase inhibitors are ongoing. There has been a long-term relationship between lipids and vascular changes involving the brain in dementia, which has been poorly understood. *In vitro*, it appears that statins reduce amyloid deposition in cell culture by around 5% a year. Thus it seems that statins may reduce the risk of dementia in the elderly, either by opposing age-related changes that lead to cognitive impairment, or by delaying its onset. The finding of Jick *et al.*[97] has been replicated,[98,99] so properly designed prevention studies are now required to elicit the mode of action and prove causality.

Unfortunately, two large studies have cast doubt on the utility of these earlier observational findings. The first used a simple telephone test at the end of the study, with no baseline for comparison, so serious conclusions cannot be drawn from these results.[100] The second was the publication of cognitive findings from the first 3 years of the PROSPER heart study.[101] This has also shown no benefit of statin over placebo as measured by simple cognitive instruments. Although disappointing, the instruments used showed significant learning effects. More-over, if the main beneficial mechanism of statins in AD is a slow reduction in amyloid deposition, then 3 years may not be long enough.

Current evidence suggests that when treating AD with AChEIs, a high baseline cholesterol level can reduce the size of any potential outcomes.[102] Thus even though current evidence does not support the routine use of statins purely for AD, their use for cardiovascular risk factors may prove to be cognitively beneficial in the long term, and AD patients with high cholesterol levels should perhaps be treated with statins regardless of their cognitive state.

Homocysteine

Elevated plasma homocysteine levels are associated with an increased risk of vascular disease and AD.[103] They may contribute to excitotoxic damage and increase amyloid toxicity, both of which would have a significant role in neurodegeneration. A meta-analysis by the Homocysteine Lowering Trialists' Collaboration suggested that using vitamin supplements, especially folic acid, could reduce plasma homocysteine levels by 25%. The enrichment of flour with folate in order to reduce neural-tube defects has already led to a mean population reduction in homocysteine levels of 7%. Aisen et al.[104] have demonstrated that high-dose vitamins can reduce these levels still lower. Long-term prospective double-blind studies are now under way to see whether such a strategy has any clinically significant effect on cognition and neurodegeneration.

Hypertension

Hypertension is common, and it is a risk factor for both AD and VaD. Two long-term treatment studies in hypertension have shown that the lowering of blood pressure in the treatment arms led to a significantly reduced incidence of both AD and VaD compared with placebo.[105,106] As only a third of hypertension cases are regularly diagnosed, better screening with more aggressive treatment could contribute to a future reduction in the incidence of dementia. If combined with other secondary preventative measures, such as smoking cessation and weight control, these represent important and achievable targets for primary care that can have significant effects later on in life.

Beta-peptide immunisation

The investigation of immunisation with pathological beta-amyloid peptide is currently suspended after problems with a T-cell-induced encephalitis in the phase II studies. These studies were attempting to generate an immune response to the amyloid plaques in the brain, and thus produce the first disease-modifying approach in AD. The rationale came from experiments with transgenic PDAPP mice, where in young mice the immunisation led to a reduction in the number of expected plaques.[107] More interestingly, the immunisation of older mice led to a reduction in amyloid burden, perhaps indicating reversal of the process. Clearly the mice did not have AD, but the human studies are now yielding information about the nature of this immune response. A post-mortem of one of the study patients has shown removal of plaques in the relevant areas, thus duplicating the mouse finding in humans.[108] This does not definitively correlate with any cognitive change, but it ensures that further research will be performed. The encephalitis that occurred may well have been caused by T-cell activation, but this can be avoided by using different epitopes of the amyloid protein.[109] New mechanisms of immunisation are thus being developed, and renewed attempts will be forthcoming.

Other treatments

Nootropics are available in Germany, the best known being *Ginkgo biloba* and piracetam. Ginkgo preparations are made from dried leaves and contain ginkgo–flavone glycosides and terpenoids. These produce antioxidant, anti-inflammatory and platelet inhibition effects. Many small studies have been performed, but five well-conducted studies were reviewed in a meta-analysis[110] which concluded that there was a small but significant improvement in cognition with ginkgo, but insufficient data to suggest functional or behavioural effects. The pharmacology, dose and exact utility of ginkgo require further research, especially as many people obtain it by over-the-counter purchase. A clinically significant drug interaction between ginkgo and trazodone, that produced coma in a patient and was reversed by flumazenil, showed that ginkgo is active at the benzodiazepine receptor as well as being antioxidant.[111]

Many small studies using piracetam (a cyclic derivative of GABA) were considered in a meta-analysis.[112] The results were difficult to extract, and although it seemed that there may be some global benefit, the current evidence does not support routine use, though further controlled studies will soon be reported.

Hydergine has been licensed for use in non-specific dementia for many years. It is a mixture of ergot peptide derivatives, and many clinical studies, with just as many designs and outcome measures, have never conclusively proved its utility, apart from a lack of adverse side-effects. A recent Cochrane Review suggests that it has some effect in global function, but recommends further research.[113]

Nerve-cell destruction seems to be secondary to activation of glial cells, so stabilisation of these glial cells may reduce the rate of AD and other dementias. Several compounds (e.g. propentofylline) have purported to have this effect, especially *in vitro*, but to date have shown too modest a therapeutic effect clinically for the regulatory authorities to pass.[114] Some of the difficulties encountered have concerned the trial methodology rather than the drug. This remains a potential area of research.

The cortical cholinergic system is diffusely spread and a long way distant from its cell bodies. As such it is dependent on nerve growth factor (NGF) to sustain it, and a reduction in NGF may be associated with AD. Studies that involved injecting NGF by cannulae into the CSF showed some effect, but this is not a practical solution. Attempts to formulate the active portion of NGF into an oral preparation that crosses the blood–brain barrier are ongoing, and methods of stimulating NGF are being investigated.

Failed treatments

Many treatments have reached clinical trial stages and failed to be licensed because of their lack of efficacy or their toxicity. Some of the better known failed treatments are summarised in Table 12.7.

A meta-analysis using both a composite test of measures and separately calculated global impression has shown acetyl-L-carnitine to be superior to placebo in patients with mild cognitive impairment and early AD.[115] This finding will need further evaluation before it can be considered an appropriate therapy.

Table 12.7 Summary of drugs that have been studied in AD and VaD, and the reasons why they failed to be licensed for clinical practice

Drug	Condition	Reason for failure
Acetyl-L-carntine	AD	No change in cognition or prognosis
Nicotine	AD	No change in cognition or prognosis
Thiamine	AD	No change in cognition or prognosis
Cycloserine	AD	Ineffective in all domains
Metrifonate	AD	Toxicity
Lazabemide	AD	Toxicity
Idebenone	AD	Development stopped due to lack of efficacy
Propentofylline	AD, VaD	Development stopped due to lack of efficacy
Pentoxifylline	VaD	Data not conclusive
Muscarinic agonists	AD	Development stopped due to lack of efficacy
Transmitter releasers	AD	Development stopped due to lack of efficacy
Selegiline	AD	Data not conclusive

Combination therapies

No data exist to support any combination of cholinesterase inhibitors. The increase in side-effects may be prohibitive, even if combining the modes of action may have some theoretical appeal. The introduction of memantine to the therapeutic arena makes it a likely choice for combination with cholinesterase inhibitors, and a 24-week, placebo-controlled US study adding it to donepezil has shown some additional benefit.[116] In this study, 404 patients were randomised. The memantine arm proved statistically superior to placebo in terms of cognition (3.4 points on the severe impairment battery), function (1.4 points on the ADCS-ADL), behaviour (3.8 points on the NPI) and global performance (0.3 points on the CIBIC). This provides evidence that the combination is safe as well as effective, and will lead to increasing consideration of combining these compounds in moderate dementia. No clinical data currently exist for memantine and other cholinesterase inhibitors, although no interaction with galantamine has been shown *in vitro*.

Vitamin E is often used in combination with other therapies in the USA. This is hoped to be combining symptomatic and potential disease modification. Table 12.8 shows how the current therapies fit into the treatment paradigms, and how they could perhaps potentially be used together. Ginkgo is often purchased by patients in Europe and taken with prescribed treatments. No prospective studies to evaluate the true validity of any of these potential combinations have yet been published.

Table 12.8 Current therapies that are either available or in development for the treatment of AD and related dementias

	Symptomatic	Disease modification	Cure
Probable – or in use	Anticholinesterase inhibitors (AChEIs): • donepezil • rivastigmine • galantamine NMDA receptor antagonists: • memantine	? AChEIs ? Vitamin E ?? Memantine ?? *Ginkgo biloba*	None
Possible – in clinical trial	Ampakines Nicotinic-like agents Other cholinesterase inhibitors Acetyl-L-carnitine	Statins Antioxidants Oestrogen NSAIDs Nootropics (e.g. piracetam) NGF stimulators Amyloid-modifying agents Vaccines	None
Possible – in clinical development	Nicotinic agonists and partial agonists Calcium-channel agents	Peptides (e.g. glucagon-like peptide) BuChEIs Tau-modifying agents Amyloid-modifying agents Gene-product manipulation Secretase blockers	? Gene/gene-product manipulation (e.g. lentiviral vector for neprilysin)

Treatment of behavioural disorders in dementia

Increasing evidence suggests that cholinesterase inhibitors ameliorate some of the behavioural problems that are often seen during the course of AD, particularly apathy and visual hallucinations.[117] This is logical, as the cholinergic system appears to be directly associated with the limbic system, which is involved in many of the symptoms that appear.

The effect is independent of improvement in cognition, and appears in differential aspects in all of the cholinesterase inhibitors tested.

Antipsychotics are the class most frequently used for treating behavioural symptoms in dementia. There is fair evidence for risperidone and olanzapine, but less for the other atypical antipsychotics. A new drug, aripiprazole, has shown good effect on the BPRS total score and psychosis subscore in a community AD sample.

The treatment of BPSD is discussed in detail in Chapter 14.

Future therapeutic options

The consistent finding in AD is the presence of neuritic amyloid plaques and neurofibrillary tangles. The amyloid cascade is the favourite explanation for the formation of plaques, and various drugs are in development to modify various steps of amyloid metabolism. These include secretase inhibitors to prevent the formation of β-amyloid, molecules to prevent amyloid accumulation, and immunisation to remove it. Several of these strategies are now reaching phase II or III clinical studies, and may be available in the fairly near future. The furthest into development is phenserine, a cholinesterase inhibitor that also binds to the APP gene and reduces the quantity of APP produced, and subsequently the amount of APP synthesised.[118] This would have a true disease-modifying effect.

Amyloid processing is part of normal metabolism. As well as being formed, it is also catabolised and removed. This means that AD is potentially due to either over-production or abnormal accumulation of pathological amyloid, and perhaps reduction in degradation. Neprilysin is a zinc metalloproteinase that may play a role in this removal. In transgenic AD mice, neprilysin mRNA levels decrease with age.[119] A lentiviral vector expressing human neprilysin has been unilaterally injected into transgenic mouse cerebrum. This produced a 50% reduction in amyloid deposition and slowing of neurodegeneration in the hippocampus and frontal cortex.[120] This finding supports the theory that neprilysin is a therapeutic option.

Other peptides are also looking promising as therapeutic options. Glucagon-like peptide (GLP) is an insulinotropic hormone that is involved in food intake regulation and stress response. GLP-1 receptors are found in the human brain, and agonists protect against apoptosis *in vitro* and modulate APP metabolism, with a subsequent reduction in cholinergic atrophy. This and related peptides appear to be a promising new avenue of exploration in AD and other neurological disorders.

The other significant pathological finding in AD is the presence of tangles composed of abnormally phosphorylated tau protein. This phosphorylation is mediated by glycogen synthetase kinase (GSK), which can be inhibited by a variety of compounds, including lithium and other new agents. Such a strategy may limit cell death, and clinical trials are imminent. Tau pathology is also known to exist in other neurodegenerative conditions, so the treatment of these tauopathies is an important area of research in other dementing diseases, such as frontotemporal dementia (FTD) and progressive supranuclear palsy (PSP).

Mild cognitive impairment (MCI)

This heterogeneous stage probably represents the first signs of impending cognitive decline, especially if it remains present after an appropriate follow-up period. When the presentation is predominantly amnestic, there is a strong association with AD. Currently there is no evidence to support treatment in this condition, although major clinical studies are imminent. However, the warning signs of MCI should lead to a review of secondary prevention strategies (e.g. cholesterol and blood pressure lowering), and also raise the index of suspicion about dementia, so that treatment with AChEIs can be initiated as early as is practicable.

Key points

- Basic scientific research is gradually unlocking some of the pathological processes in dementia, particularly AD, and this is providing interesting theoretical treatment opportunities. This began with the symptomatic treatment effect of the AChEIs, and is now revealing opportunities through altering disease progression by amyloid and tau modification. This may be via the alteration of amyloid metabolism or via the influence of other neuropeptides. Whatever the future, for the first time true therapeutic options for AD, VaD and DLB already exist, mostly through improvement of cholinergic function, but with the promise of better to come.
- Matching the clinical phenotypes to protein pathology will increase the need to understand the true aetiological nature of what we see in the clinics, as therapeutics will become increasingly specific. The diagnoses that currently exist may need re-evaluating and reclassifying according to the emerging biological findings. Treatment will almost certainly need to be initiated earlier, and as very few medical conditions respond to just one therapy, AD and other dementias will probably prove to require combinations of therapy. These already need consideration, given the current choices and a desire to maximise the benefit of the dementia treatments that we have at present.
- It seems that amyloid deposition occurs with ageing, as does cerebrovascular disease, and that perhaps the ratio of the two determines the clinical phenotype. Primary and secondary preventive strategies for cerebrovascular disease have been shown to reduce the incidence of dementia. Coupled with emerging amyloid-reducing strategies, further success in the treatment of AD and related dementias is a reasonable expectation, although quite what the aetiological role of tau disorder plays has yet to be clearly established, especially as it is the tangles that

correlate with disease progression, not the amyloid plaques. However, amyloid may play a key role in driving the abnormal tau metabolism that is currently seen, in which case a therapy for both basic neuropathological findings in AD may be closer than expected.

References

1 Sano M, Ernesto C, Thomas RG *et al.* (1997) A controlled trial of selegiline, alpha-tocopherol, or both as treatment for Alzheimer's disease. *NEJM.* **336**: 1216–22.

2 Schenk DB, Seubert P, Lieberburg I and Wallace J (2000) Beta-peptide immunization – a possible new treatment for Alzheimer disease. *Arch Neurol.* **57**: 934–6.

3 Bartus RT, Dean RL, Beer B and Lippa AS (1982) The cholinergic hypothesis of geriatric memory dysfunction. *Science.* **217**: 408–17.

4 Cameron I, Curran S, Newton P, Petty D and Wattis J (2000) Use of donepezil for the treatment of mild–moderate Alzheimer's disease: an audit of the assessment and treatment of patients in routine clinical practice. *Int J Geriatr Psychiatry.* **15**: 887–91.

5 Evans M, Ellis A, Watson D and Chowdhury T (2000) Sustained cognitive improvement following treatment of Alzheimer's disease with donepezil. *Int J Geriatr Psychiatry.* **15**: 50–3.

6 Matthews HP, Korbey J, Wilkinson DG and Rowden J (2000) Donepezil in Alzheimer's disease: eighteen-month results from Southampton Memory Clinic. *Int J Geriatr Psychiatry.* **15**: 713–20.

7 Livingston G and Katona C (2000) How useful are cholinesterase inhibitors in the treatment of Alzheimer's disease? A number needed to treat analysis. *Int J Geriatr Psychiatry.* **15**: 203–7.

8 Bullock R (1998) Drug treatment for early Alzheimer's disease. *Adv Psychiatr Treat.* **4**: 126–34.

9 Harvey RJ (1999) A review and commentary on a sample of 15 UK guidelines for the drug treatment of Alzheimer's disease. *Int J Geriatr Psychiatry.* **14**: 249–56.

10 National Institute for Clinical Excellence (2001) *Guidance for the Use of Donezepil, Rivastigmine and Galantamine for the Treatment of Alzheimer's Disease.* National Institute for Clinical Excellence, London.

11 Rogers SL and Friedhoff LT (1996) The efficacy and safety of donepezil in patients with Alzheimer's disease: results of a US multicentre, randomized, double-blind, placebo-controlled trial. The Donepezil Study Group. *Dementia.* **7**: 293–303.

12 Rogers SL, Doody RS, Mohs RC *et al.* (1998) Donepezil improves cognition and global function in Alzheimer disease: a 15-week, double-blind, placebo-controlled study. *Arch Intern Med.* **158**: 1021–31.

13 Rogers SL, Farlow MR, Doody RS, Mohs R and Friedhoff LT (1998) A 24-week, double-blind, placebo-controlled trial of donepezil in patients with Alzheimer's disease. Donepezil Study Group. *Neurology.* **50**: 136–45.

14 Burns A, Rossor M, Hecker J *et al.* (1999) The effects of donepezil in Alzheimer's disease – results from a multinational trial. *Dement Geriatr Cogn Disord.* **10**: 237–44.

15 Tariot P, Cummings JL, Katz IR *et al.* (2001) A randomized, double-blind, placebo-controlled study of the efficacy and safety of donepezil in patients with Alzheimer's disease in the nursing home setting. *J Am Geriatr Soc.* **49**: 1590–9.

16 Winblad B, Engedal K, Soininen H *et al.* (2001) A 1-year, randomized, placebo-controlled study of donepezil in patients with mild to moderate AD. *Neurology.* **57**: 489–95.

17 Mohs RC, Doody RS, Morris JC *et al.* (2001) A 1-year, placebo-controlled preservation of function survival study of donepezil in AD patients. *Neurology.* **57**: 481–8.

18 Feldman H, Gauthier S, Hecker J, Vellas B, Subbiah P and Whalen E (2001) A 24-week, randomized, double-blind study of donepezil in moderate to severe Alzheimer's disease. *Neurology.* **57**: 613–20.

19 Geldmacher DS, Provenzano G, Mcrae T, Mastey V and Ieni JR (2003) Donepezil is associated with delayed nursing home placement in patients with Alzheimer's disease. *J Am Geriatr Soc.* **51**: 937–44.

20 Birks J and Melzer D (2000) *Donepezil for Mild and Moderate Alzheimer's Disease. Cochrane Library. Issue 4.* Update Software, Oxford.

21 Amici S, Lanari A, Romani R, Antognelli C, Gallai V and Parnetti L (2001) Cerebrospinal fluid acetylcholinesterase activity after long-term treatment with donepezil and rivastigmine. *Mech Ageing Dev.* **122**: 2057–62.

22 Forette F, Anand R and Gharabawi G (1999) A phase II study in patients with Alzheimer's disease to assess the preliminary efficacy and maximum tolerated dose of rivastigmine (Exelon (R)). *Eur J Neurol.* **6**: 423–9.

23 Corey-Bloom BJ, Anand R, Veach J, Panikkar A and McKeith IG (1998) A randomized trial evaluating the efficacy and safety of ENA 713 (rivastigmine tartrate), a new acetylcholinesterase inhibitor, in patients with mild to moderately severe Alzheimer's disease. *Int J Geriatr Psychopharmacol.* **1**: 55–65.

24 Rosler M, Anand R, Cicin SA *et al.* (1999) Efficacy and safety of rivastigmine in patients with Alzheimer's disease: international randomised controlled trial. *BMJ.* **318**: 633–40.

25 Schneider LS, Anand R and Farlow MR (1998) Systematic review of the efficacy of rivastigmine for patients with Alzheimer's disease. *Int J Geriatr Psychopharmacol.* **1 (Suppl. 1)**: S26–34.

26 Birks J, Iakovidou V and Tsolaki M (1999) *Rivastigmine for Alzheimer's Disease. Cochrane Library. Issue 4.* Update Software, Oxford.

27 Farlow MR, Hake A, Messina J, Hartman R, Veach J and Anand R (2001) Response of patients with Alzheimer's disease to rivastigmine treatment is predicted by the rate of disease progression. *Arch Neurol.* **58**: 417–22.

28 Maelicke A, Samochocki M, Jostock R *et al.* (2001) Allosteric sensitization of nicotinic receptors by galantamine, a new treatment strategy for Alzheimer's disease. *Biol Psychiatry.* **49**: 279–88.

29 Kewitz H (1997) Pharmacokinetics and metabolism of galantamine. *Drugs Today.* **33**: 265–72.

30 Rainer M (1997) Galanthamine in Alzheimer's disease – a new alternative to tacrine? *CNS Drugs.* **7**: 89–97.

31 Kewitz H and Berzewski H (1994) Galantamine, a selective non-toxic acetylcholinesterase inhibitor is significantly superior over placebo in treatment of SDAT. *Neuropsychopharmacology.* **10**: 130S.

32 Wilkinson D, Murray J, Addala D *et al.* (2001) Galantamine: a randomized, double-blind-dose comparison in patients with Alzheimer's disease. *Int J Geriatr Psychiatry.* **16**: 852–7.

33 Rainer M (1997) Clinical studies with galanthamine. *Drugs Today.* **33**: 273–9.

34 Rockwood K, Mintzer J, Truyen L, Wessel T and Wilkinson D (2001) Effects of a flexible galantamine dose in Alzheimer's disease: a randomised, controlled trial. *J Neurol Neurosurg Psychiatry.* **71**: 589–95.

35 Raskind MA, Peskind ER, Wessel T and Yuan W (2000) Galantamine in AD – a 6-month randomized, placebo-controlled trial with a 6-month extension. *Neurology.* **54**: 2261–8.

36 Wilcock GK, Lilienfeld S and Gaens E (2000) Efficacy and safety of galantamine in patients with mild to moderate Alzheimer's disease: multicentre randomised controlled trial. *BMJ.* **321**: 1445–9.

37 Tariot PN, Solomon PR, Morris JC, Kershaw P, Lilienfeld S and Ding C (2000) A 5-month, randomized, placebo-controlled trial of galantamine in AD. The Galantamine USA-10 Study Group. *Neurology.* **54**: 2269–76.

38 Olin J and Schneider LS (2001) *Galantamine for Alzheimer's Disease. Cochrane Library. Issue 2.* Update Software, Oxford.

39 Rizzo J, Chang SB and Ofman J (2002) Comparison of adverse reaction reports for rivastigmine and donepezil using the FDA's adverse event reporting system. *Neurobiol Aging.* **23**: 439.

40 Greenberg SM, Tennis MK, Brown LB *et al.* (2000) Donepezil therapy in clinical practice – a randomized crossover study. *Arch Neurol.* **57**: 94–9.

41 Davis KL, Mohs RC and Marin D (1999) Cholinergic markers in elderly patients with early signs of Alzheimer's disease. *JAMA.* **281**: 1401–6.

42 Schneider LS and Farlow MR (1995) Predicting response to cholinesterase inhibitors in Alzheimers' disease – possible approaches. *CNS Drugs.* **4**: 114–24.

43 Bullock R and Connolly C (2002) Switching cholinesterase inhibitor therapy in Alzheimer's disease – donepezil to rivastigmine, is it worth it? *Int J Geriatr Psychiatry.* **17**: 288–9.

44 Auriacombe S, Pere JJ, Loria-Kanza Y and Vellas B (2002) Efficacy and safety of rivastigmine in patients with Alzheimer's disease who failed to benefit from treatment with donepezil. *Curr Med Res Opin.* **18**: 129–38.

45 Emre M (2002) Switching cholinesterase inhibitors in patients with Alzheimer's disease. *Int J Clin Pract.* **S127**: 64–72.

46 Davidsson P, Blennow K, Andreasen N, Eriksson B, Minthon L and Hesse C (2001) Differential increase in cerebrospinal fluid – acetylcholinesterase after treatment with acetylcholinesterase inhibitors in patients with Alzheimer's disease. *Neurosci Lett.* **300**: 157–60.

47 Arendt T, Bruckner MK, Lange M and Bigl V (1992) Changes in acetylcholinesterase and butyrylcholinesterase in Alzheimer's disease resemble embryonic development – a study of molecular forms. *Neurochem Int.* **21**: 381–96.

48 O'Brien KK, Saxby BK, Ballard CG *et al.* (2003) Regulation of attention and response to therapy in dementia by butyrylcholinesterase. *Pharmacogenetics.* **13**: 231–9.

49 Wilcock G, Howe I, Coles H *et al.* (2003) A long-term comparison of galantamine and donepezil in the treatment of Alzheimer's disease. *Drugs Aging.* **20**: 777–89.

50 Wilkinson DG, Passmore AP, Bullock R *et al.* (2002) A multinational, randomised, 12-week, comparative study of donepezil and rivastigmine in patients with mild to moderate Alzheimer's disease. *Int J Clin Pract.* **56**: 441–6.

51 Jones RW, Soininen H, Hager K *et al.* (2004) A multinational, randomised, 12-week study comparing the effects of donepezil and galantamine in patients with mild to moderate Alzheimer's disease. *Int J Geriatr Psychiatry.* **19**: 58–67.

52 Togashi H, Kimura S, Matsumoto M, Yoshioka M, Minami M and Saito H (1996) Cholinergic changes in the hippocampus of stroke-prone spontaneously hypertensive rats. *Stroke.* **27**: 520–5.

53 Gottfries CG, Blennow K, Karlsson I and Wallin A (1994) The neurochemistry of vascular dementia. *Dementia.* **5**: 163–7.

54 Snowdon DA, Greiner LH, Mortimer JA, Riley KP, Greiner PA and Markesbery WR (1997) Brain infarction and the clinical expression of Alzheimer disease – the Nun Study. *JAMA.* **277**: 813–17.

55 Erkinjuntti T, Kurz A, Gauthier S, Bullock R, Lilienfeld S and Damaraju CV (2002) Efficacy of galantamine in probable vascular dementia and Alzheimer's disease combined with cerebrovascular disease: a randomised trial. *Lancet.* **359**: 1283–90.

56 Moretti R, Torre P, Antonello RM and Cazzato G (2001) Rivastigmine in subcortical vascular dementia: a comparison trial on efficacy and tolerability for 12 months follow-up. *Eur J Neurol.* **8**: 361–2.

57 Black S, Roman GC, Geldmacher DS *et al.* (2003) Efficacy and tolerability of donepezil in vascular dementia: positive results of a 24-week, multicenter, international, randomized, placebo-controlled clinical trial. *Stroke.* **34**: 2323–30.

58 Wilkinson D, Doody R, Helme R *et al.* (2003) Donepezil in vascular dementia: a randomized, placebo-controlled study. *Neurology.* **61**: 479–86.

59 Perry R, McKeith I and Perry E (1997) Lewy body dementia – clinical, pathological and neurochemical interconnections. *J Neur Transm Suppl.* **51**: 95–109.

60 Lebert F, Pasquier F, Souliez L and Petit H (1998) Tacrine efficacy in Lewy body dementia. *Int J Geriatr Psychiatry.* **13**: 516–19.

61 Shea C, MacKnight C and Rockwood K (1998) Donepezil for treatment of dementia with Lewy bodies: a case series of nine patients. *Int Psychogeriatr.* **10**: 229–38.

62 McKeith I, Del Ser T, Spano P *et al.* (2000) Efficacy of rivastigmine in dementia with Lewy bodies: a randomised, double-blind, placebo-controlled international study. *Lancet.* **356**: 2031–6.

63 Lebert F, Pasquier F and Petit H (1995) The use of carbamazepine in senile dementia of Lewy body: a case study. *Alzheimer Dis.* **1 (Suppl. 1)**: 51.

64 Boeve BF, Silber MH and Ferman E (1998) Further data supporting underlying Lewy body disease in the RBD/dementia syndrome. *Neurobiol Aging.* **19**: 5205.

65 Moutoussis M and Orrell W (1996) Baclofen therapy for rigidity associated with Lewy body dementia. *Br J Psychiatry.* **169**: 795.

66 Bullock R and Cameron A (2002) Rivastigmine for the treatment of dementia and visual hallucinations associated with Parkinson's disease: a case series. *Curr Med Res Opin.* **18**: 258–64.

67 Winblad B and Poritis N (1999) Memantine in severe dementia: results of the M-9-BEST study (benefit and efficacy in severely demented patients during treatment with memantine). *Int J Geriatr Psychiatry.* **14**: 135–46.

68 Reisberg B, Doody R, Stoffler A, Schmitt F, Ferris S and Mobius HJ (2003) Memantine in moderate-to-severe Alzheimer's disease. *NEJM.* **348**: 1333–41.

69 Orgogozo JM, Rigaud AS, Stoffler A, Mobius HJ and Forette F (2002) Efficacy and safety of memantine in patients with mild to moderate vascular dementia: a randomized, placebo-controlled trial (MMM 300). *Stroke.* **33**: 1834–9.

70 Wilcock G, Mobius HJ and Stoffler A (2002) A double-blind, placebo-controlled multicentre study of memantine in mild to moderate vascular dementia (MMM500). *Int Clin Psychopharmacol.* **17**: 297–305.

71 Frei B (1994) Reactive oxygen species and antioxidant vitamins: mechanisms of action. *Am J Med.* **97**: S5–13.

72 Benzi G and Moretti A (1995) Are reactive oxygen species involved in Alzheimer's disease? *Neurobiol Aging.* **16**: 661–74.

73 Behl C, Davis J, Cole GM and Schubert D (1992) Vitamin E protects nerve cells from amyloid beta-protein toxicity. *Biochem Biophys Res Commun.* **186**: 944–50.

74 Mark SD, Wang W, Fraumeni JF *et al.* (1996) Lowered risks of hypertension and cerebrovascular disease after vitamin mineral supplementation: the Linxian Nutrition Intervention Trial. *Am J Epidemiol.* **143**: 658–64.

75 Steiner M, Glantz M and Lekos A (1995) Vitamin E plus aspirin compared with aspirin alone in patients with transient ischemic attacks. *Am J Clin Nutr.* **62**: S1381–4.

76 Doody RS, Stevens JC, Beck C *et al.* (2001) Practice parameter: management of dementia (an evidence-based review). Report of the Quality Standards Subcommittee of the American Academy of Neurology. *Neurology.* **56**: 1154–66.

77 Masaki KH, Losonczy KG, Izmirlian G *et al.* (2000) Association of vitamin E and C supplement use with cognitive function and dementia in elderly men. *Neurology.* **54**: 1265–72.

78 Tang MX, Jacobs D, Stern Y *et al.* (1996) Effect of oestrogen during menopause on risk and age at onset of Alzheimer's disease. *Lancet.* **348**: 429–32.

79 Henderson VW, Paganini-Hill A, Miller BL *et al.* (2000) Estrogen for Alzheimer's disease in women: randomized, double-blind, placebo-controlled trial. *Neurology.* **54**: 295–301.

80 Mulnard RI, Cotman CW, Kawas C *et al.* (2000) Estrogen replacement therapy for treatment of mild to moderate Alzheimer disease: a randomized controlled trial. *JAMA.* **283**: 1007–15.

81 Wang PN, Liao SQ, Liu RS *et al.* (2000) Effects of estrogen on cognition, mood and cerebral blood flow in AD: a controlled study. *Neurology.* **54**: 2061–6.

82 Shaywitz BA and Shaywitz SE (2000) Estrogen and Alzheimer disease: plausible theory, negative clinical trial. *JAMA.* **283**: 1055–6.

83 Mcewen BS and Alves SE (1999) Estrogen actions in the central nervous system. *Endocr Rev.* **20**: 279–307.

84 Xu HX, Gouras GK, Greenfield JP *et al.* (1998) Estrogen reduces neuronal generation of Alzheimer beta-amyloid peptides. *Nature Med.* **4**: 447–51.

85 Asthana S, Craft S, Baker LD *et al.* (1999) Cognitive and neuroendocrine response to transdermal estrogen in postmenopausal women with Alzheimer's disease: results of a placebo-controlled, double-blind, pilot study. *Psychoneuroendocrinology.* **24**: 657–77.

86 Thal LJ, Thomas RG, Mulnard R, Sano M, Grundman M and Schneider L (2003) Estrogen levels do not correlate with improvement in cognition. *Arch Neurol.* **60**: 209–12.

87 Mcgeer PL, Schulzer M and Mcgeer EG (1996) Arthritis and anti-inflammatory agents as possible protective factors for Alzheimer's disease: a review of 17 epidemiologic studies. *Neurology.* **47**: 425–32.

88 Breitner JCS and Zandi PP (2001) Do nonsteroidal anti-inflammatory drugs reduce the risk of Alzheimer's disease? *NEJM.* **345**: 1567–8.

89 Anthony JC, Breitner JCS, Zandi PP *et al.* (2000) Reduced prevalence of AD in users of NSAIDs and H_2-receptor antagonists: the Cache County Study. *Neurology.* **54**: 2066–71.

90 Landi F, Cesari M, Onder G, Russo A, Torre S and Bernabei R (2003) Non-steroidal anti-inflammatory drug (NSAID) use and Alzheimer disease in community-dwelling elderly patients. *Am J Geriatr Psychiatry.* **11**: 179–85.

91 Broe GA, Grayson DA, Creasey HM *et al.* (2000) Anti-inflammatory drugs protect against Alzheimer disease at low doses. *Arch Neurol.* **57**: 1586–91.

92 Halliday GM, Shepherd CE, McCann H *et al.* (2000) Effect of anti-inflammatory medications on neuropathological findings in Alzheimer disease. *Arch Neurol.* **57**: 831–6.

93 Aisen PS, Davis KL, Berg JD *et al.* (2000) A randomized controlled trial of prednisone in Alzheimer's disease. *Neurology.* **54**: 588–93.

94 Mackenzie IRA (2000) Anti-inflammatory drugs and Alzheimer-type pathology in aging. *Neurology.* **54**: 732–4.

95 Scharf S, Mander A, Ugoni A, Vajda F and Christophidis N (1999) A double-blind, placebo-controlled trial of diclofenac/misoprostol in Alzheimer's disease. *Neurology.* **53**: 197–200.

96 Eriksen JL, Sagi SA, Smith TE *et al.* (2003) NSAIDs and enantiomers of flurbiprofen target gamma-secretase and lower A beta 42 *in vivo. J Clin Invest.* **112**: 440–9.

97 Jick H, Zornberg GL, Jick SS, Seshadri S and Drachman DA (2000) Statins and the risk of dementia. *Lancet.* **356**: 1627–31.

98 Wolozin B, Kellman W, Ruosseau P, Celesia GG and Siegel G (2000) Decreased prevalence of Alzheimer disease associated with 3-hydroxy-3-methyglutaryl coenzyme A reductase inhibitors. *Arch Neurol.* **57**: 1439–43.

99 Rockwood K, Kirkland S, Hogan DB *et al.* (2002) Use of lipid-lowering agents, indication bias, and the risk of dementia in community-dwelling elderly people. *Arch Neurol.* **59**: 223–7.

100 Collins R, Armitage J, Parish S, Sleight P and Peto R (2003) MRC/BHF Heart Protection Study of cholesterol-lowering with simvastatin in 5963 people with diabetes: a randomised placebo-controlled trial. *Lancet.* **361**: 2005–16.

101 Shepherd J, Blauw GJ and Murphy MB (2002) Pravastatin in elderly individuals at risk of vascular disease (PROSPER): a randomised controlled trial. *Lancet.* **360**: 1623–30.

102 Borroni B, Pettenati C, Bordonali T, Akkawi N, Di Luca M and Padovani A (2003) Serum cholesterol levels modulate long-term efficacy of cholinesterase inhibitors in Alzheimer disease. *Neurosci Lett.* **343**: 213–15.

103 McCaddon A, Hudson B and Davies G (2001) Homocysteine and cognitive decline in healthy elderly. *Dement Geriatr Cogn Disord.* **12**: 309–13.

104 Aisen PS, Egelko S, Andrews H *et al.* (2003) A pilot study of vitamins to lower plasma homocysteine levels in Alzheimer disease. *Am J Geriatr Psychiatry.* **11**: 246–9.

105 Forette F, Seux ML, Staessen JA *et al.* (2002) The prevention of dementia with antihypertensive treatment. *Arch Intern Med.* **162**: 2046–52.

106 PROGRESS Collaborative Group (2001) Randomised trial of a perindopril-based blood-pressure-lowering regimen among 6105 individuals with previous stroke or transient ischaemic attack. *Lancet.* **358**: 1033–41.

107 Schenk D, Barbour R, Dunn W *et al.* (1999) Immunization with amyloid-beta attenuates Alzheimer disease-like pathology in the PDAPP mouse. *Nature.* **400**: 173–7.

108 Nicoll JAR, Wilkinson D, Holmes C, Steart P, Markham H and Weller RO (2003) Neuropathology of human Alzheimer disease after immunization with amyloid-beta peptide: a case report. *Nature Med.* **9**: 448–52.

109 Orgogozo JM, Gilman S, Dartigues JF *et al.* (2003) Subacute meningoencephalitis in a subset of patients with AD after A beta 42 immunization. *Neurology.* **61**: 46–54.

110 Oken BS, Storzbach DM and Kaye JA (1998) The efficacy of *Ginkgo biloba* on cognitive function in Alzheimer disease. *Arch Neurol.* **55**: 1409–15.

111 Galluzzi S, Zanetti O, Binetti G, Trabucchi M and Frisoni GB (2000) Coma in a patient with Alzheimer's disease taking low-dose trazodone and *Ginkgo biloba. J Neurol Neurosurg Psychiatry.* **68**: 679–80.

112 Flicker L and Grimley Evans J (2004) *Piracetam for Dementia or Cognitive Impairment. Cochrane Library. Issue 2.* Update Software, Oxford.

113 Olin J, Schneider LS, Novit A and Lucsak S (2004) *Hydergine for Dementia. Cochrane Library. Issue 4.* Update Software, Oxford.

114 Rother M, Erkinjuntti T, Roessner M, Kittner B, Marcusson J and Karlsson I (1998) Propentofylline in the treatment of Alzheimer's disease and vascular dementia: a review of phase III trials. *Dementia Geriatr Cogn Disord.* **9 (Suppl. 1)**: 36–43.

115 Montgomery SA, Thal LJ and Amrein R (2003) Meta-analysis of double-blind randomized controlled clinical trials of acetyl-L-carnitine versus placebo in the treatment of mild cognitive impairment and mild Alzheimer's disease. *Int Clin Psychopharmacol.* **18**: 61–71.

116 Tariot PN, Farlow MR, Grossberg GT, Graham SM, McDonald S and Gergel I (2004) Memantine treatment in patients with moderate to severe Alzheimer disease already receiving donepezil – a randomized controlled trial. *JAMA.* **291**: 317–24.

117 Cummings JL (2000) Cholinesterase inhibitors: a new class of psychotropic compounds. *Am J Psychiatry.* **157**: 4–15.

118 Shaw KTY, Utsuki T, Rogers J *et al.* (2001) Phenserine regulates translation of beta-amyloid precursor protein mRNA by a putative interleukin-1 responsive element, a target for drug development. *Proc Natl Acad Sci USA.* **98**: 7605–10.

119 Apelt J, Ach K and Schliebs R (2003) Aging-related down-regulation of neprilysin, a putative beta-amyloid-degrading enzyme, in transgenic Tg2576 Alzheimer-like mouse brain is accompanied by an astroglial upregulation in the vicinity of beta-amyloid plaques. *Neurosci Lett.* **339**: 183–6.

120 Marr RA, Rockenstein E, Mukherjee A *et al.* (2003) Neprilysin gene transfer reduces human amyloid pathology in transgenic mice. *J Neurosci.* **23**: 1992–6.

Chapter 13

Pharmacogenetics and the treatment of Alzheimer's disease

Clive Holmes and Michelle C McCulley

Introduction

Pharmacogenetics is the study of the hereditary basis for individual variation in drug response. Thus some patients will respond well to a drug, while others will respond poorly to the same medication. Likewise, a drug might be toxic to some patients but not to others. These problems are inherent in a wide variety of treatment areas in medicine. However, as a consequence of incurring adverse side-effects, poor compliance is a particular problem in psychiatry. Elderly patients with their well-documented, age-related disturbances of metabolism and polypharmacy are particularly susceptible.

Drug treatment of the cognitive deficits and neuropsychiatric features of Alzheimer's disease (AD) is confounded by a lack of efficacy and by adverse effects. However, of all the psychiatric illnesses that affect the elderly, AD is the one condition that is most likely to benefit from pharmacogenetics research in the near future. This is simply because more is known about the genetic contribution to AD than for any other elderly psychiatric condition. This chapter will therefore focus on the pharmacogenetics approach to the treatment of AD, but many of the principles involved are clearly also relevant to other elderly psychiatric illnesses.

Pharmacogenetics and pharmacogenomics

It is important to emphasise that although the presence of some genetic variants may predict the occurrence of disease and may form the basis for the development of new treatments, variants in other genes (e.g. those involved in drug metabolism) may predict treatment response but not necessarily the occurrence of the disease. The first strategy, of identifying these disease-related susceptibility genes, is known as discovery genetics or pharmacogenetics. The second strategy, of identifying genes or gene families not known to be genetically related to disease for use as pharmacological targets, is known as discovery genomics or pharmacogenomics. Pharmacogenomics is rapidly evolving. Although current research is focusing on the effects that known genetic polymorphisms have on existing drug metabolism and action, in the future it is likely that the focus will move towards the discovery of new drug response genes and the development of novel molecules to target these genes.

The advantage of discovery genetics is that, by definition, these genes are relevant to the patient's genetic contribution to the disease, whilst pharmacogenomics results in a need to validate these targets, to find the function of the gene and to find a relevant disease or clinical indication. Pharmacogenomic strategies are currently aimed at data trawling through human genome databases to identify genes that can be expressed and their products examined for functional significance. Validation of these genetic variants is heavily reliant on screening technologies such as differential gene expression or proteomics. These techniques examine different levels or patterns of gene expression or different levels of protein expression in animal tissue. The striking differences in the two approaches are highlighted by the strong likelihood that apolipoprotein E (ApoE), a well-established susceptibility gene for AD, is unlikely to have been discovered using a pharmacogenomics approach, as it is not expressed in rat neurons and would not therefore have been seen as a valid target. Conversely, the importance of genetic variation in various drug-metabolising enzymes or neuroreceptors in determining treatment response is unlikely to have been apparent from a pharmacogenetics approach.

Pharmacogenetics and pharmacogenomics will eventually streamline drug development to the point that patients with apparently similar disease phenotypes but different genotypes will receive the most appropriate drug for them with maximal effectiveness and minimal side-effects. In order to achieve this, it is clear that we will need an individualised genetic profile in order to match the right drug to the right person. To this end, single nucleotide polymorphism (SNP) mapping is pointing the way towards attaining the goal of truly individualised therapies.

Pharmacogenetics

Direct support for a genetic component to AD comes from the recognition of a small number of patients who inherit the disease largely before the age of 65 years in a clear autosomal dominant pattern. To date, mutations in three genes, namely amyloid precursor protein (APP), presenilin 1 (PS1) and presenilin 2 (PS2), have been described which lead to this early form of AD. Pathogenic APP, PS1 and PS2 mutations have been shown to alter the proteolytic processing of APP, giving rise to increased production of the β-42 form of amyloid protein which forms the core of neuritic plaques and which has been shown to be neurotoxic to cells in culture.[1]

In AD that develops after the age of 65 years, no clear autosomal dominant patterns have been established. However, a wide range of different candidate genes have been proposed, variations in which have been associated with an increased risk of developing AD. Of these candidates, the most substantially corroborated genetic risk factor remains that of the presence of the common polymorphism ApoE ϵ4. The role of ApoE in the molecular pathogenesis of AD has yet to be clearly established, but the inheritance of one or two ApoE ϵ4 alleles may result in enhanced aggregation and/or decreased clearance of β-amyloid.[2]

Current treatments

To date, only one study has looked at the influence of the rare genetic mutations in APP, PS1 and PS2 on treatment response.[3] PS1-related genotypes all responded to therapy with CDP-choline, piracetam and anapsos in a similar manner;

whereas patients with a defective PS2 gene exon 5 (PS2+ patients) always showed a poorer therapeutic response than PS2– patients. These data suggest that the therapeutic outcome in AD exhibits a genotype-specific pattern.

The ApoE genotype has been extensively examined with regard to treatment response to cholinesterase inhibitors on the basis that ApoE ϵ4 may influence choline acetyltransferase (ChAT) activity in the hippocampus of subjects with AD. One of the first pharmacogenetic studies[4] of AD examined the effect of the ApoE ϵ4 allele on cholinomimetic drug responsiveness in a group ($n=40$) of AD patients who completed a double-blind, 30-week clinical trial of the cholinesterase inhibitor tacrine. The results showed that over 80% of ApoE ϵ4-negative AD patients showed marked improvement after 30 weeks as measured by the Alzheimer's Disease Assessment Scale (ADAS), whereas 60% of ApoE ϵ4 carriers had ADAS scores that were worse than baseline values. These results supported the concept that ApoE ϵ4 played a crucial role in the cholinergic dysfunction associated with AD and might be a prognostic indicator of poor response to therapy with acetylcholinesterase inhibitors in AD patients. However, a later and much larger study of 460 subjects on variable doses of tacrine only found a trend towards a greater treatment effect in the ApoE ϵ4-negative patients using a variety of global indicators of change.[5] Indeed, a further follow-up study only showed significant findings in women.[6]

Further largely negative findings have been obtained in studies of donepezil. Thus ApoE genotyping was performed on 117 patients with mild to moderate Alzheimer's disease who were included in a 36-week open-label trial of donepezil therapy.[7] Patients were treated blindly with regard to ApoE genotype. Outcome measures were Alzheimer's Disease Assessment Scale – Cognitive Component (ADAS-Cog), the Mini-Mental State Examination (MMSE), Instrumental Activities of Daily Living (IADL), and the Caregiver-rated Clinical Global Impression of Change. An intention-to-treat analysis did not reveal significant differences between the responses of ApoE ϵ4– and ApoE ϵ4+ carriers according to the ADAS-Cog ($P=0.28$). No differences were found between the responses of men and women ($P=0.81$), and there was no significant interaction between genotype and gender ($P=0.09$). Other outcome measures all exhibited similar patterns of change to those seen using the ADAS-Cog. Consequently, these results do not support the hypothesis that the ApoE genotype and gender are predictors of the response to donepezil in AD patients.

Another study of 107 AD subjects taking galantamine also failed to show an effect of ApoE genotype and treatment response in the short term (3 months), but suggested that it may affect response over the longer term (up to 12 months).[8]

Overall, then, these results fail to show any convincing evidence that known genetic risk factors have a major influence on existing treatments aimed at inhibition of acetylycholinesterase.

Future treatments

Direct genetic manipulation to minimise the effects of these disease variants using therapeutic gene transfer in AD is not considered to be part of pharmacogenetics or pharmacogenomics,[9] and it remains a largely theoretical concept. However, it is worth noting that the technical prerequisites are being developed at an astonishing rate.[10] Two basic procedures, namely the *ex-vivo* and *in-vivo* approaches, have been developed. In the *ex-vivo* procedure the transgene is introduced into the cells by a viral vector *in vitro* which is then grafted into the organism. This approach may enable the replacement of neurotransmitters or neurotrophic growth factor by grafting in modified primary neuronal, stem or progenitor cells. In the *in-vivo* approach the gene is delivered into the organism by a viral vector for *in-situ* transduction of the target brain cell. The latter approach has a more immediate application in understanding the role of genetic risk factors in animal models, rather than a direct role in the treatment of AD.

Indirect genetic manipulation uses our knowledge of the pathogenetic mechanisms to point to what would appear to be the most relevant molecules to play a crucial role in the occurrence of the disease. Indeed so mainstream are these approaches that it is sometimes forgotten that most of the future treatment prospects in AD have their foundations in pharmacogenetics. Thus the involvement of β-amyloid and in particular the β-42 fragment in families who have inherited early autosomal dominant AD has resulted in a number of preventive strategies aimed at the early steps of the biological cascade in AD. These could include the use of compounds that inhibit β-amyloid production by reducing the activity of enzymes (including β or γ secretase), or that cleave β-amyloid from APP, or the use of inhibitors of β-amyloid aggregation or fibrillisation. Based largely on studies of Down's syndrome patients[11] and transgenic mice[12] that express mutant APP and/or PS1, it has also been postulated that β-42 accumulation and the consequent neuritic plaque formation is associated with microglia activation, reactive astrocytosis and a widespread inflammatory response. It is thought that this inflammatory response coupled with the direct toxicity arising from oligomeric and fibrillar β-amyloid produces the structural and consequent neurochemical changes seen in AD. In addition, it is thought that the effects of this inflammatory and neurotoxic process are then further compounded by the excess generation of free radicals and peroxidative injury, which causes further damage to neurons.[13] It follows from this schema that drugs that interfere with one or a number of these processes could lead to arrest or delay in the progression of the disease.

Pharmacogenomics

In the same way that common variation in genes can be associated with disease (e.g. APOE ϵ4 associated with AD), common genetic variation can also be associated with treatment response. Thus new DNA technologies allow extensive analysis of the genetic code, and make it possible to identify candidate genes that might influence the effectiveness of a drug. This is achieved by looking for polymorphisms (changes in the DNA sequence of genes between individual people or chromosomes) which correlate with a certain clinical outcome. Polymorphisms are by definition genetic variants that occur in the population with a frequency of at least 1%. Most people think of genetic mutations as being harmful, but most polymorphisms simply contribute to individual diversity, including variability in affinity for drugs or drug metabolism. Until recently the existence of known polymorphisms in candidate genes for treatment response has been the focus of research. Thus patients who carry genetic variants in drug-metabolising enzymes or, more recently, genetic variants in neuroreceptors have been assessed with regard to their differential treatment response. However, in the future it is clear that most variability in treatment response will be assessed using SNP profiling.

Genetic variation determining current treatment response

The first pharmacogenomic associations were discovered in the 1950s with adverse events in patients taking primaquine, succinylcholine and isoniazid being found to be due to deficiencies of glucose-6-phosphate dehydrogenase, serum cholinesterase and N-acetyl transferase, respectively. Indeed the majority of pharmacogenomic differences characterised to date still represent variability in drug-metabolising enzymes, some of which are more prevalent in certain ethnic groups (e.g. a lack of tolerance of alcohol in Japanese subjects due to a higher frequency of a genetic polymorphism in aldehyde dehydrogenase). Over 100 polymorphic traits in drug-metabolising enzymes have been identified that explain the variability in response to a large number of CNS drugs (e.g. succinylcholine) as well as non-CNS drugs (e.g. isoniazid and the antimalarials). In these situations the differential treatment response may be a direct result of genetic differences in drug metabolism resulting in different plasma concentrations of the drug in different patients, despite their receiving the same dosage.

However, the activity of CNS drugs can also be influenced by genetic alterations that affect the drug target molecule. These include neurotransmitter receptors, neurotransmitter transporters and other receptors and enzymes involved in psychiatric disorders. Association studies investigating the relationship between genetic polymorphisms in metabolic enzymes and neurotransmitter receptors and psychiatric treatment outcome provide a step towards the individualisation of psychiatric treatment by enabling the selection of the most beneficial drug in terms of its efficacy and low side-effect profile.

Drug metabolism

Virtually all drugs are metabolised by phase I followed by phase II metabolising enzymes. There are at least several hundred such enzymes in the human genome, including 49 human cytochrome P450 genes. Cytochrome P450 enzymes control metabolic phase I reactions and participate in the metabolism of the majority of psychiatric drugs. These enzymes are located in the membrane of the endoplasmic reticulum, mainly in the liver, and are responsible for the oxidative metabolism of drugs and other compounds such as prostaglandins, fatty acids and steroids.

Cytochrome P450 phase I metabolising enzymes include CYP2D6, CYP1A2, CYP3A4, CYP2C9 and CYP2C19, which are most commonly involved in the metabolism of psychiatric drugs. Side-effects are likely to be greater when a number of drugs are metabolised by the same cytochrome P450 system, particularly if they are not metabolised by other P450 systems. The elderly are particularly vulnerable in this context because of polypharmacy and higher rates of physical morbidity, as well as age-related changes in renal excretion. The risk of adverse drug reactions is further compounded in those individuals who have a genetically determined lower enzyme level and thus are poorer drug metabolisers. For example, approximately 7% of people show low levels of activity for the CYP2D6 system, which has more than 70 mutant alleles and is involved in the metabolism of commonly used antipsychotics and antidepressants, including haloperidol, olanzapine, chlorpromazine and paroxetine.[14] Depending on the allele that has been inherited, the individual may have poor, extensive, intermediate or ultra-rapid metabolism.[15] However, although there are clear genetic differences both in metabolism and in side-effect profiles, including an excess of tardive dyskinesia following neuroleptic treatment, no differences have been found between variants in CYP2D6 and treatment response. Likewise, about 12% of the population are genetically predisposed to have lower levels of CYP1A2 activity, the enzyme system responsible for metabolising fluvoxamine, clozapine and tacrine, among other drugs. The frequency of poor metabolisers in the population also varies significantly with regard to ethnicity for the cytochrome P450 enzymes. Thus 2% of Caucasians compared with 20% of Japanese are poor metabolisers for the CYP2C9/19 system, whose main substrates include tricyclic antidepressants, diazepam and clozapine.[16]

In addition to cytochrome P450 enzymes, phase II conjugation enzymes may also play a part in the disruption of the metabolic process (e.g. enzymes such as N-acetyl transferase and thiopurine methyltransferase). Thus the development of isoniazid-related peripheral neuropathy can be tracked to patients with certain alleles of a polymorphic gene for the liver enzyme N-acetyltransferase 2, who are slow acetylators of the drug. Such individuals are at increased risk of neuropathy because the concentration of isoniazid in their blood remains higher for longer.

It is interesting to note that although genetic association studies have shown that metabolic variants may theoretically influence the required dose for a therapeutic level, the clinical significance appears to be limited to side-effects rather than treatment response.

Receptor pharmacogenomics

In AD not only do we have multiple genes that are causative (i.e. directly involved in initiating the amyloid cascade, such as mutations in PS1), but we also have multiple genetic influences on the perpetuation and progression of these initial changes that may not be seen as directly causal (e.g. the cytokine inflammatory cascade). The final outcome of these changes is the disruption of a variety of neurochemical systems, particularly acetylcholine, glutamate and serotonin, which gives rise to the variable clinical symptoms that we see in AD and which remain the focus of our current symptomatic treatments. Genetic variation in these neurochemical systems may extenuate, or in some cases offer some protection against, these neurodegenerative losses.

There has been some research investigating the effect of genetic variants in dopaminergic and serotonergic receptors in order to find polymorphisms that influence treatment response. For example, significant associations have been found between polymorphisms in serotonin type 2A receptors and response to long-term clozapine and risperidone treatment in patients with schizophrenia.[17,18] Arranz et al. used genetic information in receptors targeted by the potent antipsychotic clozapine to predict drug response with a 78% success rate.[19] To date, there have been no reports on the potential for these variants to determine the variability in treatment response in behavioural and psychological symptoms in AD. However, a number of reports have shown that genetic variation in neuroreceptors can influence the presentation of behavioural and psychological symptoms in AD.[20] As well as treatment response, adverse events have also been associated with genetic variants in potassium and sodium ion channel receptors in individuals who are predisposed to death from cardiac repolarisation that may occur in stressful circumstances or which can be triggered by drugs such as tricyclic antidepressants and chlorpromazine.

SNP mapping and the development of individual pharmacogenetics

The vast majority of genetic variation in humans is in the form of SNPs. SNPs are present in the human genome with an average frequency of around 1 per 1000 base pairs, with more than 1 000 000 SNPs already documented on the human genome database.[21] SNPs may be directly associated with a disease, or they may occur so close to a causative polymorphism that they are highly likely to be inherited together with that polymorphism through successive generations (a process known as linkage disequilibrium). Likewise, SNPs can be used to mark treatment response and side-effect profiles. By applying SNP linkage disequilibrium mapping to patients in phase II clinical trials, it may be possible to select areas of the genome that are in linkage disequilibrium with treatment response or high side-effect profiles. These SNP maps could then be used to identify, by homing in on this area of the genome with even denser SNP maps, the actual genes responsible for efficacy or adverse events. Detailed analysis of specific genes could also provide generic SNP profiles to compare with a specific individual's SNP profile in order to estimate their likelihood of treatment response or adverse events.

For individualised drug therapy to become a reality, it is clear that a greater understanding of the complex pathways and interactions involved in disease presentation and treatment is required. In addition, it is clear that technologies such as chip-based SNP profiling need to be further developed for wider application. In conclusion, pharmacogenomics is clearly in its infancy, but we are already beginning to see the impact of pharmacogenetics, and it is likely that our genetic make-up will be used to enable the generation of personalised prescriptions within the next ten years.

Key points

- The identification of disease-related susceptibility genes is known as discovery genetics or pharmacogenetics.
- The identification of genes, not known to be genetically related to disease, for pharmacological targets is known as discovery genomics or pharmacogenomics.
- The clinical significance of genetic variation in drug metabolism appears to be largely related to side effects rather than the clinical efficacy of drugs.
- In addition to a greater undersanding of the complex pathways involved in the aetiology of Alzheimer's disease, individualised drug therapy will be largely dependent upon technologies such as chip-based single polymorphism profiling.

References

1 Lambert MP, Barlow AK, Chromy BA *et al.* (1998) Diffusible, nonfibrillar ligands derived from A-beta 1–42 are potent central nervous system neurotoxins. *Proc Natl Acad Sci USA.* **95**: 6448–53.

2 Schmechel DE, Saunders AM, Strittmatter WJ *et al.* (1993) Increased amyloid beta-peptide deposition in cerebral cortex as a consequence of apolipoprotein E genotype in late-onset Alzheimer disease. *Proc Natl Acad Sci USA.* **90**: 9649–53.

3 Cacabelos R, Alvarez A, Fenandez-Novoa L and Lombardi VR (2000) A pharmaco-genomic approach to Alzheimer's disease. *Acta Neurol Scand.* **102 (Suppl. 176)**: 12–19.

4 Poirier J, Delisle MC, Quirion R *et al.* (1995) Apolipoprotein E4 allele as a predictor of cholinergic deficits and treatment outcome in Alzheimer disease. *Proc Natl Acad Sci USA.* **92**: 12260–4.

5 Farlow MR, Lahiri DK, Poirier J *et al.* (1996) Apolipoprotein E genotype and gender influence response to tacrine therapy. *Ann NY Acad Sci.* **802**: 101–10.

6 Farlow MR, Lahiri DK, Poirier J *et al.* (1998) Treatment outcome of tacrine therapy depends on apolipoprotein genotype and gender of subjects with Alzheimer's disease. *Neurology.* **50**: 669–77.

7 Rigaud AS, Traykov L, Latour F *et al.* (2002) Presence or absence of at least one epsilon 4 allele and gender are not predictive for the response to donepezil treatment in Alzheimer's disease. *Pharmacogenetics.* **12**: 415–20.

8 MacGowan SH, Wilcock GK and Scott M (1998) Effect of gender and apolipoprotein E genotype on response to anticholinesterase therapy in Alzheimer's disease. *Int J Geriatr Psychiatry.* **13**: 625–30.

9 Roses AD (2000) Pharmacogenetics and the practice of medicine. *Nature.* **405**: 857–65.

10 Carter JE and Schuchman EH (2001) Gene therapy for neurodegenerative diseases: fact or fiction? *Br J Psychiatry.* **178**: 392–4.

11 Isacson O, Seo H, Lin L *et al.* (2002) Alzheimer's disease and Down's syndrome: roles of APP, trophic factors and ACh. *Trends Neurosci.* **25**: 79–84.

12 Tan J, Town T, Crawford F *et al.* (2002) Role of CD40 ligand in amyloidosis in transgenic Alzheimer's mice. *Nat Neurosci.* **5**: 1288–93.

13 Harris ME, Hensley K, Butterfield DA *et al.* (1995) Direct evidence of oxidative injury produced by the Alzheimer's beta-amyloid peptide (1–40) in cultured hippocampal neurons. *Exp Neurol.* **131**: 193–202.

14 Bertilsson L, Dahl ML, Dalen P *et al.* (2002) Molecular genetics of CYP2D6: clinical relevance with focus on psychotropic drugs. *Br J Clin Pharmacol.* **53**: 111–22.

15 Nebert DW and Dieter MZ (2000) The evolution of drug metabolism. *Pharmacology.* **61**: 124–35.

16 Katona CL (2001) Psychotropics and drug interactions in the elderly patient. *Int J Geriatr Psychiatry.* **16 (Suppl. 1)**: S86–90.

17 Arranz M, Collier D, Sodhi M *et al.* (1995) Association between clozapine response and allelic variation in 5HT$_{2A}$ receptor gene. *Lancet.* **346**: 281–2.

18 Lane HY, Chang YC, Chiu CC *et al.* (2002) Association of risperidone treatment response with a polymorphism in the 5-HT$_{(2A)}$ receptor gene. *Am J Psychiatry.* **159**: 1593–5.

19 Arranz MJ, Munro J, Birkett J *et al.* (2000) Pharmacogenetic prediction of clozapine response. *Lancet.* **355**: 1615–16.

20 Holmes C (2002) Genotype and phenotype in Alzheimer's disease. *Br J Psychiatry.* **180**: 131–4.

21 Sachidanandam R, Weissman D, Schmidt SC *et al.* (2001) A map of human genome sequence variation containing 1.42 million single nucleotide polymorphisms. *Nature.* **409**: 928–33.

Chapter 14

The role of drug therapy in the management of behavioural and psychological symptoms of dementia

Roger Bullock

Introduction

Up to 80% of patients with Alzheimer's disease (AD) may experience behavioural changes during the course of their disease.[1] These may occur throughout the disease, with a tendency to increase as it progresses. The term *behavioural and psychological symptoms of dementia (BPSD)* is the collective name for many of the behaviours that occur, and is defined as 'symptoms of disturbed perception, thought content, mood or behaviour that frequently occur in patients with dementia'.[2] They are associated with increased patient and caregiver stress, and are a predictor of institutionalisation and reduction in ability to perform activities of daily living.[3] The main components are summarised in Table 14.1. Most of these symptoms are treatable, many of them responding more than the cognitive and functional domains in dementia.

Table 14.1 Behavioural and psychological components of BPSD

Behavioural symptoms	Psychological symptoms
Physical aggression	Anxiety
Screaming	Depression
Restlessness	Hallucinations
Agitation	Delusions
Wandering	Misidentifications
Inappropriate behaviour	Apathy
Disinhibition	Psychosis of AD
Hoarding	
Cursing	
Shadowing	

These behaviours may actually be more frequent in dementia with Lewy bodies

(DLB), Parkinson's disease dementia and vascular dementia. Thus collectively they are an important area to treat, although to date no pharmaceutical products are actually specifically licensed to do this.

Instead, drug prescribing in patients with BPSD has evolved over the years in a haphazard and anecdotal way. One reason for this is poor psychopathological history taking, with consequent grouping of any elicited symptoms into areas of more familiar psychiatric nosology. This has led to patients being treated with antipsychotics, antidepressants and benzodiazepines, even when the individual symptom may not actually be expected to respond in any classical way. As a result, patients have been exposed to a variety of drugs, some of which are actually harmful – through their side-effects, interactions with other drugs, or acceleration of the underlying disease through toxic effects on the cholinergic system.

When considering BPSD, it must always be remembered that behaviour is a form of communication, and that when it presents it has to be placed in context in terms of the following:

- environment
- difficulties that the person is encountering (e.g. pain, constipation, urinary tract infection or loss of verbal communication)
- the person's understanding of their situation
- historic reasons for the behaviour (e.g. dislike of certain foods expressed by throwing the plate away)
- reactions of people to the person and his or her behaviour.

Any reversible elements identified at the initial assessment should be addressed before resorting to drug treatment. Instead, what has frequently happened is that antipsychotics have been used for the sake of speed, even when there is no evidence to support their use. This injudicious use of drugs, especially in nursing and residential institutions, has led to some disquiet,[4] with accusations of chemical coshes being used. Recent developments linking the use of risperidone and olanzapine to cerebrovascular adverse events has added to the disquiet and led to these drugs not being recommended in this patient group, especially in any individuals with pre-existing cerebrovascular disease. Some studies show quite widespread usage, way above what the prevalence figures predict would be required.[5] In the USA, these fears have led to a mandatory requirement that the use of non-pharmacological treatments be documented before any drugs are used. A study looking at the relevance of the medication used in nursing homes in the USA showed that 80% was justified and reported side-effects were minimal. This is a good result, but it does mean that 20% of people still actually receive drugs that are both unnecessary and potentially harmful.

Aetiological considerations

One problem in initiating the most appropriate treatment has been the difficulty in understanding the true nature of the neurobiological correlates for the behaviours that are observed. Disruption of the fronto-cortical circuits due to cholinergic loss may produce delusional symptoms that respond to cholinergic enhancement.[6] The amygdala and limbic system have cholinergic inputs and are linked to some of the BPSD that is seen. These cholinergic neurons seem to be particularly rich in butyrylcholinesterase, which may explain why rivastigmine (a dual acetyl- and butyrylcholinesterase inhibitor) appears to have a good profile in treating many of the commonly observed behaviours. The reticular activating system (sleep and arousal) also has cholinergic afferents, and these seem to be affected in DLB, where fluctuating attention is a feature of the illness and rapid eye movement (REM) sleep disorder is common. In all of these examples, restoration of cholinergic integrity may have a positive effect on symptoms arising as a result of any disease process. The relationship between cholinergic loss in DLB and visual hallucinations has been clearly demonstrated, to the extent that the presence of hallucinations predicted response in a study of rivastigmine in DLB.[7]

Dopamine, noradrenaline and serotonin have altered levels in certain areas of the brain in AD, although the relevance of this to clinical symptoms is unclear. Polymorphisms at the serotonergic and dopaminergic receptors may also influence the appearance of certain symptoms, but much more work is needed to improve our understanding of the role of genetics and how they contribute to the neurobiology of the behaviours that emerge. This may enable specific targeting of treatments, rather than the blunter methods of selection currently in use.

There is increasing evidence of disruption of the neuroendocrine system in AD. Around 50% of patients fail the dexamethasone depression test, suggesting that sleep disturbance and disturbance of diurnal rhythms are likely. In addition, imbalances of neuropeptides in the hypothalamus may indicate loss of inhibitory control due to failure of feedback mechanisms from stress systems. This could lead to agitation, restlessness and stress-related symptoms.

Neuropathological associations of psychotic disorders include low neuronal counts in the parahippocampal gyrus, region CA1 of the hippocampus, dorsal raphe and the locus ceruleus. High plaque counts in the presubiculum and occipital cortex are associated with delusions and hallucinations, as is a high tangle density in the parietal lobe and frontal cortex.

Measurement issues

Measuring behavioural symptoms poses certain methodological issues. Most information is obtained through history taking and so is delivered from the carer's perspective, whether in clinical settings or research. Rarely is behaviour observed directly for any significant time period, especially as a follow-up, and this makes it difficult to interpret the results of the interventions. Carers report according to how they feel, so behaviours that may not be particularly troubling on one occasion may be deemed unbearable on another. Also the frequency and severity of behaviours make a difference. A single severe episode may have more effect than frequent minor ones, and vice versa. This variability can make interpretation of results in clinical trials difficult – hence the continued debates over the current evidence.

Many scales have been designed to capture the behaviours that occur. No one instrument has all of the features needed to cover the area completely, but two in particular have been used extensively in clinical studies. These are the Behave-AD,[8] which is predominantly a structured psychiatric interview that measures the presence and severity of symptoms, and the Neuropsychiatric Inventory (NPI),[9] which is a checklist of the possible behaviours and their severity and frequency.

The scales are useful both in clinical trials and in individual patients, although care must be taken when interpreting total scores – the individual item scores are perhaps more informative.

Pharmacological treatment of BPSD

Cholinesterase inhibitors

There is now evidence that these drugs do have an effect on psychotic symptoms in Alzheimer's disease, especially visual hallucinations and delusions, as well as the anxiety and apathy that often coexist. These drugs have an advantage in that they do not harm the underlying disease, and in many cases they are treating the cognitive decline and disorders of activities of daily living (ADL) as well (see Chapter 12).

Most of the data available on cholinesterase inhibitors are derived from secondary outcome measures in trials designed to look at cognition, and the patients who enter these trials usually have minimal behavioural disorders. No studies randomising cholinesterase inhibitors specifically for use in behavioural disorders have yet been published. As a result, any findings to date are not conclusive.

Donepezil

The early studies of donepezil did not measure any specific behavioural effect. A 1-year Nordic study of donepezil vs. placebo in 286 patients with mild to moderate AD did not differentiate between the two groups in terms of behaviour (as assessed by the NPI), although cognition and ADL were both significantly improved with donepezil.[10] A nursing-home study of 208 nursing-home residents with more advanced AD again failed to separate the NPI total scores, although there was significantly less agitation on donepezil than on placebo.[11] The Moderate-Severe Alzheimer's Disease (M-SAD) was a placebo-controlled study in community-dwelling patients with moderate to severe AD.[12] Here both groups fared better than baseline, and at weeks 4 and 24 the donepezil group scored better on the total NPI score than the placebo group (the result was driven by an improvement in apathy, anxiety and depression). Several smaller open-label studies have yielded inconsistent results, some reporting increased behavioural problems with donepezil.[13,14]

In an open-labelled study of 17 patients with DLB, donepezil had a positive effect on behaviour.[15] However, half of the group on donepezil showed worsening of their parkinsonian symptoms, and this has been described in case reports as well.[16] A total of 30 patients with Down's syndrome were randomised for 24 weeks to donepezil or placebo.[17] Although cognition deteriorated less on donepezil, the total NPI score was worse.

Thus the evidence for the efficacy of donepezil in BPSD is not convincing. Apathy, anxiety and depression seem to respond better than any other symptoms. There is little evidence to support the use of donepezil specifically for any other behaviour.

Rivastigmine

In early studies, the behavioural aspects of the global score were significantly better in the patients on rivastigmine than in those taking placebo.[18] Three similar open-labelled nursing-home studies have all shown improvements in behaviour on rivastigmine. Cummings showed a decrease of 3.25 in mean total NPI scores in 173 residents.[19] Agitation, anxiety, delusions, hallucinations, irritability, aberrant motor activity and night-time behaviour improved in 58% of the patients, and 50% of patients showed more than a 30% reduction in their total score. Another US study reported similar findings,[20] and in Europe 50% of patients with behavioural symptoms at baseline showed improvement on every domain in the NPI at 6 months.[21] In this study, 93% of patients who did not have symptoms at baseline did not develop new symptoms during the active phase.

The best data for rivastigmine in BPSD come from a study of DLB.[22] This placebo-controlled study of 120 patients reported a mean reduction in total NPI score of 7.3 which was significantly better than placebo. Apathy, indifference, anxiety, delusions, hallucinations and aberrant motor activity improved, and the four key features of DLB, namely delusions, hallucinations, apathy and depression, were improved significantly compared with placebo.

In Parkinson's dementia, an open-labelled study with rivastigmine showed improvement on the NPI.[23] In vascular dementia, patients randomised to cardioaspirin showed significant worsening on the NPI and required more neuroleptics compared with a rivastigmine group.[24]

Thus there is some randomised evidence to suggest that rivastigmine has some effect on BPSD, particularly hallucinations, delusions, abberant motor activity, anxiety and apathy. It has been suggested that this effectiveness may be due to the inhibition of butyrylcholinesterase (BuChE) as well as acetylcholinesterase. BuChE is found in amounts in the amygdala and key areas of the limbic system,[25] so it could be postulated that rivastigmine offers more selective improvements in these areas.

Galantamine

In the original study by Tariot[26] in patients with mild to moderate AD, there was a clear dose–response effect of galantamine in preventing the emergence of behavioural symptoms during the 5-month treatment period. In a study of patients with vascular dementia and AD with cerebrovascular disease, galantamine showed a significant improvement in behavioural symptoms (on the NPI) over placebo, with anxiety and apathy showing individually significant improvements.

In general, the NPI has remained stable at around baseline in all of the galantamine studies, often well into longer-term follow-up. Galantamine has an allosteric action on nicotinic receptors, improving their sensitivity (*see* Chapter 12). Presynaptic nicotinic receptors modulate many other transmitter systems and maintain their integrity. This may account for the way in which galantamine helps to preserve some of the systems in which failure leads to emergence of some BPSD.

Summary

Cholinesterase inhibitors do appear to exert a consistent effect on apathy, anxiety and perhaps depression, with a lesser but significant effect on aberrant motor activity and disinhibition. Rivastigmine seems to have an effect on psychosis that is not seen with the other cholinesterase inhibitors, and galantamine appears to have a delaying effect on the emergence of these behaviours. More research needs to be done to clarify how these drugs truly help with individual BPSD symptoms, but it would seem that already being on them for their cognitive effects must confer benefit with regard to some of the commonly observed behavioural symptoms as well.

NMDA antagonists

The only licensed product is memantine (*see* Chapter 12). It showed no difference compared with placebo with regard to behaviour when measured on the NPI in a 6-month randomised study in severe AD.[27] There was a statistical trend towards a reduction in the presentation of agitation, but there were some isolated instances of psychosis.

However, in a study that added memantine or placebo to patients on donepezil, significant decreases in agitation, irritability and delusions were noted,[28] demonstrating that memantine is one of the few compounds to show a significant reduction in agitation in this patient group.

Antipsychotics

Classical antipsychotics

These have traditionally been given for a wide variety of symptoms, many of which are not psychotic. Sedating side-effects exert a calming influence, which may solve some immediate problems, but the older typical antipsychotics are harmful, often with marked anticholinergic side-effects. As a result, there is increasing evidence that they accelerate the illness, resulting in extra memory loss, further functional decline and an increased rate of falls.[29] They also produce marked extrapyramidal side-effects, especially tardive dyskinesia (*see* Chapter 9). Jeste *et al.*[30] showed that 66% of patients developed tardive dyskinesia over a period of 3 years' exposure to a typical antipsychotic, compared with 2% of those on risperidone.

These effects are reduced if low doses are used, but some reports suggest that low-dose typical antipsychotics such as haloperidol do not even work,[31,32] and that when they do it is for aggression, not agitation. One large meta-analysis of typical antipsychotics showed that only 18% of the drugs given had a defined treatment effect, and the rest had no more than placebo.[33] Given this finding, it is appropriate that patients with dementia should not receive these older drugs, and if they do have true psychotic symptoms, atypical drugs with no anticholinergic activity should be preferred. This has been borne out in the Older Person's National Service Framework in the UK, which suggests that atypical antipsychotics are most appropriate for use in this patient group.

Atypical antipsychotics

Risperidone
The then limited adverse side-effect profile of risperidone led to interest in its use in those patients who exhibited psychotic and agitated symptoms in dementia. Until 1998, most of the literature on risperidone for this group of elderly patients consisted of non-comparative trials, case studies, small controlled trials or retrospective reviews.

Since then, De Deyn et al.,[34] Katz et al.[35] and Brodaty et al. [36] have independently reported successful studies. They were each large, comparative, 12-week, placebo-controlled, double-blind, randomised, multi-centre trials of risperidone use in the treatment of elderly patients living in nursing homes and suffering from Alzheimer's dementia, vascular dementia or mixed dementia. These trials demonstrated that risperidone at an average dose of 1 mg/day is at least as effective as haloperidol in treating behavioural symptoms as measured by the Behave-AD (particularly aggression), and that it is superior to placebo. Neither was it associated with cognitive decline. The study by Katz et al. was followed by a 1-year non-comparative open-label extension phase reported by Jeste et al.[37] This revealed that the clinical benefits obtained were maintained for treatment periods of up to 1 year, and the incidence of tardive dyskinesia was only 2.6% (5% of that seen with conventional antipsychotics).

There were no clinically relevant abnormalities in laboratory tests, vital signs or electrocardiogram results. However, an increased incidence of cerebrovascular events in the risperidone group compared with placebo, albeit in very small numbers, has led to some concerns, especially in patients with pre-existing significant cerebrovascular disease. This has led to non-recommendation of risperidone for this condition in some countries (including the UK). The studies showed efficacy of risperidone at doses ranging from 0.5 mg to 4.0 mg daily, but extrapyramidal side-effects became a problem at doses above 2 mg. Thus risperidone at a dose of 0.5 mg/day to 1 mg/day was the optimal dose for the full range of target symptoms, including aggression, agitation and psychosis.

Behavioural symptoms such as agitation, aggression and psychosis may occur in more than 80% of patients with AD during the course of their illness.[38] Dementia patients may also present with a cluster of negative symptoms,[39] which are clinically similar to those described in subjects with chronic schizophrenia.

A retrospective study by Negron and Reichman[40] showed that risperidone was efficacious in the treatment of clinically significant positive symptoms and also negative symptoms in AD, and that it was generally very well tolerated. Importantly, the improvement in negative symptoms with risperidone appeared to be independent of the response with regard to positive symptoms. In contrast, clinical observations by Raheja et al.[41] showed that the symptoms of dementia that closely resemble the negative symptoms of schizophrenia did not respond well to risperidone.

Risperidone is available in many forms, including tablet, liquid, quick-dissolving tablets and now a long-acting injectable. The minimum blood level of risperidone achieved with this last method of delivery is 2 mg, which may be too high in patients with dementia. No controlled data exist, but case reports will undoubtedly inform future practice. However, the problem with cerebrovascular adverse events may now limit the usage of risperidone, although it remains licensed for short-term use in psychotic conditions under specialist guidance, and should still be considered an effective treatment under those conditions.

Olanzapine

A multi-centre, double-blind, placebo-controlled, 6-week study designed to assess the efficacy and safety of olanzapine in the treatment of psychotic and behavioural symptoms in 206 elderly patients with AD was performed in nursing-care facilities by Street et al.[42] This study concluded that low-dose olanzapine (5 and

10 mg/day) was significantly superior to placebo and well tolerated in treating agitation/aggression and psychosis in elderly patients with AD. Paradoxically, in this study the lowest dose (5 mg/day) appeared to have the greatest effect. This inverse dose response is puzzling, as it is not the usual scenario. However, this efficacy was achieved at the cost of a 25% incidence of sedation and 26% incidence of gait disturbance, both of which are undesirable in this population. Satterlee et al. [43] designed an 8-week, multi-centre, double-blind trial to assess the efficacy of olanzapine in patients aged 65 years or older with psychotic and behavioural manifestations associated with AD. Patients ($n = 238$) were randomly assigned to olanzapine (1 to 8 mg/day) or placebo. This study concluded that the olanzapine-treated group did not differ significantly from the placebo group with regard to efficacy.

A retrospective analysis of olanzapine in a hospitalised group of patients with refractory behavioural problems had a side-effect rate of 38%, most of the side-effects being anticholinergic in nature.[44] The same study did show significant improvements in 60% of treated patients, so it would seem that olanzapine will be useful in this patient group, but further definitive research is needed to show how best to use it. The anticholinergic profile is a cause for concern, and although it is reported to be clinically insignificant, it does seem to have clinical manifestations.

The efficacy at the cost of side-effects has led to reduced use of olanzapine in this population. When cerebrovascular adverse events were also found to be more common than in patients on placebo, olanzapine was not recommended for use in this patient group – a decision that was supported by the manufacturers. It is therefore only under very unusual circumstances that this compound will now be used in this patient group.

Quetiapine

As yet there are no published placebo-controlled studies of the use of quetiapine in elderly demented patients. An exploratory analysis performed by Yeung et al.[45] on the subsets of 78 patients with AD from the open-label trial by Tariot et al. [46] in elderly patients with psychosis of varied causes suggested that quetiapine may be useful in the treatment of psychotic patients with AD who exhibit hostile or aggressive behaviour. Because of its very low side-effect profile and its supposed 'motor friendliness', it is often also used in patients with Parkinson's disease. More definitive studies are needed to allow firm recommendations to be made, but the ability to start with very low doses, the flexible dosing and the tolerability profile are making it a popular choice. At present no data have been published to suggest that it suffers from the same cerebrovascular adverse-event profile as risperidone and olanzapine.

Clozapine

A small, open-label, withdrawal study conducted by Oberholzer et al.[47] reported that, at a mean dose of 41 mg/day (range 12.5–75 mg/day), clozapine was a useful alternative treatment for demented geriatric patients with paranoid or socially disturbing behaviour who had developed severe side-effects with classical neuroleptics. However, the use of this drug was restricted to a hospital setting because of the need of haematological monitoring.

A retrospective chart review by Salzman *et al.*[48] suggested that clozapine is possibly useful in controlling behavioural disruption in older patients, but the elderly may be at greater risk of developing leukopenia. There are no published placebo-controlled studies of the use of clozapine in elderly patients with dementia.

Aripiprazole

Aripiprazole is a partial agonist at the dopamine receptor, and through this interesting mode of action it restores abnormal dopaminergic function, whether it be high (through competitive inhibition) or low (through its partial agonism). A trial in community patients using the NPI as a primary outcome showed no effect over a very high placebo response, even though the treated group had a 68% response rate.[49] However, on individual items reflecting psychosis in the Brief Psychiatric Rating Scale (BPRS),[50] significant effects were demonstrated. Two conclusions can be drawn from this. First, aripiprazole may prove useful in treating the psychotic symptoms of BPSD. Secondly, by using the NPI carer-rated scale to measure this BPSD entity, rather than the psychiatrist interview in the BPRS, the study obtained an unfairly negative result. Two further nursing-home studies are shortly to be reported. To date, tolerability has seemed very good in the elderly, and no increase in cerebrovascular adverse events has so far been reported.

Aripiprazole became available in the USA and in Europe from mid-2004. Current doses are either 10 mg or 15 mg, which may be relatively high for use in dementia, although the tablets are scored. A 5 mg tablet is anticipated. Clinical evidence will start to appear as the drug is used, which in the absence of the currently worrying side-effects seen with other antipsychotics it almost certainly will be.

Amisulpiride, ziprasidone and zotepine

There is no specific evidence that any of these drugs work in dementia, and any usefulness is extrapolated from data for younger adults. Given that they have less potential for harm than typical antipsychotics, they could be considered where other atypicals have not helped. Amisulpiride is a pure D_2 antagonist with very few side-effects or drug interactions. It can be started at very low doses, which is useful with this patient group. Neither ziprasidone nor zotepine are available in the UK.

Practical considerations with antipsychotics

The first such consideration is cost. The newer drugs are more expensive, which has proved a barrier to their use. However, the doses required in the elderly are low, which reduces the expense considerably. For example, risperidone is often effective at doses of 0.5 to 1.5 mg. This equates to £100 to £300 per annum – much less than the general perception. This is reduced further if the drugs are reviewed at 16 weeks and discontinued. Some patients may need higher doses, but this is not the norm.

The next issue is whether the antipsychotics are the most appropriate choice, even for the psychotic symptoms. These symptoms may occur as a result of the disease process, so an alternative strategy is to use cholinesterase inhibitors to boost cholinergic function as described previously. The cholinergic toxicity encountered with typical antipsychotics may negate the effects of anticholine-sterase inhibitors, and so they should not be used in combination.

A third consideration is safety. The elderly, especially those with dementia, are very sensitive to antipsychotics, so these drugs should really only be used if they are clearly indicated. Patients with DLB are particularly at risk. Deaths have occurred in DLB patients as a result of antipsychotic use, and although this is more of a problem with the older drugs, it can occur with any of the newer drugs as well. This is especially worrying when the illness can present with such vivid psychotic symptoms. It is generally considered that patients with these symptoms in DLB should be given a cholinesterase inhibitor, usually rivastigmine, as first-line therapy.

The recent reporting of cerebrovascular adverse events adds to safety concerns. These events almost certainly occur with typical antipsychotics as well, and although they have not yet been demonstrated in all atypical antipsychotics, they are feared to be a class effect. Unfortunately, no mechanism of action to explain why this happens has yet been elucidated, so no measures can be adopted to prevent it. The recommendation is caution in patients with cerebrovascular risk factors. This is problematic, given that most elderly patients are at some risk, and it is those with the most cerebrovascular disease that often show the more noticeable behavioural changes. However, it should be stated that these drugs are not contraindicated, so where they are the best available option they should continue to be used, with documentation of any risks.

The fourth issue is duration of treatment. Although the behaviours are often of limited duration, they can overlap and interact. No data support the optimum length of treatment, although studies that have withdrawn treatment at 6 weeks have seen symptoms return. The accepted view is that the need for continued treatment should be reviewed, initially quite frequently and certainly at 2 and 4 weeks. This is to balance benefit against side-effects. Most antipsychotics should have been withdrawn by 16 weeks.

The final consideration is an ethical one. Typical antipsychotics do cause more harm than atypical ones in this patient group, so can their continued use now be justified? More importantly, all too often treatment is used in these patients for other people's benefit. Care must be taken to ensure that the right person is being treated by the most appropriate method, which also means the proper use of antipsychotics whenever indicated, especially for aggression.

Combination with cholinesterase inhibitors

Although this is common practice, there is little trial evidence to support it. An open-label, 20-week study of rivastigmine plus risperidone, compared with each individually, in a mixed dementia group showed that using the NPI as an outcome measure, the combination was superior to either drug on its own.[51] Several case reports of the combination of other cholinesterase inhibitors with risperidone exist, adding to the safety data but not the efficacy data.

Antidepressants

Many patients with dementia appear to have depressive episodes (*see also* Chapter 8), although many of these do not reach research level criteria for major depression, and the symptoms fluctuate spontaneously over time. Separating depressive symptoms from the apathy and anxiety that occur in the illness can be difficult. Specific scales such as the Cornell Depression Scale have been designed specifically for use in dementia.[52] These can identify true cases. As a result of over-inclusive diagnosis, many more patients receive antidepressants than are depressed, but this often seems appropriate. What can be a problem is the choice of antidepressant and the reason why it is given.

Tricyclic antidepressants should not generally be used in dementia, as the anticholinergic side-effects are potentially harmful, exacerbating the dementia and causing confusional episodes. They are sometimes used in primary care for their sedative effect, but like the old antipsychotics, these drugs do cause significant side-effects and cannot really be justified as a first-line therapy, especially in view of the fact that they do not always work (studies with maprotoline[53] and imipramine[54] have proved negative).

Serotonergic drugs (selective serotonin reuptake inhibitors, SSRIs) are commonly used in all stages of dementia. A study with citalopram showed efficacy over placebo, although methodological issues perhaps made the results less reliable.[55] Adding sertraline to donepezil produced some added benefit in treating affective symptoms.[56] However, in general the available data are not definitive. SSRIs may have a role in the treatment of aggression in dementia, and *post-mortem* evidence suggests that this symptom could be a result of failure of the serotonergic system. Studies of the use of citalopram in aggression have produced a positive effect, and it is reasonable to use this class of drugs to treat aggression, especially as they have no harmful effects. Unfortunately, they are not sedating, so minor tranquillisation may be required as well. This is preferable to using the sedative tricyclics, whose other side-effects are too harmful.

Post-mortem studies have suggested that clinical depression in dementia is also the result of failure of the noradrenergic system. It would therefore be wise to select drugs which boost noradrenaline (e.g. reboxetine and moclobemide) or have a mixed action (e.g. mirtazapine), rather than a serotonergic drug alone. The only large study of the use of an antidepressant in dementia employed moclobemide.[57] A total of 511 patients were randomised, and moclobemide proved more effective than placebo on the Hamilton Depression Scale.

Trazodone (a mixed-action drug) is used by many as a tranquilliser for aggression, and some controlled evidence now supports this. However, it has an interaction with ginkgo that may cause deep sleep for several hours, so carers should be warned.[58]

Mood stabilisers

Mood stabilisers have been used to treat agitation and aggression in dementia, and more recently have been associated with the treatment of 'manic' phenomena.[59,60] There is increasing evidence of their effectiveness, with sizeable studies using carbamazepine[61] and sodium valproate. In the USA they are licensed for the BPSD indication, but this is not so in the UK. Lithium and carbamazepine are now used far less often than sodium valproate (available either generically or as divalproex sodium). Divalproex sodium is formulated as a slow-release drug and has far less side-effects due to its consistent plasma levels. It is still essentially sodium valproate, and whether slow-release valproate will have similar tolerability in this patient group needs to be evaluated. Lamotrigine is also being used for this indication, but there are no controlled data to support this.

Overall the use of this class is increasing, especially for non-psychotic, driven behaviours such as pacing and abnormal vocalisations (including screaming), but only after depression, obsessive-compulsive disorder and pain have been excluded. As mood stabilisers do not have any harmful effect on the underlying disease, this seems reasonable. In fact, lithium and valproate also inhibit glycogen synthase kinase (the enzyme that phosphorylates tau), so they may actually have an additional protective effect (*see also* Chapter 15). There are some monitoring and safety issues associated with mood stabilisers, but the outcomes seem to justify the use, many of the small studies having an NNT (number needed to treat) of 2–6 (*see also* Chapter 8).

Benzodiazepines and related compounds

Anxiety commonly occurs in dementia, but often for reasons associated with the cognitive difficulties and cholinergic loss. It seems to respond well to cholinesterase inhibitor treatment, regardless of which drug is used. A specific rating scale for anxiety in dementia exists.[62] In cases where difficulties and concerns are detected, they initially need to be addressed by social and environmental intervention. Early AD patients should always be offered cholinesterase inhibitors, if they are not already on them, prior to any other medication. Benzodiazepines can be utilised for their anxiolytic effect in short-term use, but it should be remembered that they do have intrinsic anticholinergic effects – to the extent that they are used to produce a model for cognitive impairment in young healthy volunteers. They need regular review in the same way as treatment of any other anxiety disorder. The evidence suggests that they are more effective than placebo for patients with dementia, but may be less effective than low-dose antipsychotics.

It is also useful to utilise their sedative properties when the circumstances are appropriate, especially as the newer psychiatric drugs do not generally have sedative properties. However, most patients do not require sedation for long, so benzodiazepine usage should always be reviewed at regular intervals. As in all patients, the benzodiazepines can have a paradoxical effect and cause disinhibition – which may also be a symptom of the disease itself.

Elderly people metabolise benzodiazepines less well as they age, increasing the expected half-life of the drug. This is a differential effect, and is not true of the entire class. Diazepam, chlordiazepoxide and nitrazepam are commonly used compounds, but in individuals over 65 years of age their metabolism can be slowed by two- to threefold, making accumulation a real problem. If possible they should not be used, and lorazepam, oxazepam and temazepam should be used preferentially, as the metabolism of these drugs is not affected by age. Intramuscular lorazepam is often used in more acute situations. It is usually well tolerated, but until recently few data supported its use. When used as a comparator to intramuscular olanzapine in an American study, it fared almost as well, only being inferior with regard to the time to produce sedation[63] – at last providing some supportive controlled data.

Buspirone has a limited anxiolytic effect, and should only be used as an anxiolytic after other avenues have failed.

Sleep disturbance and day–night reversal are common problems, but no evidence exists as to what is best practice. Hypnotics are frequently used, often non-benzodiazepine (e.g. zopiclone or zolpidem). Trazodone is also often selected for its sedative mode of action and flexible titration. Some patients have REM sleep disturbance (e.g. waking from dreams and not being able to distinguish between where these end and reality begins) or become very disturbed while sleeping in bed. Low doses of clonazepam (0.5 mg) will suppress REM sleep and can alleviate these symptoms. The use of high-dose zopiclone (up to 30 mg) for day–night reversal has been reported in a Canadian journal.

Other drugs

Anticholinergic drugs (e.g. procyclidine) should be avoided where possible in patients with cognitive decline. They are not needed with atypical antipsychotics. Graduate patients who are already on such drugs for extrapyramidal side-effects should continue with them, but the dose should be reduced as much as possible. Similar medications used for incontinence and Parkinson's disease should also be discontinued if possible. These drugs impede cognition and can cause confusional states. If older antipsychotics are not initiated, anticholinergic drugs will not be needed.

Cimetidine has been reported to be useful in managing hypersexuality in a case report,[64] but this is by no means a mainstream use of a drug that is frankly anticholinergic. Cyproterone and depot norethisterone have also been used anecdotally to good effect, but no controlled data exist.

Methylphenidate has been used to treat driven behaviours in several individual case reports, but not in significant numbers or controlled studies. This also applies to electroconvulsive therapy.

A guideline for the management of BPSD

Stage 1

An assessment of the physical state of the patient is needed to exclude pain, constipation, retention of urine, etc. Patients with dementia can get ill as well, and in a US nursing-home study it was found that 25% of persistent 'moaners' had a fractured hip. Delirium must always be excluded, especially if there has been a sudden onset of agitation. This management stage would hopefully be initiated by the primary care doctor prior to referral, and should be included in any shared care arrangement.

Stage 2

The psychosocial environment should be assessed, and an Antecedent Behaviour Consequence (ABC) evaluation used to obtain the relevant information – and perhaps even solve the problem. Behavioural interventions (suitably matched to the behaviour) can then be attempted if the carer is able and willing. This stage is best suited to nursing or psychology staff, who could ideally make the initial assessment after specialist referral, provided that possible physical problems have been excluded. They can also use the assessment to educate caregivers.

Stage 3

If the behaviour proves to be intransigent, drug therapy should be considered. The classes of drug to be used are indicated in Figure 14.1. Drugs should be given in low doses and slowly built up to an effective dose. All patients should be reviewed regularly in the first 2 weeks of treatment to balance effect vs. harm. At 4 weeks a decision should be made as to whether to continue. By 16 weeks most patients will need a full review to ensure that they still need to continue the drug therapy. Many of the treatment choices are straightforward enough to be incorporated into protocols that could be used for primary care and nurse prescribing.

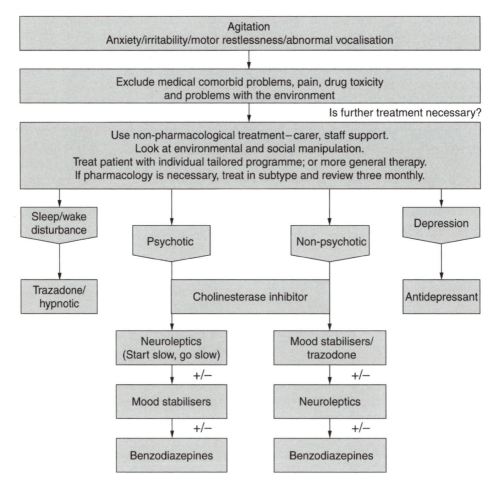

Figure 14.1 Treatment algorithm for agitation in dementia.

Key points

- The use of pharmacological agents in BPSD must always be preceded by a thorough physical and environmental assessment, and any suitable non-pharmacological interventions.
- Antiopsychotics have proven efficacy in aggression and psychosis, but not in other areas of BPSD. Therefore their use should be confined to these areas where possible.
- Increasing safety concerns, particularly concerning cerebrovascular adverse events, have started to limit antipsychotic use. Serious events can be reduced through careful patient selection.
- Cholinesterase inhibitors have an increasing role in some of the behaviours frequently encountered – particularly apathy, anxiety and visual hallucinations.
- Memantine looks to have a positive effect on agitation – and is the only agent so far to show this. This adds to its rationale to be used in combination with cholinesterase inhibitors as the disease progresses.
- Antidepressants can be used for depression, though no one has been demonstrated superior to another.
- There is a range of treatments that can be used in combination that can be matched to specific behaviours. Clinicians need to think in terms of symptoms as well as overall disease – particularly as dementia progresses.

References

1 Jost BC and Grossberg GT (1996) The evolution of psychiatric symptoms in Alzheimer's disease: a natural history study. *Am J Geriatr Psychiatry* 4: 383–4.
2 Cummings JL (1997) Behavior as an efficacy outcome. *Alzheimer Dis Assoc Disord.* 11: R5–6.
3 Kaufer D, Catt K, Pollock B and DeKosky S (1998) Assessing the effects of donepezil in Alzheimer's patients and its impact on caregivers. *J Am Geriatr Soc.* 46: 198.
4 Furniss L, Craig SKL and Burns A (1998) Medication use in nursing homes for elderly people. *Int J Geriatr Psychiatry.* 13: 433–9.
5 Draper BM (2000) The mental health of older people in the community. *Med J Aust.* 173: 80–2.
6 Cummings JL and Masterman DL (1998) Assessment of treatment-associated changes in behavior and cholinergic therapy of neuropsychiatric symptoms in Alzheimer's disease. *J Clin Psychiatry.* 59: 23–30.
7 Wesnes KA, McKeith IG, Ferrara R *et al.* (2002) Effects of rivastigmine on cognitive function in dementia with Lewy bodies: a randomised placebo-controlled international study using the cognitive drug research computerised assessment system. *Dementia Geriatr Cogn Disord.* 13: 183–92.
8 Sclan SG, Saillon A, Franssen E, HugonotDiener L, Saillon A and Reisberg B (1996) The behavior pathology in Alzheimer's disease rating scale (BEHAVE-AD): reliability and analysis of symptom category scores. *Int J Geriatr Psychiatry.* 11: 819–30.
9 Cummings JL, Mega M, Gray K, Rosenberg TS, Carusi DA and Gornbein J (1994) The Neuropsychiatric Inventory: comprehensive assessment of psychopathology in dementia. *Neurology.* 44: 2308–14.

10 Winblad B, Engedal K, Soininen H *et al.* (2001) A 1-year, randomized, placebo-controlled study of donepezil in patients with mild to moderate AD. *Neurology.* **57**: 489–95.

11 Tariot P, Cummings JL, Katz IR *et al.* (2001) A randomized, double-blind, placebo-controlled study of the efficacy and safety of donepezil in patients with Alzheimer's disease in the nursing home setting. *J Am Geriatr Soc.* **49**: 1590–9.

12 Feldman H, Gauthier S, Hecker J, Vellas B, Subbiah P and Whalen E (2001) A 24-week, randomized, double-blind study of donepezil in moderate to severe Alzheimer's disease. *Neurology.* **57**: 613–20.

13 Dunn NR, Pearce GL and Shakir SA (2000) Adverse effects associated with the use of donepezil in general practice in England. *J Psychopharmacol.* **14**: 406–8.

14 Bouman WP and Pinner G (1998) Violent behavior associated with donepezil. *Am J Psychiatry.* **155**: 1626–7.

15 Minett TS, Thomas A, Wilkinson LM *et al.* (2003) What happens when donepezil is suddenly withdrawn? An open-label trial in dementia with Lewy bodies and Parkinson's disease with dementia. *Int J Geriatr Psychiatry.* **18**: 988–93.

16 Shea C, MacKnight C and Rockwood K (1998) Donepezil for treatment of dementia with Lewy bodies: a case series of nine patients. *Int Psychogeriatr.* **10**: 229–38.

17 Prasher VP, Huxley A and Haque MS (2002) A 24-week, double-blind, placebo-controlled trial of donepezil in patients with Down syndrome and Alzheimer's disease – pilot study. *Int J Geriatr Psychiatry.* **17**: 270–8.

18 Rosler M, Anand R, Cicin SA *et al.* (1999) Efficacy and safety of rivastigmine in patients with Alzheimer's disease: international randomised controlled trial. *BMJ.* **318**: 633–40.

19 Cummings JL (2003) Use of cholinesterase inhibitors in clinical practice: evidence-based recommendations. *Am J Geriatr Psychiatry.* **11**: 131–45.

20 Etemad B, Anand R and Hartman R (2001) Behavioral and cognitive benefits of rivastigmine in nursing home patients with Alzheimer's disease and related dementias: a 26-week follow-up. *Ann Neurol.* **50**: S44–5.

21 Bullock R (2001) Rivastigmine and behaviour – a European nursing home study. *Rapid Report.* **2**: 2–3.

22 McKeith I, Del Ser T, Spano P *et al.* (2000) Efficacy of rivastigmine in dementia with Lewy bodies: a randomised, double-blind, placebo-controlled international study. *Lancet.* **356**: 2031–6.

23 Reading PJ, Luce AK and McKeith IG (2001) Rivastigmine in the treatment of parkinsonian psychosis anti-cognitive impairment: preliminary findings from an open trial. *Movement Disord.* **16**: 1171–4.

24 Moretti R, Torre P, Antonello RM and Cazzato G (2001) Rivastigmine in subcortical vascular dementia: a comparison trial on efficacy and tolerability for 12 months follow-up. *Eur J Neurol.* **8**: 361–2.

25 Darvesh S, Grantham DL and Hopkins DA (1998) Distribution of butyrylcholinesterase in the human amygdala and hippocampal formation. *J Comp Neurol.* **393**: 374–90.

26 Tariot PN, Solomon PR, Morris JC, Kershaw P, Lilienfeld S and Ding C (2000) A 5-month, randomized, placebo-controlled trial of galantamine in AD. The Galantamine USA-10 Study Group. *Neurology.* **54**: 2269–76.

27 Reisberg B, Doody RS, Stoffler A *et al.* (2004) Memantine in moderate to severe Alzheimer's disease. *NEJM.* **348**: 1333–41.

28 Tariot P, Farlow MR, Grossberg GT *et al.* (2004) Memantine treatment in patients with moderate to severe Alzheimer's disease already receiving donepezil: a randomised controlled trial. *JAMA.* **291**: 317–24.

29 McShane R, Keene J, Gedling K, Fairburn C, Jacoby R and Hope T (1997) Do neuroleptic drugs hasten cognitive decline in dementia? Prospective study with necropsy follow-up. *BMJ.* **314**: 266–70.

30 Jeste DV, Caligiuri MP, Paulsen JS *et al*. (1995) Risk of tardive dyskinesia in older patients – a prospective longitudinal study of 266 outpatients. *Arch Gen Psychiatry*. **52**: 756–65.

31 Devanand DP, Marder K, Michaels KS *et al*. (1998) A randomized, placebo-controlled dose-comparison trial of haloperidol for psychosis and disruptive behaviors in Alzheimer's disease. *Am J Psychiatry*. **155**: 1512–20.

32 Teri L, Logsdon RG, Peskind E *et al*. (2000) Treatment of agitation in AD – a randomized, placebo-controlled clinical trial. *Neurology*. **55**: 1271–8.

33 Schneider LS, Pollock VE and Lyness SA (1990) A meta-analysis of controlled trials of neuroleptic treatment in dementia. *Am J Geriatr Psychiatry*. **38**: 553–63.

34 De Deyn PP, Rabheru K, Rasmussen A *et al*. (1999) A randomised trial of risperidone, placebo and haloperidol for behavioural symptoms of dementia. *Neurology*. **53**: 946–55.

35 Katz IR, Jeste DV, Mintzer JE, Clyde C, Napolitano J and Brecher M (1999) Comparison of risperidone and placebo for psychosis and behavioral disturbances associated with dementia: a randomized, double-blind trial. *J Clin Psychiatry*. **60**: 107.

36 Brodaty H, Ames D, Snowdon J *et al*. (2003) A randomised placebo-controlled trial of risperidone for the treatment of aggression, agitation and the psychosis of dementia. *J Clin Psychiatry*. **62**: 134–43.

37 Jeste DV, Okamoto A, Napolitano J, Kane JM and Martinez RA (2000) Low incidence of persistent tardive dyskinesia in elderly patients with dementia treated with risperidone. *Am J Psychiatry*. **157**: 1150–5.

38 Sweet RA and Pollock BG (1998) New atypical antipsychotics: experience and utility in the elderly. *Drugs Aging*. **12**: 115–27.

39 Doody RS, Massman P, Mahurin R and Law S (1995) Positive and negative neuropsychiatric features in Alzheimer's disease. *J Neuropsychiatry Clin Neurosci*. **7**: 54–60.

40 Negron AE and Reichman WE (2000) Risperidone in the treatment of patients with Alzheimer's disease with negative symptoms. *Int Psychogeriatr*. **12**: 527–36.

41 Raheja RK, Bharwani I and Penetrante AE (1995) Efficacy of risperidone for behavioral disorders in the elderly: a clinical observation. *J Geriatr Psychiatry Neurol*. **8**: 159–61.

42 Street JS, Scott Clark W, Gannon KS *et al*. (2000) Olanzapine treatment of psychotic and behavioral symptoms in patients with Alzheimer disease in nursing care facilities. *Arch Gen Psychiatry*. **57**: 968–76.

43 Satterlee W, Reams S, Burns PR *et al*. (1995) A clinical update on olanzapine treatment in schizophrenia and in elderly Alzheimer's disease patients. *Psychopharmacol Bull*. **31**: 534.

44 Solomons K and Geiger O (2000) Olanzapine use in the elderly: a retrospective analysis. *Can J Psychiatry*. **45**: 151–5.

45 Yeung PP, Tariot PN, Schneider LS, Salzman C and Rak IW (2000) Quetiapine for elderly patients with psychotic disorders. *Psychiatr Ann*. **30**: 197–201.

46 Tariot PN, Salzman C, Yeung PP, Pultz J and Rak IW (2000) Long-term use of quetiapine in elderly patients with psychotic disorders. *Clin Ther*. **22**: 1068–84.

47 Oberholzer AF, Hendriksen C, Monsch AU, Heierli B and Stahelin HB (1992) Safety and effectiveness of low-dose clozapine in psychogeriatric patients: a preliminary study. *Int Psychogeriatr*. **4**: 187–95.

48 Salzman C, Vaccaro B and Lieff J (1995) Clozapine in older patients with psychosis and behavioral disruption. *Am J Geriatr Psychiatry*. **3**: 26–33.

49 De Deyn PP, Jeste D and Auby P (2003) *Aripiprazole in dementia of the Alzheimer's type*. Unpublished paper.

50 Overall JE and Gorham DR (1962) The Brief Psychiatric Rating Scale. *Psychol Rep*. **10**: 799–812.

51 Weiser M, Davidson M, Rotmensch H *et al*. (2002) A pilot, randomized, open-label trial assessing safety and pharmacokinetic parameters of co-administration of rivastigmine with risperidone in dementia patients with behavioral disturbances. *Neurobiol Aging*. **23**: 633.

52 Alexopoulos GS, Abrams RC, Young RC and Shamoian CA (1988) Cornell Scale for Depression in Dementia. *Biol Psychiatry.* **23**: 271–84.

53 Fuchs A, Hehnke U, Erhart C *et al.* (1993) Video rating analysis of effect of maprotiline in patients with dementia and depression. *Pharmacopsychiatry.* **26**: 37–41.

54 Reifler BV, Teri L, Raskind M *et al.* (1989) Double-blind trial of imipramine in Alzheimer's disease patients with and without depression. *Am J Psychiatry.* **146**: 45–9.

55 Nyth AL and Gottfries CG (1990) The clinical efficacy of citalopram in treatment of emotional disturbances in dementia disorders: a Nordic multicentre study. *Br J Psychiatry.* **157**: 894–901.

56 Finkel SI, Mintzer JE, Dysken M, Krishnan KR, Burt T and McRae T (2004) A randomized, placebo-controlled study of the efficacy and safety of sertraline in the treatment of the behavioral manifestations of Alzheimer's disease in outpatients treated with donepezil. *Int J Geriatr Psychiatry.* **19**: 9–18.

57 Roth M, Mountjoy CQ, Amrein R *et al.* (1996) Moclobemide in elderly patients with cognitive decline and depression: an international double-blind, placebo-controlled trial. *Br J Psychiatry.* **168**: 149–57.

58 Galluzzi S, Zanetti O, Binetti G, Trabucchi M and Frisoni GB (2000) Coma in a patient with Alzheimer's disease taking low-dose trazodone and *ginkgo biloba. J Neurol Neurosurg Psychiatry.* **68**: 679–80.

59 Lott AD, McElroy SL and Keys MA (1995) Valproate in the treatment of behavioral agitation in elderly patients with dementia. *J Neuropsychiatry Clin Neurosci.* **7**: 314–19.

60 Tariot PN, Schneider LS, Mintzer JE *et al.* (2001) Safety and tolerability of divalproex sodium in the treatment of signs and symptoms of mania in elderly patients with dementia: results of a double-blind, placebo-controlled trial. *Curr Ther Res Clin Exp.* **62**: 51–67.

61 Tariot PN, Erb R, Podgorski CA *et al.* (1998) Efficacy and tolerability of carbamazepine for agitation and aggression in dementia. *Am J Psychiatry.* **155**: 54–61.

62 Krasucki C, Ryan P, Ertan T, Howard R, Lindesay J and Mann A (1999) The FEAR: a rapid screening instrument for generalized anxiety in elderly primary care attenders. *Int J Geriatr Psychiatry.* **14**: 60–8.

63 Meehan KM, Wang HE, David SR *et al.* (2002) Comparison of rapidly acting intramuscular olanzapine, lorazepam, and placebo: a double-blind, randomized study in acutely agitated patients with dementia. *Neuropsychopharmacology.* **26**: 494–504.

64 Wiseman SV, McAuley JW, Freidenberg GR and Freidenberg DL (2000) Hypersexuality in patients with dementia: possible response to cimetidine. *Neurology.* **54**: 2024.

Chapter 15

Treatment of delirium

E Jane Byrne

Introduction

The treatment of any condition is based on diagnosis, although on occasion in the absence of clear diagnosis it may be pragmatic. Although the concept of delirium stretches back at least two and a half thousand years,[1] there is still a degree of disagreement about the diagnostic features of delirium in the major nosological systems. The importance of subtypes of delirium has been recognised for 20 years and may be a contributing factor to the under-recognition of delirium in treatment settings. However, there is good concordance in the literature on the mortality and morbidity associated with delirium, and consistency in the literature on prevalence and incidence. There is also a high level of agreement about the underlying principles of management, although the evidence base is somewhat patchy. It is encouraging that in the last 10 years there has been a renewed interest in delirium in old people and recognition of its importance in clinical practice. The pioneer of work in this hitherto neglected area is Lipowski, whose books on delirium remain among the standard texts. More recent reviews and publications pay homage to his pioneering work.[2–4]

Definitions

DSM-IV and ICD-10 criteria for definition of delirium are listed in Tables 15.1 and 15.2. The two systems agree with regard to disturbances in consciousness, changes in cognition and fluctuation over time. ICD-10 includes psychomotor disturbances and emotional disturbances as core symptoms. The two systems also differ in their comments about the duration of delirium.

ICD-10 notes that delirium rarely lasts more than 6 months, whereas DSM-IV comments that in 15% of cases delirium may last up to and beyond 30 days. However, DSM-IV does acknowledge that delirious states in older people are more likely to be prolonged.

Table 15.1 DSM-IV criteria for delirium

(a) Disturbance of consciousness (i.e. reduced clarity of awareness of the environment, with reduced ability to focus, sustain or shift attention).

(b) A change in cognition (such as memory deficit, disorientation, language disturbance) or the development of a perceptual disturbance that is not better accounted for by a pre-existing established or evolving dementia.

(c) The disturbance developed over a short period of time (usually hours to days) and tends to fluctuate during the course of the day.

(d) Where the delirium is due to a *general medical condition*, there is evidence from the history, physical examination or laboratory findings that the disturbance is caused by the direct physiological consequences of a general medical condition.

Where the delirium is due to *substance intoxication*, there is evidence from the history, physical examination or laboratory findings of either 1 or 2:

1 The symptoms in criteria (a) and (b) developed during substance intoxication

2 Medication uses – aetiologically related to the disturbance.

Where the delirium is due to *substance withdrawal*, there is evidence from the history, physical examination or laboratory findings that the symptoms in criteria (a) and (b) developed during or shortly after the withdrawal syndrome.

Where delirium is due to *multiple aetiologies*, there is evidence from the history, physical examination or laboratory findings that the delirium has more than one aetiology (e.g. more than one aetiological general medical condition, a general medical condition plus substance intoxication, or medication side-effects).

(e) Delirium not otherwise specified – this category should be used to diagnose a delirium that does not meet the criteria for any of the specific types of delirium described above. Examples include a clinical presentation of delirium that is suspected to be due to a general medical condition or substance use, but for which there is insufficient evidence to establish a specific aetiology, or where delirium is due to causes not listed (e.g. sensory deprivation).

Table 15.2 ICD-10 diagnostic criteria for delirium

For a definite diagnosis, symptoms, mild or severe, should be present in each of the following areas:

(a) Impairment of consciousness and attention (ranging from clouding to coma), reduced ability to direct, focus, sustain and shift attention.

(b) Global disturbance of cognition (perceptual distortions, illusions and hallucinations – most often visual; impairment of abstract thinking and comprehension, with or without transient delusions, but typically with some degree of incoherence; impairment of immediate recall and of recent memory, but with relatively intact remote memory; disorientation for time as well as, in more severe cases, for place and person).

(c) Psychomotor disturbances (hypo- or hyperactivity and unpredictable shifts from one to the other; increased reaction time; increased or decreased flow of speech; enhanced startle reaction).

(d) Disturbance of the sleep–wake cycle (insomnia or, in more severe cases, total sleep loss or reversal of the sleep–wake cycle; daytime drowsiness; nocturnal worsening of symptoms; disturbing dreams or nightmares, which may continue as hallucinations after awakening).

(e) Emotional disturbances (e.g. depression, anxiety or fear, irritability, euphoria, apathy or wandering, perplexity).

A unitary syndrome?

The inclusion of psychomotor changes in ICD-10 acknowledges the now validated concept of subtypes of delirium. This concept, which was first described by Engel and Romano, correlating clinical psychological and EEG data in patients with delirium, was published in 1959.[5] Their work was further elucidated by Lipowski, and the concept of hyperactive–hyperalert, hypoactive–hypoalert and mixed types is now well recognised and has been validated by Camus et al.[6] Implicit in these observations is the likelihood that the hypoactive–hypoalert type is less likely to be recognised, although this has yet to be definitively demonstrated by research studies. Although Camus et al.[7] found few differences in terms of outcome or aetiology between the subtypes, others have observed differences in morbidity according to subtype.[8]

Prevalence of delirium

The prevalence of delirium varies according to the population that is studied. There have been only two studies in the community. A community survey of mental health problems found a prevalence of 1.1% of those aged over the age of 55 years and 13.6% of those aged over 85 years,[9] similar to the rate found in the oldest old in Finland.[10] In treatment settings either in hospital populations or in nursing homes, prevalence rates for dementia are much higher.[11] The prevalence rates for older medical inpatients range from 5% to 80%, with the majority of studies ranging from 10% to 20%. Inpatient prevalence rates for post-operative delirium range from 5% to 52%, with the majority of studies showing a prevalence higher than 23% of patients. Incidence rates of delirium in elderly medical inpatients range from 5% to 10%, whereas the range for similar patients in surgical settings is up to 20%. Although the studies differ in their methods of case identification and in other respects, such as the average age of the population studied, there is little doubt that the prevalence and incidence of delirium are high in the older population in hospital.[11]

Duration of dementia

A meta-analysis of studies of delirium showed the duration in older patients to be on average about 3 weeks.[12] Subsequent research has confirmed that delirium in older patients is prolonged.[13,14] These findings contrast with a typical liaison consultation referral for old age psychiatry when, if delirium is not resolved within a week, this is thought to be unusual. In a minority of patients delirium may be extremely prolonged. Marcantonio et al.[13] found that 6% of hip fracture patients had a persistent delirium at 6 months after surgery, and Kelly et al.[14] found that delirium persisted until death or hospital discharge in 72% of cases and at 3-month follow-up in 25% of cases. In a seminal study, Levkoff et al.[15] found that only 69% of DSM-III-diagnosed hospitalised patients no longer met the criteria for delirium at the 6-month follow-up.

Certain aetiological factors, such as infarction in the territory of the right middle cerebral artery, may be associated with prolongation and delirium.[16]

Mortality and morbidity of delirium

Both mortality and morbidity are increased by the presence of delirium in older people. The mortality rates associated with delirium are variable. A review of studies of delirium up to 1993 found a mortality rate of 14.2 within 1 month of admission.[12] Kelly *et al.*[14] suggest that mortality rates are particularly high in delirious patients admitted from nursing homes, with a mortality rate of 18% at 1 month and 47% at 3 months. However, O'Keefe and Lavan did not find an independent association of delirium with mortality (after adjustment for other factors).[8] Morbidity associated with delirium includes increased lengths of hospital stay, poor functional outcome, and increased risk of institutionalisation.[2] One study found that the subtype of delirium is related to outcome, and that the

Table 15.3 Causes of delirium (only independent associations are listed[17])

Predisposing causes of delirium
Older age
Male gender
Visual impairment
Severity of dementia
Depression
Functional dependence
Immobility
Hip fracture
Dehydration
Alcoholism
Severity of physical illness
Stroke
Metabolic abnormalities

Precipitating causes
Sedative hypnotics
Narcotics
Severe acute illness
Urinary tract infection
Hypernatraemia
Hypoxaemia
Shock
Anaemia
Pain
Physical restraint
Bladder catheter use
Introgenic event
Orthopaedic surgery
Cardiac surgery
Duration of cardiopulmonary bypass
Non-cardiac surgery
Intensive-care-unit admission
High number of hospital procedures

length of hospital stay was significantly longer in the hypoactive variant,[8] whereas another found few differences in terms of outcome relating to subtype.[17]

Identification of risk factors

The identification of delirium may be aided by a knowledge of those factors which predispose to or precipitate delirium.[11,16,17] These are summarised in Tables 15.3 and 15.4. Increased age is one of the commonest reported predisposing risk factors for the development of delirium. The reasons for this are complex but include the increased likelihood of comorbid conditions known to predispose to delirium, such as dementia, multiple physical illnesses, increased use of prescribed medication, changes in pharmacodynamics and increased physical frailty.

Table 15.4 Odds ratios for precipitating causes of delirium

Study	Factor	Odds ratio (95% CI)
Elie et al.[24]	Dementia	5.2 (4.2, 6.3)
	Medical illness	3.8 (2.2, 6.4)
	Alcohol abuse	3.3 (1.9, 5.5)
	Depression	1.9 (1.3, 2.6)
Aldemir et al.[25]	Respiratory disease	30.6 (9.5–98.4)
	Infections	18 (3.5–90.8)
	Fever	14.3 (4.1–49.3)
	Anaemia	5.4 (1.6–17.8)
	Hypotension	19.8 (5.3–74.3)
	Hypocalcaemia	30.9 (5.8–163.2)
	Hyponatraemia	8.2 (2.5–26.4)
	Azotaemia	4.6 (1.4–15.6)
	Increased liver function tests	6.3 (1.2–32.2)
	Hyperarmylesaemia	43.4 (4.2–442.7)
	Metabolic acidosis	4.5 (1.1–17.7)
	Hyperbilirubinaemia	8.7 (2.0–37.7)

Identification of those older people who are at higher risk for delirium is a laudable treatment principle. However, in practice such an approach is often overtaken by events. This does not negate its potential usefulness. Table 15.3 lists those factors that have been found to be independently associated with the risk of delirium.[18] Lipowski[1] also described four facilitating factors which he defined as 'conditions which are neither necessary nor sufficient but only contributory' to delirium. These include psychosocial stress, sleep deprivation, sensory underload or overload and immobilisation. Such factors may be found in intensive-care units (ICUs). The role of these factors in ICUs remains contentious. However, sensory impairment and immobility are listed in one review as independent predisposing causes,[18] rather than as facilitating factors as suggested by Lipowski.[1] In order to treat delirium, it first has to be recognised. An educational programme can improve the detection of delirium by junior doctors.[19] However, whether such an approach improves outcome has yet to be established. Conn and Lieff[20] concluded from a literature review that diagnosis of delirium can be aided by using DSM-IV criteria, the Delirium Symptom Interview[21] or the confusion assessment method.[22] Two randomised controlled trials designed to prevent delirium have recently been published. Marcantonio et al. (2001)[23] randomised consenting patients in an orthopaedic surgical unit to treatment as usual or proactive consultation by a geriatrician. The intervention group had a significantly lower rate of delirium, but there was no difference in the length of hospital stay. Similar findings were reported by Inoye et al.[17] in their intervention, which consisted of standardised protocols for the management of six risk factors for delirium, namely cognitive impairment, sleep deprivation, immobility, visual impairment, hearing impairment and dehydration. They too found a lower rate of delirium in the intervention group. However, the severity of the delirium and the recurrence rates did not differ between the two groups.

Principles of management

There is general agreement about the principles of management of delirium,[1,4,26,27] namely identifying and treating the underlying cause, supportive measures and somatic interventions. These reviews also recommend that this approach should be set in the context of ongoing monitoring of the condition, whether by the use of standard instruments or nursing observations, and that it should include information and support for the patient's family.

Identifying the underlying causes

The plural of cause in the above sub-heading is used advisedly. A multiplicity of causes is frequently reported in the literature.[28] The interaction of predisposing and precipitating factors has been incorporated into a useful model of vulnerability.[29] This model suggests that people who at baseline have a number of predisposing factors are more likely to develop delirium on exposure to any minor precipitating factors. Physicians seem to be unaware of the culminative nature or importance of minor precipitating factors. For example, the older person with dementia who also has a minor degree of anaemia and infection and metabolic disturbances is frequently categorised as having no apparent cause for their delirium. Table 15.4 lists the odds ratios for precipitating factors for delirium derived from the meta-analysis by Elie et al.[24] and the study by Aldemir et al.[25] of 818 patients admitted to a surgical ICU. Elie et al.[24] found that the commonest precipitating factors for delirium in older people were dementia, medication, medical illness, increased age and male gender.

Basic principles of assessment in delirium are no different to those for the assessment of any medical condition – that is, history, examination and investigation. It is useful to obtain a history of the current complaint from a number of informants, including relatives, formal carers and physicians and surgeons where relevant. The history should be directed at identifying both predisposing and precipitating factors. I concur with the regretful statement of Meagher that 'unfortunately routine cognitive assessment is less common in the technological world of modern medicine, and knowledge of a patient's prior cognitive status is often minimal'.[27]

Examination

This must include examination of both mental status and physical status. Unfortunately, inexperienced examiners can be misled by the frequent presence of symptoms such as depression in delirious older people. Farrell and Ganzini[30] found that 41.8% of people referred for the evaluation of depression were in fact delirious. The referring physicians had considered delirium in only 3 out of 28 cases. In geriatric medicine it is probably more common that a test of cognitive function is routinely administered. However, what is perhaps not so widely appreciated is the importance of qualitative as well as quantitative observations. Vagueness, distractibility and fluctuating mood may be indicators of delirium that can be missed by inexperienced observers. The very nature of delirium, with its changeability over time, is also a source of misdiagnosis. This changeability over time is often best illustrated in the nursing record rather than the medical notes. Another confounding variable is the frequent coexistence of delirium with dementia. The history of the current state in this situation then becomes paramount.

Screening tests for delirium may improve recognition. Such screening methods include standardised diagnostic criteria such as DSM, the confusion assessment method and brief bedside tests such as clockface drawing.[4,20] The latter may be useful not only for detecting delirium but also for monitoring the progress of the condition.[31]

Investigations

Routine investigations that are agreed on by most authorities include full blood count and erythrocyte sedimentation rate, blood chemistry, urine analysis, ECG, chest X-ray and EEG.[4,31] Additional investigations should be ordered on the basis of these preliminary screening tests and of clinical examinations. The use of EEG is controversial, particularly as the investigation requires being quiescent for up to 20 minutes. However, one study produced some preliminary evidence that quantitative EEG is more discriminating and has the advantage of being quicker than conventional EEG, and may be particularly important in monitoring the progress of the delirium.[32] Not infrequently one is presented with a situation where the underlying causes have been identified and treated but the patient has not recovered from their delirium. In this situation, quantitative EEG has been shown to detect abnormalities in cerebral functioning that persist beyond the resolution of the underlying aetiology. Once the underlying aetiology or aetiologies have been identified, measures can be introduced to treat these conditions.

Supportive measures

Supportive measures can be considered under the following categories:

- psychological measures
- environmental measures
- somatic measures.

Psychological measures

The experience of our patients may guide us in this respect. In a landmark study, a systematic evaluation was performed on 50 older people who developed delirium during hospital admission and who were able to be interviewed after that experience.[33] Around 80% of this sample recalled their experiences frequently in great detail. Qualitative research techniques suggested that patients found themselves in a borderland of understanding and non-understanding, experiencing as reality impressions of all kinds that came to mind, mixing the past and present. Earlier anecdotal reports[34,35] describe the recall of psychotic experiences and distortions of reality beyond that which would be expected from the profound disturbances in awareness and consciousness that are characteristic of delirium.

They also point to the importance of continuous monitoring and 'psychological approaches to management', and they attest to the value of informing relatives and other carers about the process and experience of delirium. Delirium is a frightening experience for both the sufferer and their carers (whether informal or formal), and the value of reassurance has been highlighted.[36,37]

Environmental measures

It is often nurses who are key in these general supportive measures for both the patient and their family. Nurses trained in the management of delirium increase recognition, improve outcome by limiting risk factors and enhance treatment.[38,39] Other supportive measures include regulation of hydration, control of pain and optimising the environment. The latter is the most challenging problem in the modern National Health Service. The nostrum of continuity of personnel, reduced noise, and aids to orientation and location (e.g. a single room) may be difficult to achieve. However, what is achievable is an increased recognition of the condition of delirium by education, and the application of good nursing practice and the principles of patient-centred care. Attention to detail, such as ensuring that hearing aids are switched on or have functioning batteries and that glasses are available and clean, does not involve complicated procedures but may often be overlooked.

Somatic interventions

It may be that, given the known association of prescribed medications with precipitation of delirium, cessation of medication is the first step. However, the implications of this need to be understood. Although psychoactive substances are an important precipitant of delirium, the reason for their prescription in the first place is often neglected and may lead to a reappearance of troublesome symptoms during the recovery phase.

This may apply particularly to anticholinergic medication such as tricyclic antidepressants. An important principle of management should be that if such medication is (and it frequently can be) the cause of delirium, those who have been treating the condition for which the medication was prescribed should be informed of the cessation of the treatment. This general caveat should apply to the cessation of all medications which have been prescribed, and consultation with the prescriber is the preferred option.

Given the frequency of adverse effects associated with drugs commonly prescribed to ameliorate the symptoms of delirium, the first decision should be whether or not these treatments are necessary. Such decisions are of necessity pragmatic and involve considerations such as the situation in which the delirium arises and the expertise of the staff who are caring for the patient.

In cases where the level of agitation is severe and prejudices care, or where environmental and supportive measures have been ineffective, somatic therapies may be considered. The disadvantage of haloperidol is its tendency to cause extrapyramidal side-effects. Its advantages are that it is available in several forms (for intravenous, intramuscular or oral administration) and has dosage flexibility. It is also unlikely to induce hypotension, in contrast to other typical antipsychotics such as chlorpromazine. Some guidelines have recommended escalating doses of haloperidol until the agitated behaviour and psychotic symptoms are controlled. This is not a recommendation that this author would advocate. The first question should be whether the patient really needs medication. Could a nurse or an environmental intervention alone improve the situation? If it is decided that medication is indicated because of the level of agitation and risk of harm, the second question should be which treatment to use and the aim of that treatment.

If control of psychotic symptoms is desired, it must be recognised that the antipsychotic effects are delayed even in the case of the most effective antipsychotics. If sedation is required, particularly for night-time sleep disturbance, there may be alternatives to the use of antipsychotics. The third important question concerns the nature of the underlying aetiology or comorbid condition. If delirium arises in dementia, it is vital that the possibility of the presence of dementia with Lewy bodies is raised, as these patients can experience severe antipsychotic sensitivity even on very low doses of either typical or atypical antipsychotics.[40]

It is fascinating to observe that in clinical practice low-potency antipsychotics (e.g. promazine) are frequently used, particularly in the evenings. For delirium that is not associated with alcohol withdrawal in older people, this author has never had to use an intravenous escalating dose regime, nor would they recommend it, but they would concur with the series of letters that followed one review.[27] These pointed out that with high doses of antipsychotics there was an increased risk not only of extrapyramidal symptoms but also of potentially more serious adverse effects, such as torsades de pointes, and that the dosage regime proposed was above the limits specified in the *British National Formulary*.[41–43] Although antipsychotics are recommended by several reviews,[4,27] there is a paucity of data on which these recommendations are based. At the time of writing, this author has not identified any randomised controlled trials of the use of antipsychotics in delirium. One double-blind controlled trial on the specific causation of AIDS delirium did find that haloperidol and chlorpromazine were superior to lorazepam.[44] In clinical practice it is the disturbance of the sleep–wake cycle that is frequently the cause of presentation to liaison consultation services for old age psychiatry. My empirical experience is that in such cases, particularly when delirium arises in the setting of pre-existing dementia, if the sleep disturbance is frequent, troublesome and potentially harmful, an alternative to antipsychotics is chlormethiazole.

A useful strategy can be to prescribe one dose (192 mg in the early evening and another dose 5 to 6 hours later if required). This is a strategy that has been particularly successful in some patients with dementia with Lewy bodies.[45]

Benzodiazepines

In the specific aetiology of alcohol withdrawal, benzodiazepines are the drug of choice. Delirium tremens is relatively rare in older people. Potential adverse effects of benzodiazepines include respiratory depression, over-sedation and paradoxical excitation. One review[26] considers benzodiazepines to be second-line agents in the management of delirium in the elderly.

Other drugs

There is a small amount of evidence to suggest that trazodone may be beneficial in some patients for treating agitation in delirium,[46] and there are a few case reports of the use of cholinesterase inhibitors in delirium treatment.[47]

Post-delirium care

Given the persistence of symptoms of delirium in older people, the fact that a delirious episode may herald the onset of dementia,[48] and the frightening nature of the experience for survivors, it is surprising that this aspect of delirium management is rarely mentioned.[4] There is a role for community teams in this respect, with continued explanation, education and psychological support for patients and their carers and follow-up, or at the very least the identification of an increased risk of dementia. One small study has shown that community follow-up reduces post-delirium morbidity (e.g. acute admissions or institutional care) compared with a treatment-as-usual group.[49]

Key points

- After many years of neglect, delirium is now receiving the attention it deserves as one of the 'greats' of geriatric medicine, and old shibboleths are being subjected to scientific scrutiny.
- The principles of management attract wide agreement, in the absence of a robust evidence base. However, this is beginning to be established, and the experiences of survivors are beginning to be explored. Until the 'Utopia' of an evidence base is established there is still a place for good clinical practice, education and empirical treatment.

References

1 Lipowski ZJ (1990) *Acute Confusional States*. Oxford University Press, New York.
2 Lyndesay J, Rockwood K and Macdonald A (2002) *Delirium in the Elderly*. Oxford University Press, Oxford.
3 Fleminger S (2002) Remembering delirium. *Br J Psychiatry.* **180**: 4–5.
4 American Psychiatric Association (1999) *Practice Guidelines for the Treatment of Patients with Delirium*. American Psychiatric Association, Washington, DC.

5 Engel C and Romano J (1959) Delirium, a syndrome of cerebral insufficiency. *J Chron Dis.* **9**: 260–77.

6 Camus V, Burtin B, Simeone I, Schwed P, Gonthier R and Dubos G (2000) Factor analysis supports the evidence of existing hyperactive and hypoactive subtypes of delirium. *Int J Geriatr Psychiatry.* **15**: 313–16.

7 Camus V, Gonthier R, Dubos G, Schwed P and Simeone I (2000) Etiological and outcome profiles in hypoactive and hyperactive subtypes of dementia. *J Geriatr Psychiatry Neurol.* **13**: 38–42.

8 O'Keeffe ST and Lavan J (1999) Clinical significance of delirium subtypes in older people. *Age Ageing.* **28**: 115–19.

9 Folstein MF, Bassett SS, Romanowski AJ and Nestadt G (1991) The epidemiology of delirium in the community: the Eastern Baltimore Mental Health Survey. *Int Psychogeriatr.* **3**: 169–79.

10 Rahkonen T, Eloniemei-Sulkava U, Halonen P *et al.* (2001) Delirium in the non-demented oldest old in the general population: risk factors and prognosis. *Int J Geriatr Psychiatry.* **16**: 415–21.

11 Lyndesay J, Rockwood K and Rolfson D (2002) The epidemiology of delirium. In: J Lyndesay, K Rockwood and A Macdonald (eds) *Delirium in the Elderly.* Oxford University Press, Oxford.

12 Cole MG and Primeau F (1993) Prognosis of delirium in elderly hospital patients. *Can Med Assoc.* **149**: 41–6.

13 Marcantonio ER, Flaker JM, Michaels M and Resnick NM (2000) Delirium is independently associated with poor functional recovery after hip fracture. *J Am Geriatr Soc.* **48**: 618–24.

14 Kelly KG, Zisselman M, Cutillo-Schmitter R, Reichard R and Payne D (2001) Severity and course of delirium in medically hospitalised nursing facility patients. *Am J Geriatr Psychiatry.* **9**: 72–7.

15 Levkoff SE, Evans DA, Liptzin B *et al.* (1992) Delirium: the occurrence and persistence of symptoms among elderly hospitalised patients. *Arch Intern Med.* **152**: 334–40.

16 Mori E and Yamadoria A (1987) Acute confusional state and acute agitated delirium. Occurrence after infarction of the right middle cerebral artery. *Arch Neurol.* **44**: 311–19.

17 Inouye SK, Bogardus ST, Charpentier PA *et al.* (1999) A multicomponent intervention to prevent delirium in hospitalised older patients. *NEJM.* **340**: 669–76.

18 Rolfson D (2002) The causes of delirium. In: J Lyndesay, K Rockwood and A Macdonald (eds) *Delirium in the Elderly.* Oxford University Press, Oxford.

19 Rockwood K, Cosway S, Stolee P *et al.* (1994) Increasing the recognition of delirium in elderly patients. *J Am Geriatr Soc.* **42**: 252–6.

20 Conn DK and Lieff S (2001) Diagnosing and managing delirium in the elderly. *Can Fam Physician.* **47**: 101–8.

21 Albert MS, Levkoff SE, Reilly C *et al.* (1992) The Delirium Symptom Interview: an interview for the detection of delirium symptoms in hospitalised patients. *J Geriatr Psychiatry Neurol.* **5**: 14–21.

22 Inouye SK, van Dyck CH, Alessi CA, Balkin S, Siegal AP and Horwitz RI (1990) Clarifying confusion: the confusion assessment method, a new method for the detection of delirium. *Ann Intern Med.* **113**: 941–8.

23 Marcantonio ER, Flacker JM, Wright RJ and Resnick NM (2001) Reducing delirium after hip fracture: a randomised trial. *J Am Geriatr Soc.* **49**: 678–9.

24 Elie M, Cole M, Primeau F and Bellavance F (1998) Delirium risk factors in elderly hospitalised patients. *J Gen Intern Med.* **13**: 204–12.

25 Aldemir M, Ozen S, Kara IH, Sir A and Bac B (2001) Predisposing factors for delirium in the surgical intensive care unit. *Crit Care.* **5**: 265–70.

26 Marcantonio E (2002) The management of delirium. In: J Lyndesay, K Rockwood and A Macdonald (eds) *Delirium in the Elderly.* Oxford University Press, Oxford.

27 Meagher DJ (2001) Delirium: optimising management. *BMJ.* **322**: 144–9.

28 Fairburn AF (2002) Delirium: an overview. In: JRM Copeland, MT Abou-Saleh and DG Blazer (eds) *Principles and Practice of Geriatric Psychiatry* (2e). Wiley, Chichester.

29 Inouye SK and Charpentier PA (1996) Precipitating factors for delirium in a hospitalised elderly person. Predictive model and inter-relationship with baseline vulnerability. *JAMA.* **275**: 852–7.

30 Farrell KR and Ganzini L (1995) Misdiagnosing delirium as depression in medically ill elderly patients. *Arch Intern Med.* **155**: 2459–64.

31 Byrne EJ (1994) *Confusional States in the Elderly*. Churchill Livingstone, Edinburgh.

32 Leuchter AF and Jacobson SA (1991) Quantitative measurement of brain electrical activity in delirium. *Int Psychogeriatr.* **3**: 231–47.

33 Andersson EM, Hallberg IR, Norberg A and Edberg AK (2002) The meaning of acute confusional state from the perspective of elderly patients. *Int J Geriatr Psychiatry.* **17**: 652–63.

34 Levin M (1968) Delirium: an experience and some reflections. *Am J Psychiatry.* **124**: 1120.

35 Schofield I (1997) A small exploratory study of the reaction of older people to an episode of delirium. *J Adv Nurs.* **25**: 942–52.

36 Jacobson S and Schreibman B (1997) Behavioural and pharmacologic treatment of delirium. *Am Fam Physician.* **56**: 2005–20.

37 Mohta M, Sethi AK, Tyagi A and Mohta A (2003) Psychological care in trauma patients. *Injury.* **34**: 17–25.

38 Zimberg M and Berenson S (1990) Delirium in patients with cancer: nursing assessment and intervention. *Oncol Nurs Forum.* **17**: 529–38.

39 Simon L, Jewell N and Brokel J (1997) Management of acute delirium in hospitalised elderly: a process improvement project. *Geriatr Nurs.* **18**: 150–4.

40 McKeith IG, Fairbairn AF, Perry RH, *et al.* (1992a) Neuroleptic sensitivity in patients with senile dementia of Lewy body type. *BMJ.* **305**: 673–8.

41 Junaid O and Junaid K (2001) *Neuroleptics in Delirium*; Bmj.com/cgi.eletters/322/7279/144

42 Ryan CJ (2001) *Neuroleptics in Delirium*; Bmj.com/cgi/eletters/

43 King DJ (2001) *Neuroleptics in Delirium*; Bmj.com/cgi/eletters

44 Breitbart W, Marotta R, Platt MM *et al.* (1996) A double-blind trial of haloperidol, chlorpromazine and lorazepam in the treatment of delirium in hospitalised AIDS patients. *Am J Psychiatry.* **153**: 231–7.

45 Byrne EJ (2000) Treatment of dementia with Lewy bodies. In: N Qizilbash, LS Schneider, H Chiu, *et al.* (eds) *Evidence-based Dementia Practice*. Blackwells, Oxford.

46 Okamoto Y, Matsuoaka Y, Sasaki T, Jitsuuiki H, Horiguchi J and Yamawaki S (1999) Trazodone in the treatment of delirium. *J Clin Psychopharmacol.* **19**: 280–2.

47 Wengel SP, Burke WJ and Roccaforte WH (1999) Donepezil for postoperative delirium associated with Alzheimer's disease. *J Am Geriatr Soc.* **47**: 379–80.

48 Rahkonen T, Luukkainen-Markkula R, Paanila S, Sivenius J and Sulkava R (2000) Delirium episode as a sign of undetected dementia among community-dwelling elderly subjects: a 2-year follow-up study. *J Neurol Neurosurg Psychiatry.* **69**: 519–21.

49 Rahkonen T, Eloniemi-Sulkava U, Paanila S, Halonen P, Sivenius J and Sulkava R (2001) Systematic intervention for supporting community care of elderly people after a delirium episode. *Int Psychogeriatr.* **13**: 37–49.

Concluding remarks

Stephen Curran and Roger Bullock

We hope that you have enjoyed reading this book. We also hope that you think we have at least partly achieved our aim of providing a synthesis of a modern scientific understanding and a thoroughly practical multi-disciplinary approach to old age psychopharmacology. Bridging the gap between theory and practice remains essential as teams expand and more people from differing disciplines contribute to the care of the older person with mental illness, including making decisions about pharmacological therapy.

Those who plan and provide services for older people with mental illness need an understanding of the issues to provide the capacity to work well with the different professionals and the relatives and carers with whom they engage if they are to achieve satisfactory results in their work, and the best outcomes for their patients and clients. Such a multi-professional approach has often been lacking in old age psychopharmacology, but with the advent of supplementary nurse and pharmacist prescribing, we hope that this book will stimulate increased interest in multi-professional working in this area, enabling all clinicians to increase their understanding of the scientific background to old age psychopharmacology.

A book of this length can never be fully comprehensive, but we hope that it will serve as a ready reference for those working in the field, and that it will perhaps inspire them to continue improving the service we offer to this uniquely vulnerable and often neglected group in our society.

Old age psychopharmacology is a rapidly developing area. We have included a few useful websites to help you keep informed about developments in this area.

The Cochrane Library
www.nelh.nhs.uk/cochrane.asp

Committee on Safety of Medicine (CSM)
www.mca.gov.uk/aboutagency/regframework/csm

United States Food and Drug Administration (USFDA)
httt:/omni.ac.uk

Medicines and Healthcare products Regulatory Agency (MHRA)
www.mca.gov.uk

National electronic Library for Health (NeLH)
www.nelh.nhs.uk

NICE
(In April 2005 NICE joined with the Health Development Agency to become the National Institute for Health and Clinical Excellence – the new organisation is still abbreviated as NICE)
www.nice.org.uk

The Royal College of Psychiatrists
www.rcpsych.ac.uk

United Kingdom Psychiatric Pharmacy Group (UKPPG)
www.ukppg.org.uk

Index

Page numbers in italics refer to figures or tables.
AD refers to Alzheimer's disease; VaD to vascular disease and dementia